THE PERFECT DEFENCE

THE ULTIMATE FULLY ILLUSTRATED SELF-DEFENCE MANUAL FOR ANYONE ANYWHERE ANY TIME

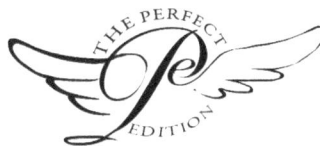

www.theperfectedition.com

Thanks.

This book was created with the help of a lot of very talented people,
some of them prefer to remain nameless for reasons that I respect and some who I would
like to name and thank here.

Sensei Bruno Carmeni, for shaping my early years and showing me how real talent is always
humble.

Stunt coordinator Dave Judge for letting me have fun doing some crazy stuff and for writing the chapter on driving skills.

Kickboxing Champion Keith Wilson, who taught me how to punch when my hand was
broken and to kick when my toes were smashed.

Actress Sirle Von Schihver who gave a light touch to such a heavy subject.

Sascha Beyer for his precious expertise in Internet security.

My children Enrico and Elena, never shy in front of the camera,
together with my wife Cristina, for being so patient and forgiving for all the times that I died.

About the author.
Franz has black belts in several Martial Arts, he practices many activities, from ice diving to
high altitude climbing and has been to war zones and other places where no one is welcome and some never come back. He has survived and rescued others many times, applying a very important principle: simplicity.

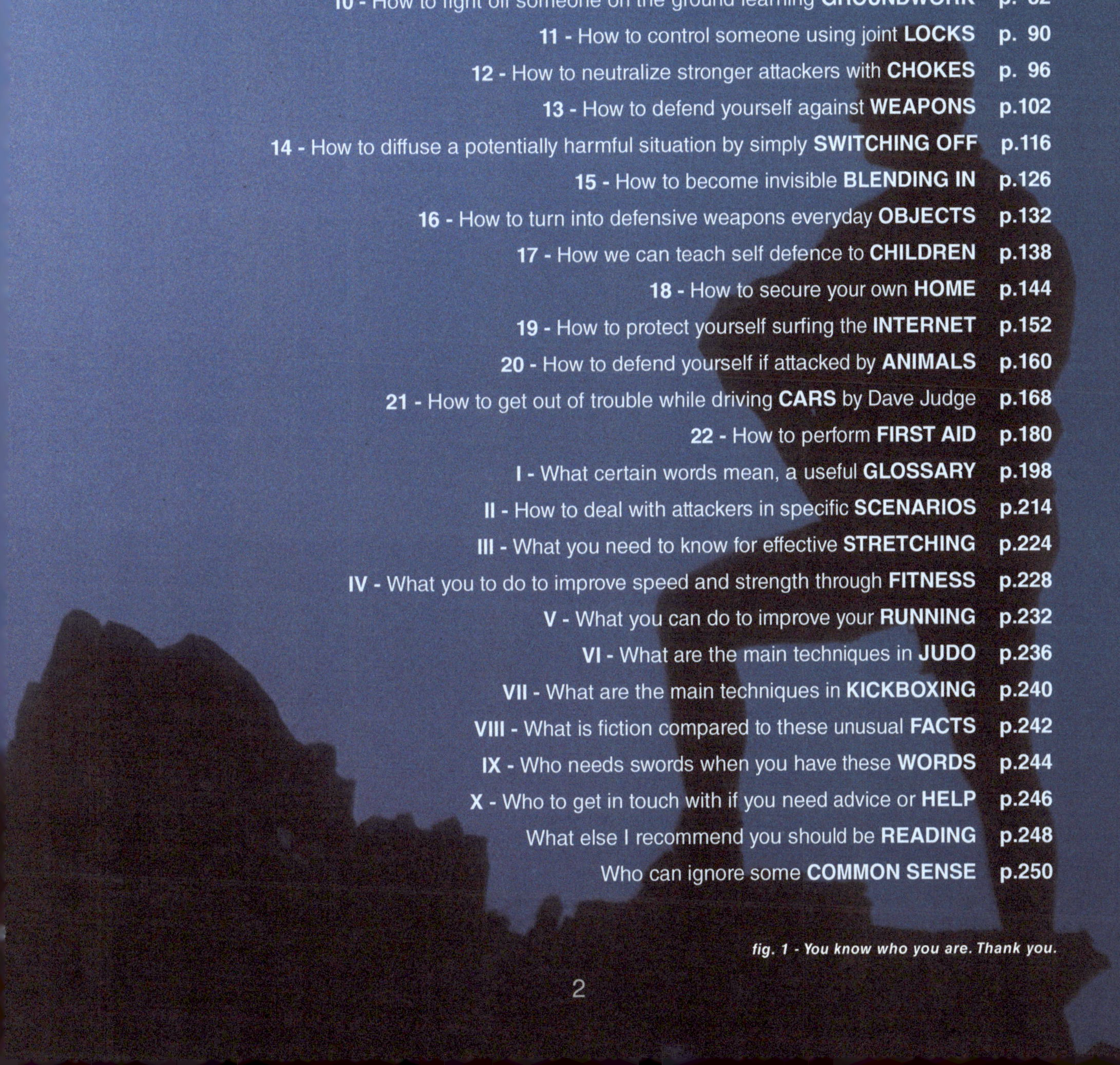

fig. 1 - You know who you are. Thank you.

Foreword by Sensei Bruno Carmeni - 8th Dan Judo

When my friend Franz showed me the draft of his book "The Perfect Defence" I thought it was just another book on self-defence, but when I started to read it I realized that it is not simply another manual crowding bookstores shelves these days.

In the modern society we are living, we all have to be ready to face different kinds of violence, physical and psychological, sexual and financial, including mobbing and stalking facing also some bad consequences caused by modern technology.

These aspects are not all taken into account in other self-defence books.

The reader after absorbing these pages will be equipped to cope with all the violence that is embedded in our lives in this century.

The author is an expert of many different self-defence methods, therefore I advise everybody, especially women, to read this carefully and use it the perfect way.

Bruno Carmeni

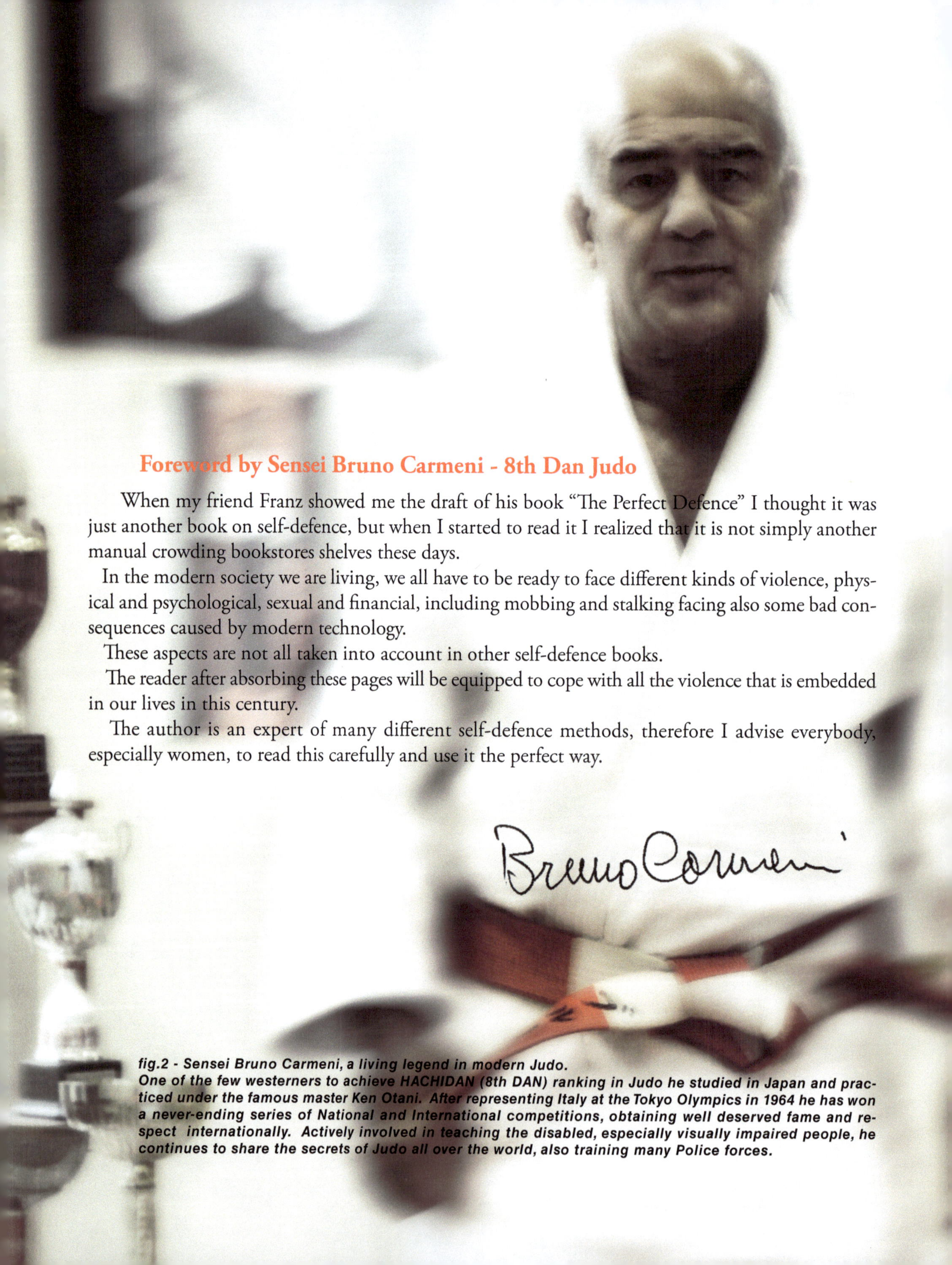

fig.2 - Sensei Bruno Carmeni, a living legend in modern Judo.
One of the few westerners to achieve HACHIDAN (8th DAN) ranking in Judo he studied in Japan and practiced under the famous master Ken Otani. After representing Italy at the Tokyo Olympics in 1964 he has won a never-ending series of National and International competitions, obtaining well deserved fame and respect internationally. Actively involved in teaching the disabled, especially visually impaired people, he continues to share the secrets of Judo all over the world, also training many Police forces.

introduction

This self-defence book is like no other. It gives everyone, irrelevant of strength, gender, training and fitness a fighting chance in any situation where they are targeted by a violent attack. However, this should not be considered a do-it-yourself book, it is still preferable that you enrol in a practical hands on course or a self-defence class at some point in the future.

Is this really the perfect self-defence? It is if you'll never use any of the techniques that you are about to learn, because it means that you have learned to avoid danger in the first place. Prevention is better than cure, and here you will learn mostly how to turn the odds in your favour. The probabilities of anyone living in the modern world becoming a victim of a crime are still quite slim, even if unfortunately there's a widespread tendency to instil unnecessary fear.

It should be noted nevertheless that in case we have to face violence we have softened that animal fighting instinct that protected man for one hundred thousands years. It is certainly true that today we are not as tough as we used to be: we walk less, we eat finer food, we are better protected from the elements, cocooned in our cars and consequentially we are not prepared to face a rough situation anymore.

LEARN THE PRINCIPLE NOT THE SEQUENCE.

This self-defence system was created considering that the average person has no martial arts background, has very little experience of contact sports, or very often has never punched, kicked or even pushed anybody, yet it employs very advanced techniques to either revive your survival instinct or at least show you what to do, choosing a technique that should come to you naturally. We call this the Perfect Defence System, or just PD. There are some people who have the mentality of fighters, they have a will to survive and not to be put down whatever happens and there are others who simply cannot bear any physical or verbal confrontation, never mind how mild it is, they just cannot cope with it.

It might be helpful reading and knowing about attacks and violent aggressions, it will prepare you and at the same time toughen up the mind and prepare you for worse.

Reading how different people managed to fight off attackers will give you strength.

You do not have to comply or submit to your fate, you can fight back, and we want to show you how. Teaching self-defence we often come across people, especially women, who have no idea of how to punch, or have never, luckily for them, been involved in even a small scuffle with their bigger brother, some have never even shouted at somebody.

It is important to bear in mind that the Perfect Defence will not turn the practitioner into a fighting machine. It takes time and a certain inclination or pre-disposition to become a good fighter and we want to emphasise that this book is not aimed at soldiers in a battle environment or at anyone who wants to go out and cause trouble or harm somebody.

The Perfect Defence has many highly effective techniques, but they work best defensively.

Some self-defence manuals strongly advocate high-kicks, restraining techniques and fancy martial arts techniques, sometimes quite gratuitously so, often forgetting that the average person doesn't have any clue on how to achieve certain advanced techniques in the first place, never mind performing a leg split.

It is also important to understand that you cannot learn to defend yourself by numbers; anyone who has been subjected to a violent attack knows too well that the assailant followed no pattern and was not lying in wait and, more often than not, there were no warning signs. It's no use trying to remember that in figure 36 of page 142 of your self-defence manual, the assailant has his forearm at 45 degrees above your head, so you have to pivot on your right front foot to the left and 15 degrees anticlockwise and duck under his right and then… you know what I am getting at especially if you have read similar material.

fig.3 - Step forward with your hands between his arms to neutralize his attack.

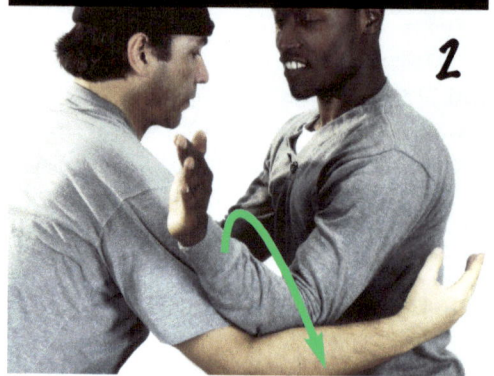

More important is understanding the sequence of actions and remembering the principles behind it, even though nevertheless there are instances when a sequence of moves IS the principle.

Within the PD system every technique is based on a principle easy to remember.

For example, if someone launches at your throat, it does not matter if you don't remember where your forearms should go or the position of your feet, what you should remember is that instead of stepping back you should step forward with your hands between his to neutralize the attack (fig. 3). Always try to remember the concept: if the technique fails the principle will take over and correct the technique without much thinking involved.

We will of course examine the deserted car park scenario (see SCENARIOS page 214) or the unwanted attention of someone sitting next to you on the bus, but to be honest, car parks nowadays are pretty safe, and a firm and loud 'keep your hands off to the 'perv' on the bus is more effective than making a fool of yourself trying to break his arm. Sometimes, if not every time, it's better to just walk away. The PD system differs in tackling realistic scenarios with simple, direct and practical techniques, knowing too well that often it is all over in less than 8 seconds. In other words, remember the principles and read the scenarios only as a sequence of events where the principle is applied and you will find that certain concepts or techniques are repeated several times throughout the book across different pages: forgive us, this is necessary to make sure that

SIMPLE, PRACTICAL TECHNIQUES TO USE QUICKLY AND EFFECTIVELY.

these principles are properly assimilated and become second nature.

The PD system also focuses on the psychological aspect on dealing with aggressive or violent behaviour in SWITCHING OFF page 116, and it is fundamental to remember that quite often you can diffuse aggressive behaviour with firm, calm commands or by ignoring provocations. In a nutshell, the PD system gives you a collection of elements and techniques that you can make yours to suit your needs.

We cannot emphasise enough that before reacting to a threat you should consider your local laws and we also want to remind you that you should apply a proportionate response to the threat.

We are totally against carrying objects on your person intending to use them as weapons.

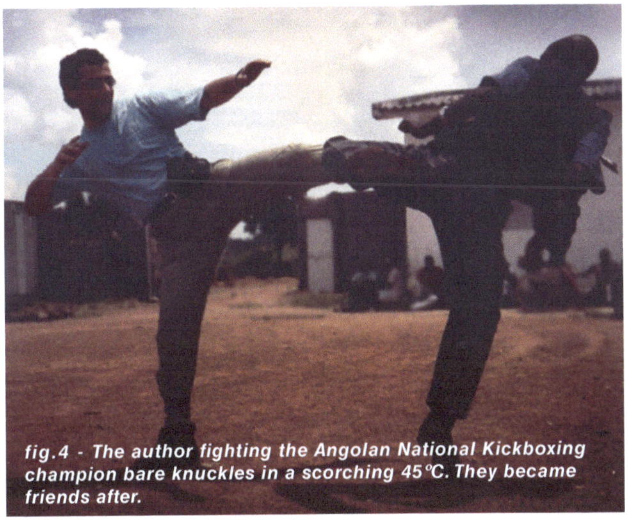

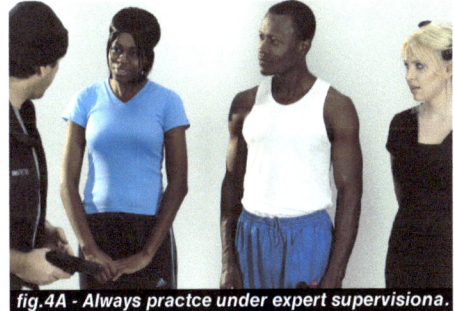

fig.4 - The author fighting the Angolan National Kickboxing champion bare knuckles in a scorching 45°C. They became friends after.

Your reaction to a 16 lb man attacking you with a knife should be different to the response used to repel a teenager attacking you in the same way. It might sound absurd but believe me, it is a different situation altogether, without underestimating either attacker.

To survive a violent situation you don't need Bruce Lee's reflexes or Tyson's strength or James Bond inventiveness, you simply need to know what to do and develop a will to react.

KNOWING WHAT TO DO IS YOUR PERSONAL DEFENCE WEAPON.

We don't expect to cover every possible situation, but all situations have something in common and we will find this common denominator but while we don't make you believe you can fight your way through a gang mobbing you, but we can certainly suggest how to avoid being involved in such situation in the first place. We don't expect you to modify your lifestyle or what you normally wear but we'll try to make you more aware and skilful in handling aggressive behaviour.

Prevention is better than cure, but we will also show you, once disaster strikes, what to do.

The final aim of the Perfect Defence system is that if confronted suddenly by an attacker, wherever you are, in whatever mood you are, you will not be mesmerized with fright, but you will react swiftly, rapidly, and efficiently. We will try to show you even how to improvise, using whatever is available to you at that particular moment.

Never forget though that every time we will illustrate a technique, you shouldn't try it by yourself on somebody who is not trained or qualified to do so, we insist that you take a course in self-defence at some stage, especially to experience physical contact. You should find out in a class situation how it actually feels to block a body blow or having someone tighten his hands around your neck, helping you to overcome the initial shock if it happens in a real situation. Finally, you must develop a will to survive, a determination

fig.4A - Always practce under expert supervisiona.

to protect yourself and not to submit passively, or defend the ones you love, at any cost. This confidence in your acquired abilities should however, not give you the irresponsible attitude to get into trouble gratuitously, thinking you can fight your way out, you will not, and you and whoever is with you will pay dearly for such an attitude. The reason

DEVELOP A WILL TO SURVIVE, DO NOT ACCEPT VIOLENCE, EVER.

is other people will be able to read in advance your challenging stance and your excessive self-confidence and react accordingly. At the same time, somebody who is trying to harm you will not expect you to respond efficiently to his aggressive behaviour, making yourself a hard target instead of an easy prey. Remember that your best defence is always to call the police or local authority, or generally call for help and even more importantly to learn how to avoid getting into trouble in the first place and that defending yourself resorting to physical action should be your last resort when no other option is available at the time.In any case, always report a crime to the authority, especially to the local Police, it might help to prevent further crimes happening in that area in the future if they know about it.

Lastly, remember that while reading this you probably have something to hand that can become a defensive weapon if you use it to whack an aggressor in the face, and this is the first lesson to learn: you always have something within reach that can help to defend yourself, and you should always be aware of your surroundings.

LEARN TO IMPROVISE WITH WHAT IS AVAILABLE TO YOU RIGHT THEN.

WARNING: BUYING THIS BOOK OR DOWNLOADING THE INFORMATION AVAILABLE MEANS THAT YOU UNDERSTAND THAT ALL THE TECHNIQUES AND ADVICE SHOWN IN THIS BOOK SHOULD NOT BE USED UNSUPERVISED, AND THAT YOU TAKE FULL RESPONSIBILITY FOR YOUR ACTIONS ACCORDING TO YOUR LOCAL GOVERNING LAWS AND THAT YOU WILL CHECK WITH YOUR DOCTOR BEFORE BEGINNING ANY EXERCISE REGIME. EVEN THOUGH ALL FITNESS EXERCISES AND ALL TECHNIQUES SHOWN ARE SAFE WE DO NOT ACCEPT ANY RESPONSIBILITY FOR INJURIES OR ILL HEALTH ARISING FROM PERFORMING THEM. BE RESPONSIBLE AND SAFE AT ALL TIME.

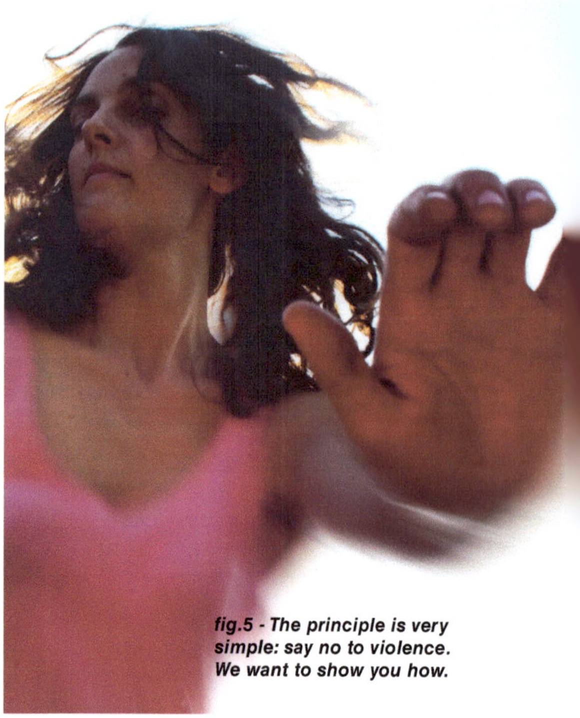

fig.5 - The principle is very simple: say no to violence. We want to show you how.

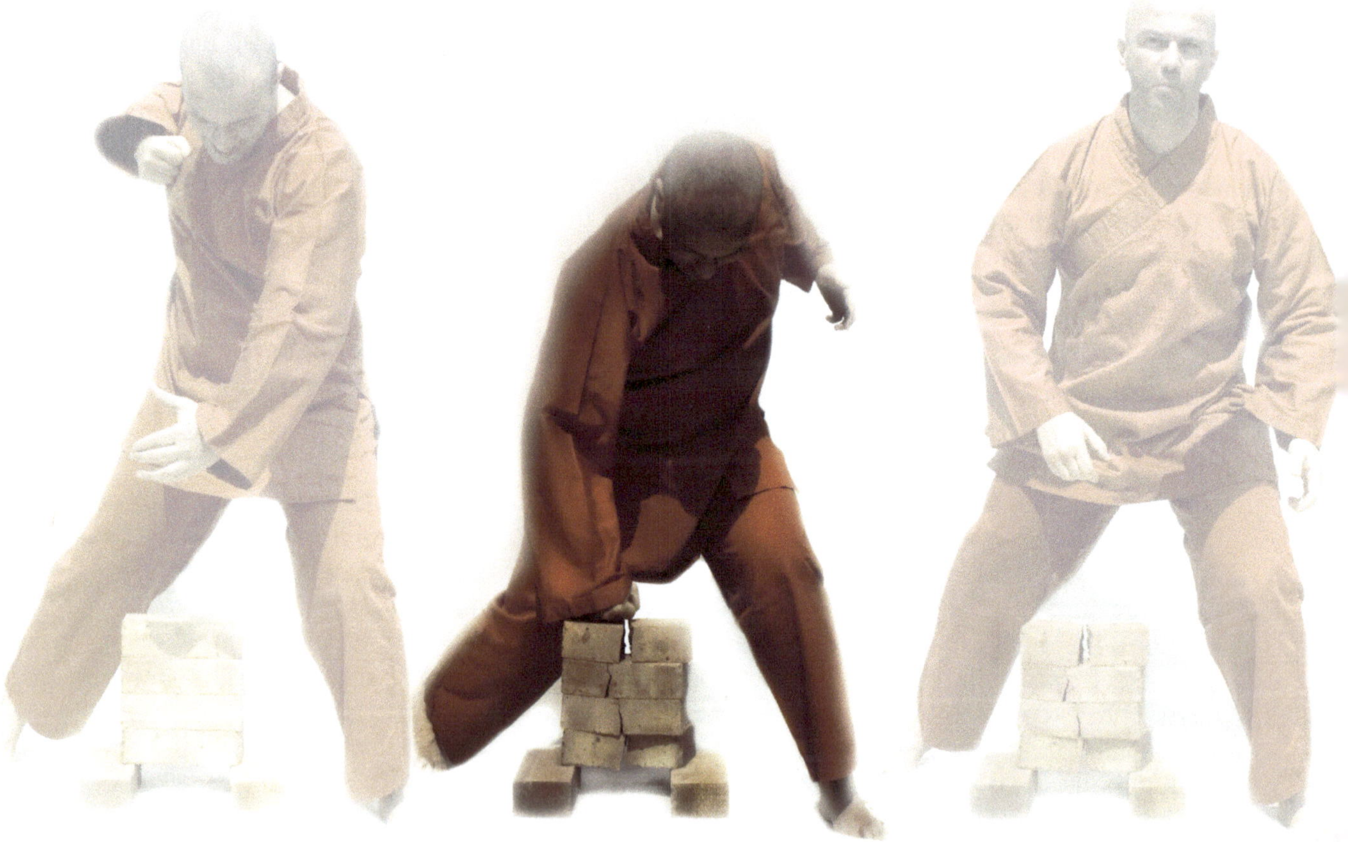

fig.6 - Don't try this at home, it takes many years of practice and sacrifices, as well as training with Shaolin Monks. Using your body to smash objects is called TAMASHIWARI in Japanese and has a long tradition. (see Glossary page 211) You can also see a video of it here: http://tinyurl.com/48t3dr or at www.theperfectdefence.com

Note: We will refer for simplicity as HE when indicating an attacker; this is because unfortunately most of the time in the real world attackers are male but also for simplicity.

The illustrations and photos are made following the same principle, this is only to simplify the roles and make them easily identifiable. We hope nobody will be offended.

The symbols below appear on the pages to emphasize concepts or to help you focus:

- KEEP A POSITIVE ATTITUDE -
- STAY RELAXED, HIDE YOUR FEAR -

- BEE VIGILANT, PAY ATTENTION -
- BE AWARE OF YOUR SURROUNDINGS -

- CALL EMERGENCY SERVICE -
- REPORT TO THE POLICE OR TO THE AUTHORITIES -

- PAUSE AND THINK -
- DO NOT PANIC -

- VERY IMPORTANT -
- DON'T FORGET! -

- WALK AWAY -
- PROCEED WITH CAUTION -

- ACT FAST -
- LIGHTNING ACTION -

- RUN AWAY FAST -

- REPEAT ACTION -
- COMBINE WITH OTHER MOVE -
- PRACTICE! -

- AGGRESSIVE ANIMALS -

- BE CAREFUL -
- CONSIDER CAREFULLY -

- WATCH OUT FOR WEAPONS! -

- RISK OF SERIOUS INJURY -
- DO NOT REHEARSE UNLESS PROPERLY SUPERVISED -

- REAL EXPERIENCE BY AUTHOR -

- RISK OF INJURY -
- REHEARSE WITH CAUTION -

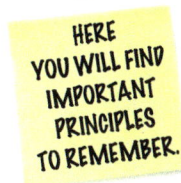

HERE YOU WILL FIND IMPORTANT PRINCIPLES TO REMEMBER.

- USEFUL MENTAL NOTES -

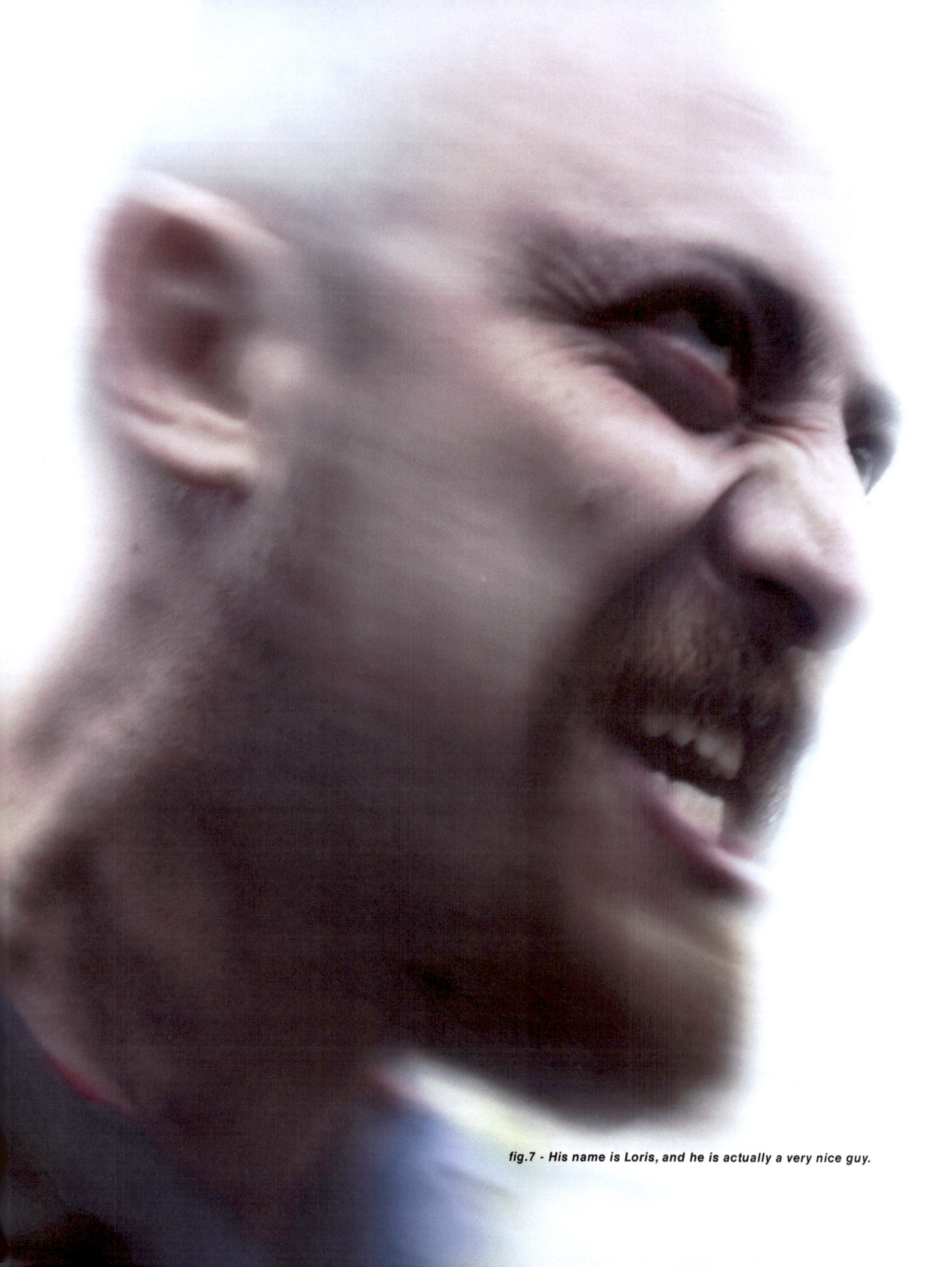

fig.7 - His name is Loris, and he is actually a very nice guy.

aggressors

Aggression is a violent action, verbal, physical and/or psychological, directed towards another person, directly or indirectly. It can happen anywhere, including your home, or your workplace, and against anything, like your valuables, for example your purse. Even when directed against objects (indirectly) it can still bear dangerous consequences for your person, for instance someone snatching your purse from a scooter might drag you onto the ground and hurt you badly.

DO NOT TOLERATE VERBAL AGGRESSION, IT VIOLATES YOUR DIGNITY.

Verbal aggression shouldn't be underestimated because more often than not it leads to physical aggression, and in any case it is degrading to the dignity of a person and should never be tolerated or justified in any way for any reason.

Aggressors are normally men, you will be pleased to know that women represent a small percentage, and normally you can divide them into known aggressors (relatives, friends, colleagues) and unknown aggressors, strangers. An unknown intruder such as a burglar is normally only interested in your valuables and will rarely resort to violence unless he feels trapped, preferring to flee. Our advice (see SCENARIOS page 214 is that if a burglar awakens you at night, make enough noise to make him aware of your presence, and make sure you don't block his escape route.

The common perception that burglars and thieves do not carry weapons should be disregarded, always assume every aggressor or intruder carries some sort of weapons, often a large screwdriver to break in. Also don't forget that nowadays you might find that the person breaking into your house is under the influence of drugs or other substances, and steals to feed his habit.

Drug users under the influence are totally unpredictable and do not have any inhibition or fear, it is better if you do not approach or tackle them unless there is no other option. The same principle applies when awakened by a wild animal up close, while sleeping in the woods for instance (see ANIMALS page 160).

Pick-pocketers and so-called professional thieves will want to accomplish their task in the least possible time without being seen, they are only interested in your valuables.

It is worth pointing out that you can always replace a valuable item, even if dear to you, but it's never worth to lose your life or sustain serious injuries to defend it. You should react to these types of aggression only if you think your well-being is at risk or that the consequences could be highly damaging.

Let's see more in detail in the case of a sexually motivated assault. A sexually motivated aggressor normally falls into the following types: the flasher, happy enough to expose his genitals to total strangers, most of the times physically harmless apart from causing obvious psychological distress.

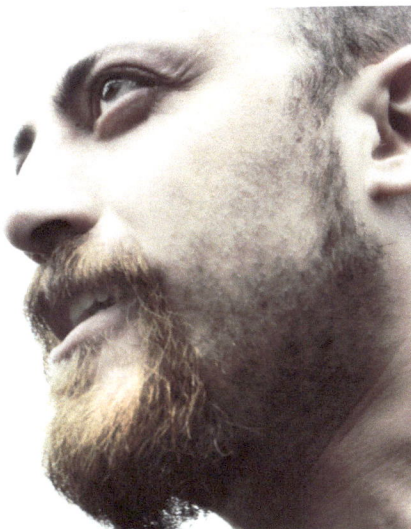

fig.7A - The smile can conceal a sudden sucker punch or a headbutt.

A SEXUALLY MOTIVATED MOLESTER CAN END UP USING PHYSICAL VIOLENCE.

Reporting the incident to the police is always a good course of action. Flashers can eventually become more physical, turning into the second type of sexual aggressor, the molester, someone who finds gratification touching some-one's intimate parts, quite often in a busy or crowded environ-ment like a bus or a train carriage. Even if your initial reaction as a victim is to physically retaliate to his action, you are better off saying in a loud but firm voice something like 'Stop, get your hands off me, or I'll call the police!'

This should be said as if you are telling off a child and will have a double-effect: stop his action and make everyone aware of what is happening without giving him the chance of calling you hysterical and pretending he wasn't doing it on purpose. For some this is still quite difficult, they feel embarrassed to let every-one know what happened. In that case stomp on his toes with a smile or kick his shin with the heel of your shoe. (fig. 8 and fig. 9) he will get the message and you will feel quite good about it believe me.

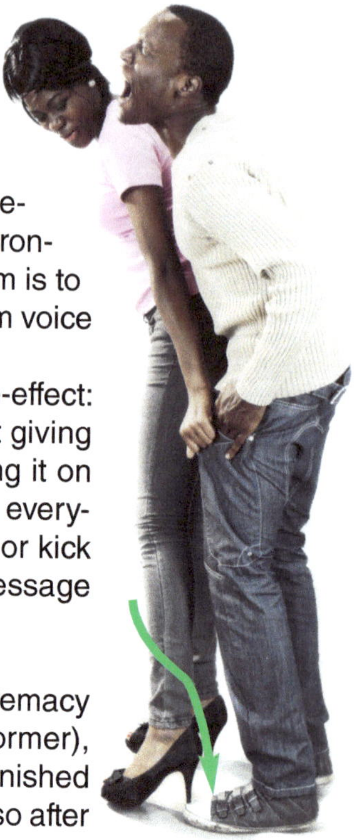

The most dangerous sexual aggressor is the rapist.

This is an aggressor motivated by a distorted desire of power and supremacy over women (or men, gay rape is as common and abominable as the former), often full of hate and rage against the victim, seen as an object to be punished and to be owned through a sexual act, often accompanied by violence also after he has obtained submission.

fig.8 - Stamp on his toes with a smile.

Aggressors do not necessarily act alone; there has been a lot of talk on the media about juvenile gangs recently, often as young as twelve, from a good family background and not motivated by poor economic status and other usual sociographic denominations.

The reasons why individually some people behave perfectly well as individuals but in a group or a gang become violent are several. We will not enter a complex psychographical and psy-chological discussion, for the simple reason that discussing this type of argument will inevitably distract us from the core problem, the actual aggression intended as a physical act of violence. Suffice to say that, for the sake of argument, the actions of a gang are motivated by a general in-security of each individual who find within the group confidence and acquire gratification by the group's strength, indulging in violent acts and bullying as a distorted sense of acquired manhood.

This particular type of aggressor will be discussed also in SWITCHING OFF, page 116.

VIOLENCE WITHIN THE FAMILY NEEDS SPECIALIZED HELP.

A complex subject is the known aggressor: the difficulty is that there is a relationship already established for a certain time in a certain environment.

A work colleague, a relative, a partner, all persons that until yesterday you knew well or thought so, and suddenly, either because of a change in personal circumstances or frustrations, turn violent maybe because of drug use, including alcohol.

The difficulty is that you should react at the earliest signs of this behaviour and should be deci-sive; if you wait too long the other person will think you are accepting their behaviour.

In the workplace, there can be situations when somebody above you in terms of job status will sub-ject you to unwanted attentions, possibly turning violent.

It can happen within a family: a violent father, or a son turned violent towards his parents are all very difficult situations to tackle, professionals that are trained to deal with these sorts of situa-tions find it very complex, and it is an aggressive behaviour regardless of social status, edu-cation or geographical position.

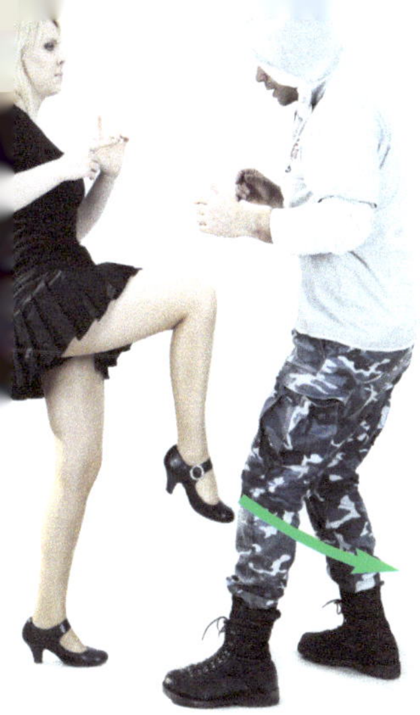

Domestic violence can begin at any stage of a relationship and may continue even once the relationship has ended. In this book we can only show you a quick fix to an imminent physical threat, you should find specialised help if you are experiencing this type of situation.

There are many Institutions, public and private, in your country that can help you. (see HELP page 246).

There are also the aggressors driven by pure malice, the ones who have as their sole idea of fun beating people up or getting people in trouble with a mate of theirs who enjoys violence.

These aggressors can be recognized by body language, they are often loud, parading like a cockerel, looking for a fight, often showing their bare arms as a sign of strength.

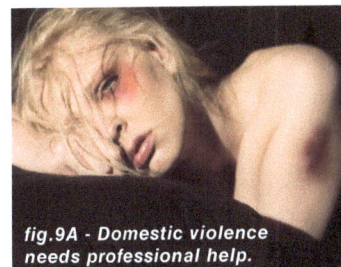

fig.9 - Kick his shin hard.

fig.9A - Domestic violence needs professional help.

They are erratic and unpredictable, looking for eye contact to start with the classic "what are you looking at?" prompt.

Depending on your given answer the situation will either escalate or resolve into nothing (see SWITCHING OFF page 116). What normally follows is a series of repeated remarks that will get shorter and almost hissing as the adrenaline kicks in, a sure sign that a fight is imminent. Splaying arms, a jerky movement of the head, normally tilting left and right and turning his body sideways are all signs that he is preparing to fight.

All aggressors set upon you in exactly the same way, through a common pattern that is known amongst criminals in general. The typical mugging or street robbery starts with a distraction, often asking you the time, directions or for a lighter.

LEARN TO SPOT VIOLENCE AS IT DEVELOPS FROM VERBAL CHALLENGE INTO PHYSICAL CONTACT.

That distraction allows an accomplice to sneak up behind you or the attacker coming closer and threatening you with a weapon. However, dialogue can also be accompanied by a more elaborate form of deception, such as an arm in a plaster, carrying heavy shopping, faking an injury or an accident, to make you open your door for instance. If you feel brave enough have a look at photos of the worst serial killers in criminal history and you will be surprised how "boy next door" they looked. Jeffrey Dhamer could have easily passed as a teacher, David Berkowitz - Son of Sam- as a local cop, Ted Bundy as a journalist and so on. (you can see a photo gallery with descriptions here: http://crime.about.com/od/serial/ig/serialkillerphotos/).

Very few aggressors look like a person up to no good.

All this often starts with a very polite tone, almost charming and friendly. After this initial approach normally violence follows, often explosive and sudden, from which people, even trained martial artists, do not recover. The main aim of this book is to learn the signs of this and to become aware and able to respond effectively, giving you a 'sixth sense" that will keep you attentive and cautious all the time, automatically without realising after a while.

This attitude, a true dormant animal instinct, will allow you to sense danger before it fully develops into a irreversible situation, the same attitude that keeps a gazelle alive in the savannah, ready to put distance between itself and the predator at the first whiff of hunting presence.

As we bring our introduction to a close, enjoy the following material and absorb what we show you and make it yours. We don't expect you to learn all the moves and all the techniques, only real practice, under proper supervision, can do that for you, but at least we can expect that you will become more informed and more aware not only of what to expect but also how to make the most of what you naturally have and what you normally carry or is available.

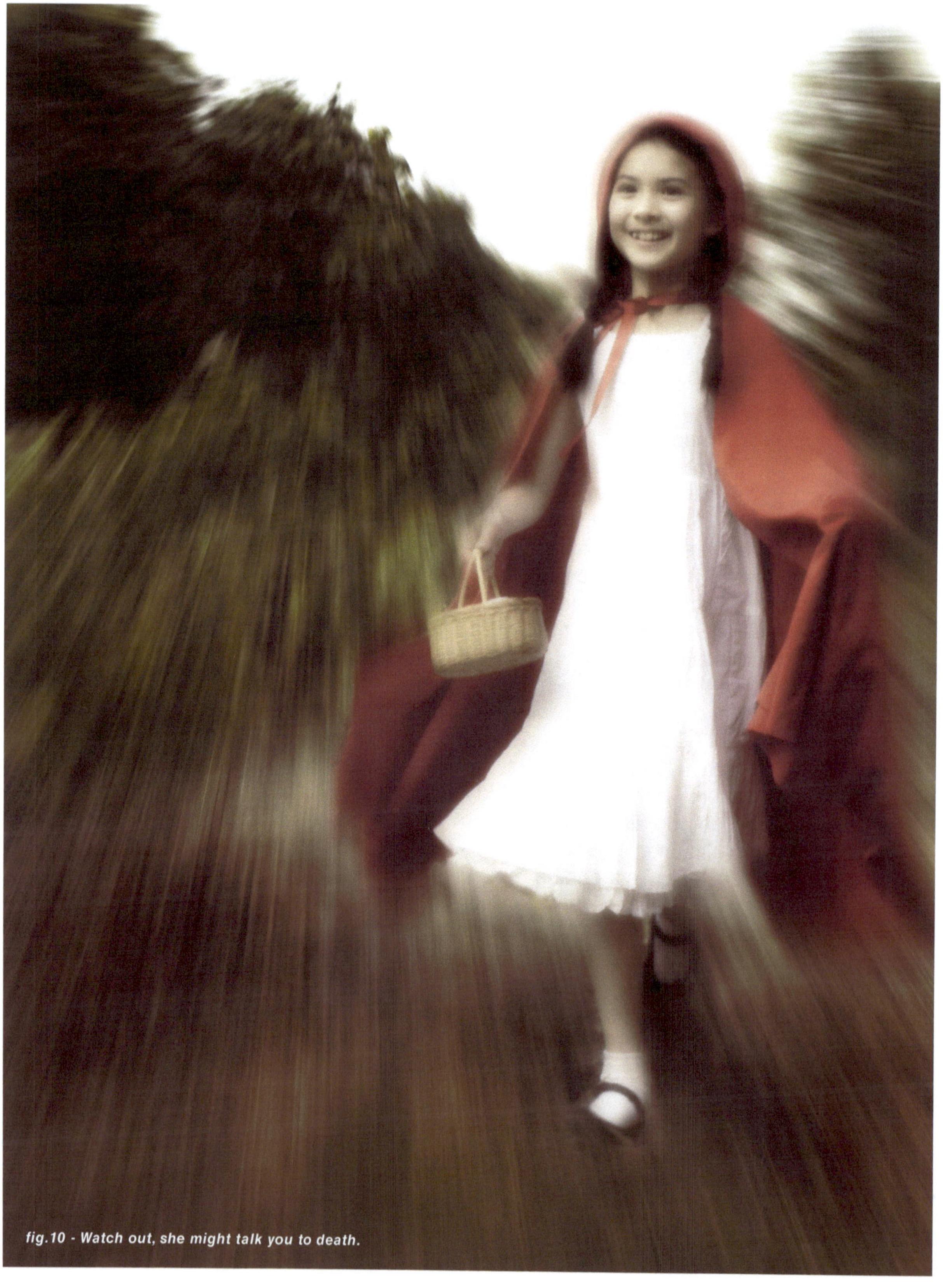

fig.10 - Watch out, she might talk you to death.

We all know the story of the big bad wolf, but do we really know why unfortunately some people end up more often than others as targets of aggressive behaviour, or violent attacks?

Women, children and elderly people seem to be the ideal prey in our society. This is only partially true; in fact statistics in many countries often show that it is mostly young males between 16 and 25 that are the subject of violent attacks in the modern world. This book is not the place to discuss why this happens but it is worth remembering that as a woman or an elderly person you are actually quite safe.

Nevertheless, both categories tend to be physically weaker compared to men and normally lesser in weight and height, making them more vulnerable.

There is also a general tendency from women to refrain from violent behaviour.

However, it is worth remembering that a woman who has self-defence knowledge has the advantage of surprising an attacker, because a man will feel superior physically.

It is also true that women are often a target because they carry their valuables in view, jewels are worn around the neck, bags are carried as a trophy or a status symbol, often containing everything inside, documents, money, keys, mobile phone, while men tend to carry their money in the pocket, their phone in the breast pocket.

BLEND IN IF YOU PREFER TO AVOID UNWANTED ATTENTION.

Men don't carry a brief case with them all the time.

This is important to understand: the first form of self-defence is not to attract unwanted attention.It's okay going to a reception or a party with your family jewels on you, but walking downtown gleaming like a Christmas tree will obviously be felt by some people as a provocation.

In BLENDING IN (page 126) we will show you some dos and don'ts, and remember that most importantly you should be aware of your environment all the time, meaning that walking around talking on your mobile phone oblivious to what happens around you is quite inappropriate.

Wear what you want where you want, but it is almost unavoidable that wearing, a mini skirt and high heels next to a building site might start a whistling concert.

A victim is the subject of an attack, and feeling victimized is a mental status that has often potentially serious consequences for anyone's psyche.

If you feel you need support because you have been a victim of a violent attack you'll find a list of useful contacts to get specialised help at page 246, HELP.

We will also examine further the psychological aspect of aggressive behaviour in SWITCHING OFF (page 116).

To understand what someone goes through during a dangerous situation let's talk about fear and how to control it.

Fear is a strong emotion that pervades the whole organism provoking physiological and psychological reactions: your heartbeat increases considerably, and so does blood circulation.

FEAR AFFECTS YOUR BODY'S ABILITY TO RESPOND EFFECTIVELY.

Breathing speeds up to cope with the increased oxygen consumption, and your blood pressure rises to compensate the extra work. Your muscles contract, including your facial muscles, giving your face a typically fearful expression. Pupils dilate, perspiration increases, you start sweating profusely, your hair stands up. This physical scenario is accompanied by a psychological status that makes you freeze.
Your movements are heavy, your legs go to jelly, and even if you want to run you just cannot move, you are frozen on the spot like a rabbit. All these reactions are normally automatic, even an experienced boxer before entering the ring still feels his legs going to jelly, and his hair standing up, a tingling sensation pervading his body.
The answer that naturally comes to the stimulus described is to run or to fight, it is a natural survival response.

Our general advice is, if you can, run, if you can't, for whatever reason, andyou are in fear for your own life, then you can only fight, and you should always go for broke. You can see already this is the main problem teaching self-defence, teaching how to overcome fear without been able to recreate it in a simulated scenario, especially considering that any training environment must take into consideration safety while demonstrating techniques.
The simulation of an attack and its appropriate response suffers from one important and very damning factor: lack of realism.

DON'T LET SHOCK BECOME PANIC.

PANIC IS THE REAL KILLER.

Attending a demonstration of martial arts or similar hand- to-hand combat techniques, it becomes clear almost immediately to the trained eye that both attacker and defender know what is going to happen next. Obviously, unless we are talking about elite commando units training where as-close-to-reality scenarios are necessary, including live fire, it is unthinkable to achieve attack/counter attack demonstrations exactly as they would happen in reality in a civilian environment, both for practical and legal reasons. One solution is to minimize the actions to take if under violent attack: it is important to keep everything simple and direct.

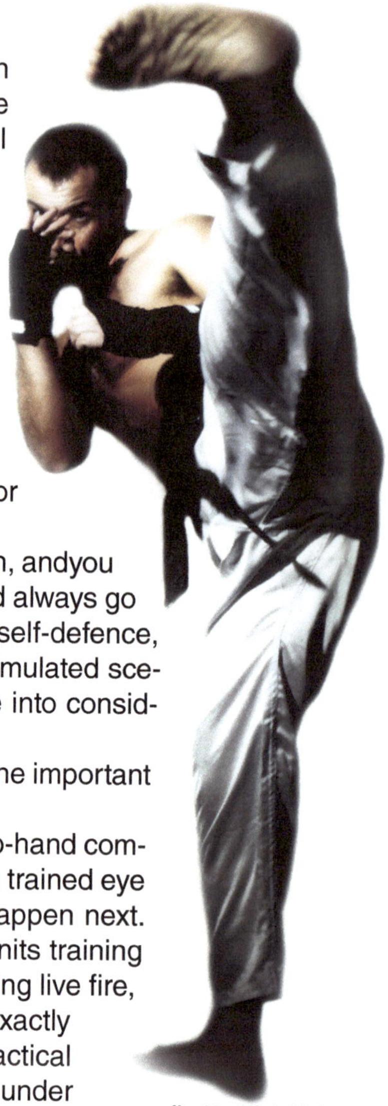

fig.11 - High kick to the chin.

For instance, a high kick to the chin (fig.11) or a spinning flying hook kick to the head (fig.41) looks spectacular and has made many martial artists movie stars but in a real situation very seldom is it effective to neutralize an attacker.
We will explore this further on in more detail, especially concentrating on simple moves.
Fundamentally it is almost impossible to recreate real fear, the most disabling factors of a real life attack. "Fear" as we have seen is a mental state that provokes disabling reactions, and it can be controlled through previous experience, training and acquired knowledge, this is why a boxer entering the ring will still feel fear but will also be able to control it.

YOU CAN LEARN TO CONTROL FEAR IF YOU EXPERIENCE IT IN TRAINING.

In the Perfect Defence system practical course, a fundamental aspect is to make sure that the participant experiences at least once how it feels to be intimidated, abused or manhandled roughly (fig.12).
Some people might object to that, but the feedback we have received afterwards has always been extremely positive and reactions to this part of the training have varied from hysterical behaviour, freezing on the spot or disproportionate physical reaction to the threat.

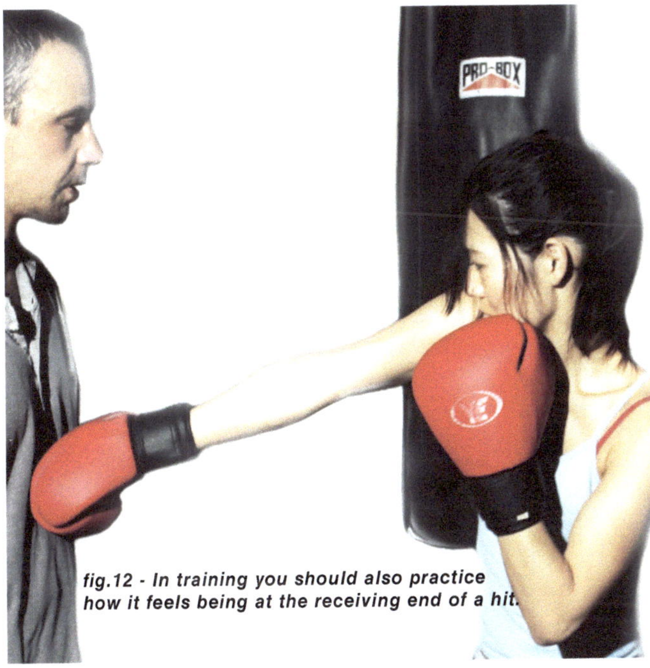

fig.12 - In training you should also practice how it feels being at the receiving end of a hit.

It is important to face the invasion of our own space and to feel somebody getting you into a headlock for instance and might help overcoming the initial shock faster when it is happening for real.

Quite often the initial attack is carried out after approaching the victim with the broadest of smiles and warm words.

At the same time there are signs that can show the real intention such as glancing around, scanning the surrounding for fear of being caught while hiding his hands in his pockets, or down the sides to conceal a knife or using something such as a plastic bag.

In any case, speed of reaction is fundamental and equally important is to experience in training some rough handling to be able to reduce the surprise and sub sequential shock of someone physically attacking you.

SPEED OF REACTION IS ACHIEVED BREAKING BARRIERS.

Reducing the initial shock of physical contact through practice increases the speed of reaction and we will keep emphasising throughout this site that speed is the most important factor in reacting to a threat, and any technique simulating the rough edges of a real attack will help you to cut down your reaction time, overcoming the shock of the new and being able to defend yourself much more effectively, without thinking but just reacting appropriately.

We will state many times over the following pages that it is always better to walk away from violence, however if you feel that you will be subjected to an attack do not wait for the first strike, but instead strike first with all you got, without hesitating.

If you are still not sure about it or you are worried about the consequences in a Court of Law remember that most Laws allow someone to strike first as a preventive measure when you have the honest belief, supported by evidence, that you were about to be attacked and decided to strike first. The first few seconds are decisive in most cases of impending physical violence, hesitation in these cases is synonymous with being hurt because you are thinking as a victim, someone who stands no chance, but all it means is that indecision equals defeat.

React and react with all you have got in the fastest, strongest most violent way that you can give, once you have hit him successfully then run as fast and as far as you can.

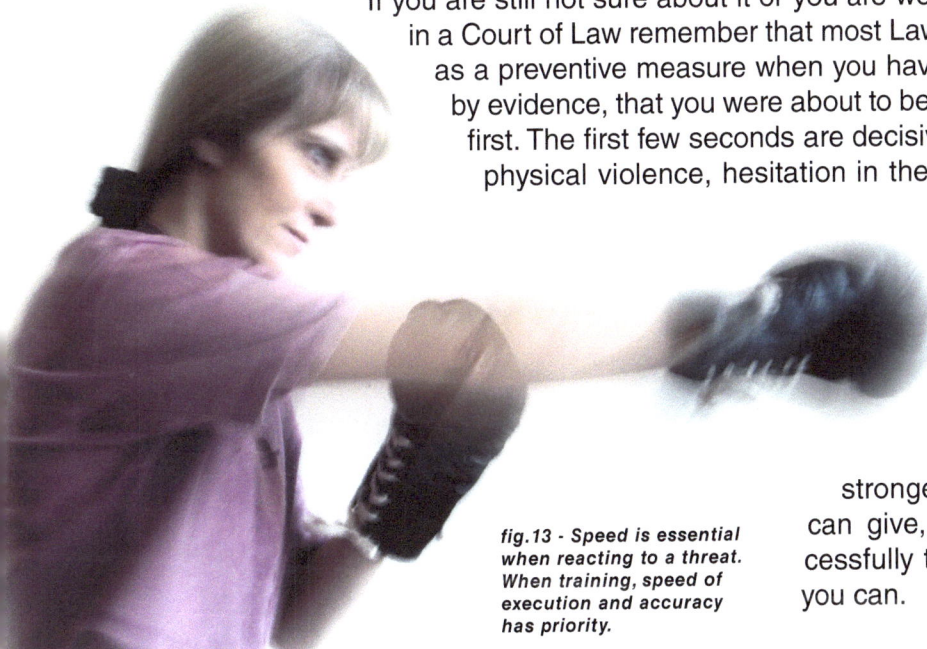

fig.13 - Speed is essential when reacting to a threat. When training, speed of execution and accuracy has priority.

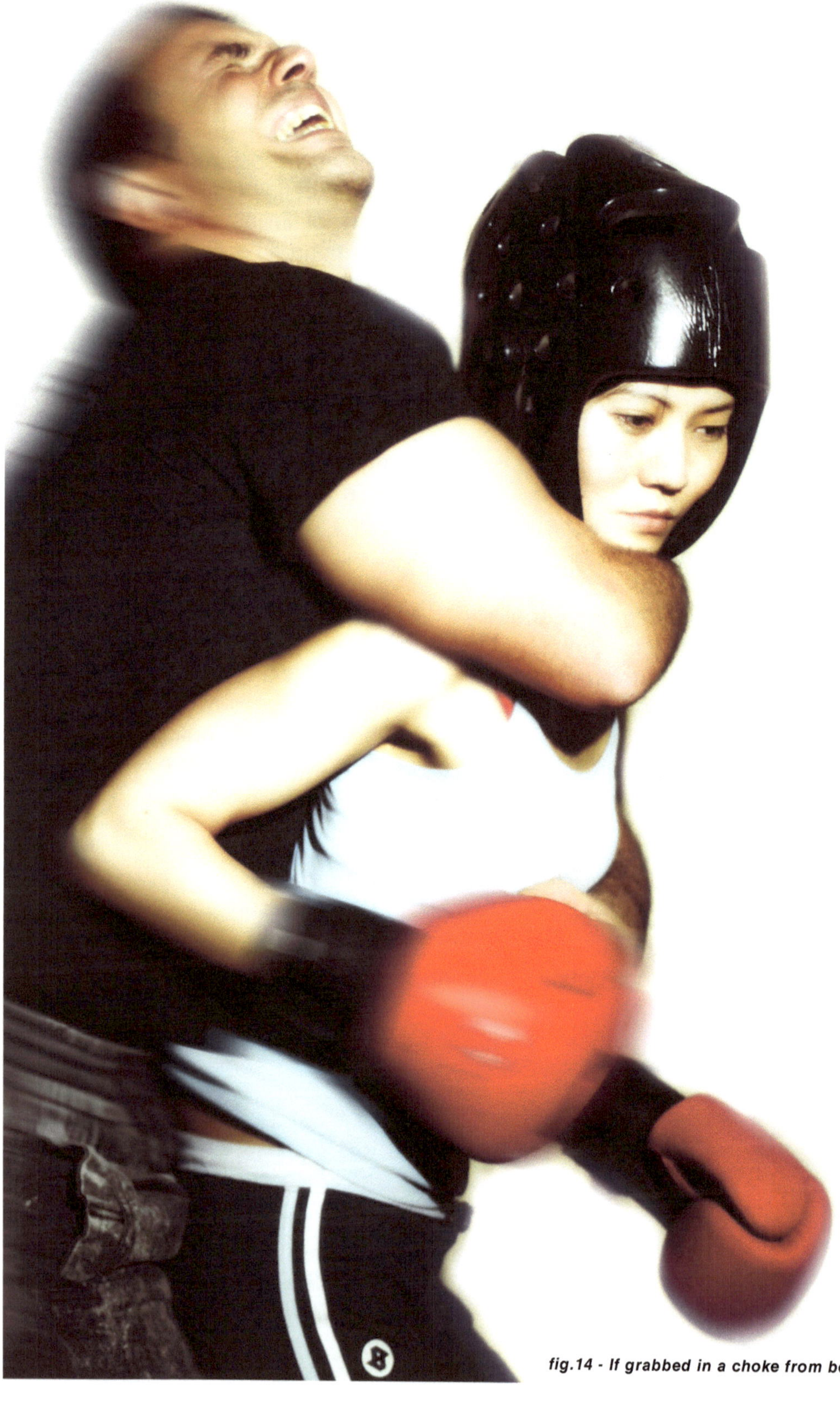

fig.14 - If grabbed in a choke from behind, use your elbows.

17

defence

Learning to defend oneself starts from avoiding ending up in a dangerous situation in the first place, in other words, prevention.

We will not fall into discussions about the fact that it shouldn't be that way and it is the authorities' duty to protect everyone at all times, everywhere, and it is the Police's job to make sure everyone can carry on with their lives without being subjected to violence.

We will only concentrate on simple and practical advice with moves that comes natural to most. In nature all animals that we commonly consider easy prey have developed a clever and simple system to minimize the risk of becoming an easy meal to their predators.

This clever system Mother Nature developed is called camouflaging or blending in.

A zebra's mantel pattern against high grass and the arctic hare's capacity of changing coat with the season, allows them to survive longer because they don't stand out, therefore the rule number one is: when in Rome, do what the Romans do.

BLEND IN IF YOU WANT TO SURVIVE, A LOW PROFILE IS THE BEST DEFENCE.

If you go around a big city, dressed like a tourist and behaving like a tourist, with all your money in the purse, your camera around your neck and a big map in your hands, it is like inviting everyone with little or no scruples to help themselves to your belongings. Use common sense, observe the environment you find yourself in, and blend in (see also BLENDING IN - page 126).

Once in their usual, familiar environment, neighbourhood or street, the majority of individuals tend to be less vigilant and are a bit more easy going, including yourself.

You know the landscape, you know some of the people, and everything is familiar.

That's why if you get attacked around the corner from where you live or on your doorsteps, the shock will be greater and suddenly home does not feel so safe anymore.

That is possibly to do with an unfortunate one in a million encounter or maybe because suddenly you have changed something and attracted attention, a little change that made you stand out in an environment where until a while ago you would go unnoticed, blending in nicely.

The usual most common advice is, as a general principle, to avoid areas poorly lit or abandoned.

Make sure that if you go somewhere you have never been before that at least somebody else knows your whereabouts, and ideally if you can go with somebody the better.

Use licensed taxis or a reputable certified company or if you drive by car always lock yourself in, even during daytime, putting your valuables on the floor in the front.

Do not put all your documents, phone, cards, car keys and house keys in one bag.

Keep at least your mobile phone on you so you can call for help even if your bag has been taken.

If you have to walk alone hold your mobile phone hidden in your hand, away from view, and pre-dial 999 or your local emergency number, so that just pressing the call button will automatically dial the number without you dialling every single number.

Try and walk with confidence, without holding your bag as if it contains a large sum.
If someone approaches you asking for information or the time, DO NOT STOP, keep walking and politely answer you don't know or that your watch is broken, or just don't answer. If you feel somebody is following you, it is quite possible that they are , therefore stop at the nearest house, ring the bell, even at a late hour, explain the situation and ask whoever answers to call a cab, or to call the police. Don't be shy, if the occupiers are decent people they'll be glad to help. Don't go inside the house unless you are absolutely sure that the occupants are trustworthy, ideally a mature or elderly couple, or someone with children (are there any toys on the front lawn or near the entrance?) in any case ask to wait on the doorstep until the cavalry arrives. If you have to wait for somebody on the street at night make sure you stay with other people until they arrive, or set yourself a cut off time to call it off and return home. There is more on preventive measures, further on and in SCENARIOS (page 214).

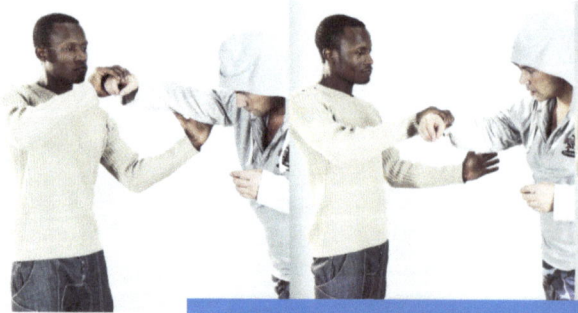

A good exercise that can be fun and lets you acquire effective defensive methods is to observe people's behaviour and think what would you do in case they turn aggressive towards you, it also keeps you mind alert without getting paranoid.
For instance: you are walking to your local shop and you see a man running towards you. Imagine for a moment what you would do to stop him snatching your purse (in fact it is more likely that he is trying to catch the bus that is just pulling over behind you).
Assuming he is really after your beautiful leather companion would you:
1) Enter the nearest shop as quickly as possible.
2) Back off to a stationary car, holding the purse as close to your chest as possible.
3) With a sudden and explosive move cross the road suddenly.
4) Step sideways and at the same time kick him on his thigh (fig.15).
This little game will help you train your brain to create elaborate solutions quickly, creating predefined patterns, to apply if this should happen for real. Here it is: you are sitting in a train.
Two young men are sitting opposite you; they had one too many drinks. What would you do if one of them suddenly sits next to you and suddenly puts his hand between your legs starting harassing you?
1) You grab his wrist moving his hand away and tell him to behave or you'll call the police.
2) You grab his wrist and apply an arm lever, (see LOCKS, page 90) pinning him to the ground (fig.16).
3) You elbow him on the chest and almost immediately punch him in the face with the back of your fist. Mind you though, this shouldn't become an obsession or more than just a mental exercise, it's just something to train your mind, considering that it could happen, even if the chances are it never will.

In any case, a calm, confident, firm response is always the best approach, and it will diffuse most potentially dangerous situations without necessarily resorting to physical action.

fig.15 - Step sideways, at the same time strike his thigh with your knee.

fig.16 - Grab his wrist and apply an arm lever. See also LOCKS page 90.

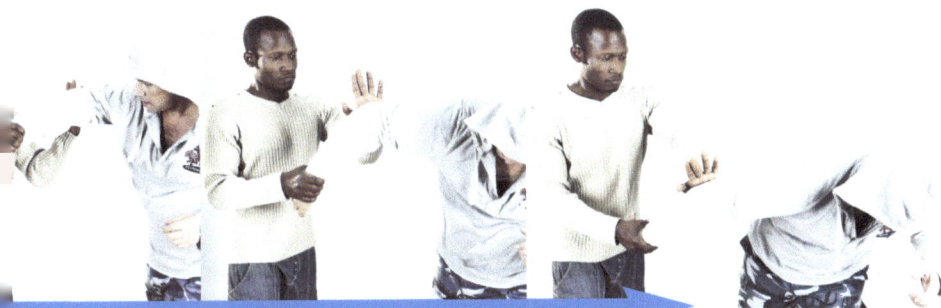

The first week I moved to London, I was on my way to a training session by Tube, the London Underground. I got into a train carriage that wasnearly empty. Sitting right opposite me there was a twenty-something nerdish look-ing male student, reading a book.

At a stop, a big man, quite scruffy looking, walked in, drunk and looking quite aggressive.

He was swearing and angry at the entire world, wearing a large coat and carrying a plastic bag. He sat next to the student, mum-bling something in-comprehensible; the student continued read-ing his book without flinching.

Suddenly, with no warning sign, the drunken man pulled out a kitchen knife about a foot long, and slowly but decisively landed the blade in the middle of the book the student was holding mut-tering obscenities. As I was about to jump on him, and put into practice years of training and real life experience with armed as-sailants, the student elegantly but firmly grabbed the man's wrist, lifting his arm and bending it towards him, and with the calmest tone said 'Come on, just behave yourself'.

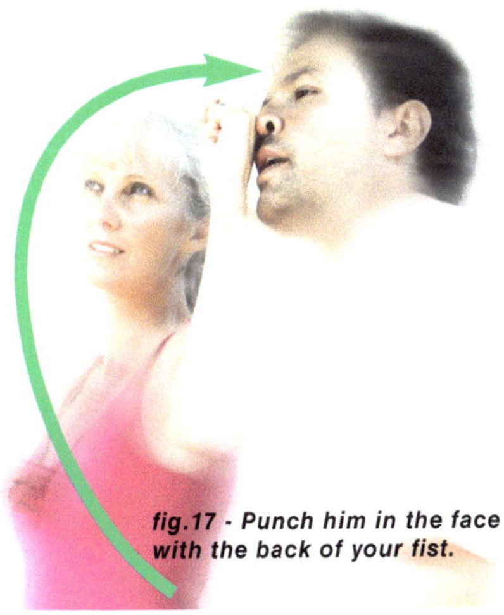

fig.17 - Punch him in the face with the back of your fist.

Like a child that has been told off, the man retreated and fell asleep on his seat. The student carried on reading totally un-phased by the whole experience. If the student's re-action had been hysterical, shouting or else, probably he would have provoked a violent reaction to the confused and intoxicated mind of the drunken man.

CONTROL YOURSELF TO BE ABLE TO CONTROL OTHERS.

Always keep a calm and controlled approach, and train your mind to react quickly.

In a real life situation, you will not be able to think, only to react, either by running or defending yourself by predetermined tried patterns, without any reasoning involved.

This book contains possible scenarios, some collected over the years from real experience which show you possible ways how to cope, but no written word on a screen can teach you how to stay calm: if you can learn to control your emotions you can learn to control your actions.

In any training the endless repetition of a single technique allows you to deploy what you have learned without too much thinking, almost as second nature, more like a rediscovered instinct.

There are many ways to achieve control and become calmer in stressful situations, probably the easiest one is to breathe slowly and deeply to allow correct oxygenation of your brain, and to learn how to feel your body, and how your body works. In other words achieve control of your actions, the opposite of panicking, where fear takes control of your reactions.

A contact sport will give you the "valve" you'll need to vent frustration as well as keeping fit while having fun (fig.17) and you can always put a picture of your boss or ex-boyfriend on your punch bag and hit the hell out of it, making you feel good, extremely good, believe me.

Prevention is still the best defence though, and you should always remember that there are peo-ple who, especially in certain environments unfortunately, prey on the weak ones.

Nightclubs or discotheque are places where people want to have fun and enjoy themselves, without worrying about conventions and constrictions, letting off frustrations and stress.
You had a tough week at work and the loud music, drinks and a crowd that is having a good time is all you want. I have worked in clubs and similar venues and one of the things that was always a concern was to keep an eye on the vulnerable, the ones who might fall easy prey to the simplest of tricks. Here are some very simple rules, which if remembered will save you more than a simple headache (see also COMMON SENSE - page 250 - for more tips).

1) Always go out in the company of trusted friends or colleagues and leave with them or with someone you have known for a while, not someone you just met, even if he seems absolutely charming.

2) Do not accept drinks from strangers, NEVER, and if you leave your drink unattended (for example when you went to the toilet, went on the dancefloor) just get a new one. It is so incredibly simple to slip something into someone's drink and the consequences can be really ugly and devastating for years.

3) Do not accept lifts or any kind of transport if you are on your own, by someone you have just met or you don't know. If you are lost ask a female member of staff or someone from the security staff of the venue to help you, that is what they are for.

4) Make sure someone else who is not there knows where you went, and approximately at what time you were planning to be back, it does not have to be your mum or brother, but a friend will do. You'll do the same for her/him next time, I am sure they will be equally grateful.

5) Don't drink yourself to the point of not knowing where you are, and if you can't help it at least be with someone who will take care of you and knows you, you can return the favour.

6) When you enter a building where there is a crowd memorise where the emergency exits are, and check which one is the shortest route to leave safely in case there is trouble and pay attention to where the security staff are usually located, you might need them.

7) Use common sense and remember that if you have a bad feeling about a situation or about someone, most of the time you are right. You can read more suggestions also in SCENARIOS (page 214).
We are going to see in the next pages various techniques in full detail that will help you if you ever are attacked, but remember that the best form of defence is prevention, acquired through knowledge because knowledge of possible danger gives you awareness.
All this makes a lot of sense but how do you become more aware?
You can become more aware simply through carefully observing your everyday surroundings. Give it more thought, see it with different eyes, ideally as if you were a criminal looking for your next victim, the easy one to prey on. Next time you go shopping or to the cinema sit in the parking lot for a few minutes and note how easy it would be for a criminal to attack or prey on someone, and see how you shouldn't behave.

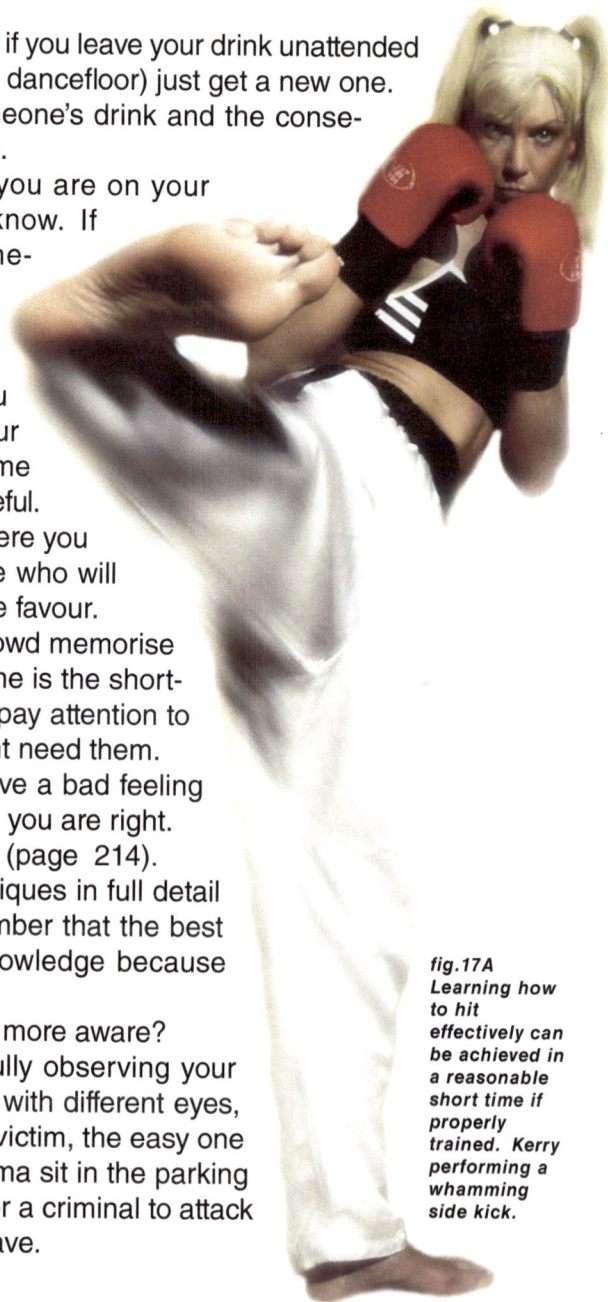

fig.17A
Learning how to hit effectively can be achieved in a reasonable short time if properly trained. Kerry performing a whamming side kick.

Women walking to and from their cars totally immersed in deep thoughts or busy chatting on their mobile phones, often look lost as they try to remember where they have parked the car. They are blissfully unaware of what happens around them as they load their shopping into the car, or while securing their child into the back seat, sometimes with the engine running in winter to heat up the car, in summer to get the air conditioning going. When would you strike? Exactly…

Muggers and robbers are always creative and inventive with ways of approaching their victims and create the right opportunity. A successful one is the so called "huggy mugging" that works like this: you have just left a pub, club or bar and are quite jolly and probably intoxicated.

Someone approaches you with a broad smile, sometimes acting drunk, possibly pretending he is being celebrating and asks you to give you a hug. Before you are able to say anything he is hugging you and other people suddenly join in, chanting, hugging and sometimes performing a little dance. By the time you realise that your wallet is gone they have already left.

Defence is mostly a preventive measure, perfect defence is when you can spot a potentially dangerous situation in time to avoid it. It is rather important that you can recognise the signs of verbal threat that can escalate into a physical attack. There are situations, especially if you are a man, that can put you more at risk.

You might come across people while with your girlfriend who love to make very unpleasant comments about your girl loud enough for everyone to hear for instance.

Move on and ignore them completely, all they are trying to do is to set you up to a fight knowing that such comments would wind you up. If you are confronted by someone who you think can turn violent and you want to have a better chance to defend yourself you should consider assuming one of the poses as shown in figure 18.

These stances are quite "normal" in the sense that they don't show a defence mechanism but at the same time put a barrier between you and a potential threat without giving away your defence.

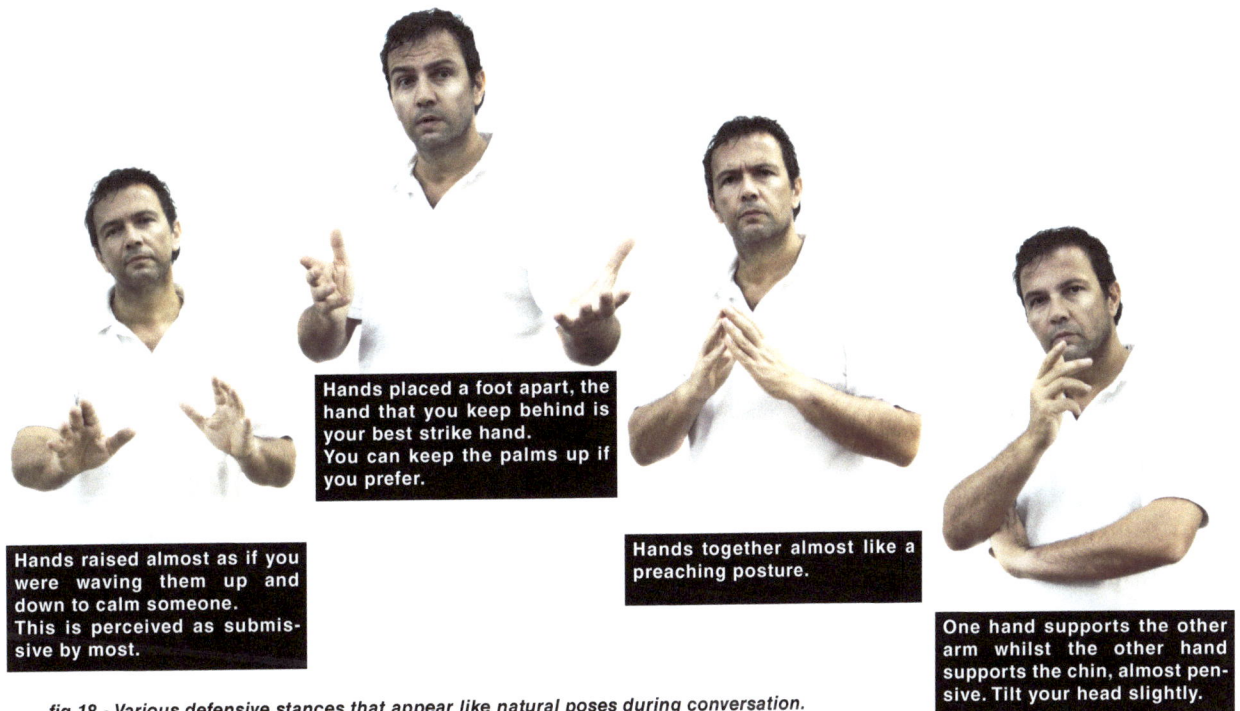

Hands placed a foot apart, the hand that you keep behind is your best strike hand. You can keep the palms up if you prefer.

Hands together almost like a preaching posture.

Hands raised almost as if you were waving them up and down to calm someone. This is perceived as submissive by most.

One hand supports the other arm whilst the other hand supports the chin, almost pensive. Tilt your head slightly.

fig.18 - Various defensive stances that appear like natural poses during conversation.

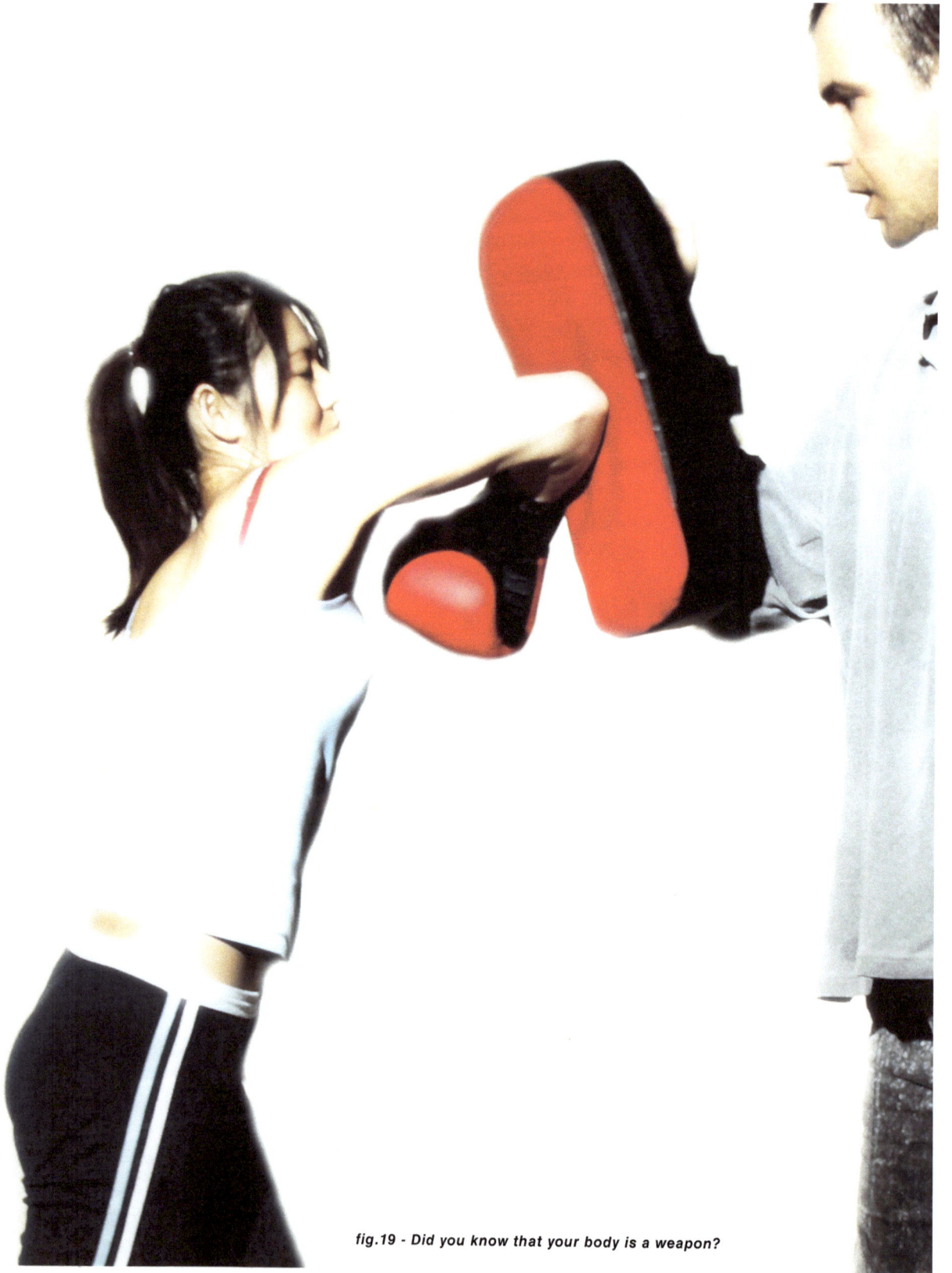

fig.19 - Did you know that your body is a weapon?

strong

Fitness should be considered an important factor to increase the efficiency in executing a technique: stamina, strength and quick reflexes will help you achieve results against a violent aggressor. A well-toned body can take 'punishment' better than an untrained one and by muscular tone we mean the general definition of a slight constant tension of the muscles (see FITNESS - page 228).

This persistent contraction of a muscle even when resting is important also to obtain a good posture and efficient blood circulation.

A well toned muscle contracts faster and allows you a prompt immediate movement when the need arises and this doesn't mean spending hours in the gym, it means walking up steps instead of taking the lift, use the car a bit less, and in general keep a healthy diet. To take just one simple step a person normally employs 200 muscles; just imagine what can be achieved with a little extra going up flights of stairs.

To imagine that technique alone will throw to the ground a heavy man is a bit naive. It is true that most Judo and Aikido techniques use the momentum of the attacker to project him to the ground (see TAKEDOWNS - page 52) but it's also true that a firm grasp and the ability to twist your body to get into a good position is also as important.

LOOK AFTER YOUR BODY AND YOUR BODY WILL LOOK AFTER YOU.

In other words, if you consider your body as a weapon, you should look after it, maintain it well and service it properly.

Stamina is the capacity to sustain fatigue for a given time, and it's stamina that allows a fighter to execute several techniques or combinations for at least 30 seconds without stopping.

Ideally, you should be able to run fast a couple of hundred meters without becoming breathless or feeling any abdominal pain (see RUNNING - page 232).

Elasticity and flexibility is something that has to be acquired through constant training and daily exercise as every dancer or martial artist knows (see STRETCHING - page 224) and it has to be kept up with constantly.

Being supple depends greatly on articulation movement and coordination.

If you find it difficult to raise your arm above your head to counteract an attack you obviously have less techniques available at your disposal.

Probably the most important articulations are the shoulders and the Cox femoral (hips joint) because they allow the biggest movement of the longest limbs.

Being supple and agile is not absolutely necessary but it certainly helps and it can be improved upon with very simple exercises.

UNDER STRESS YOU WILL ALWAYS REACT ACCORDING TO HOW WELL YOU HAVE TRAINED.

Good articulation mobility, will allow you to rotate your body more efficiently to deflect an attack, as well as easily move into a good position to strike back.

A top physical preparation requires constant commitment, without many compromises, especially at competition level. This shouldn't be used as an excuse, try at least to dedicate a few minutes a day, or at least twice a week, and practice some of the very simple exercises contained in the tables (STRETCHING - page 224 and FITNESS - page 228). Our body is quite amazing: it has been designed to withstand aggressive factors such as heat, cold, sharp blows and so forth but at the same time, we are not as well protected as most animals are.

USE YOUR HEAD IN EVERY SENSE AND EVERY WAY.

In actual fact, we are one of the weakest creatures on earth and very vulnerable if left alone and naked in the wild, nevertheless you can use parts of your body to strike an attacker acquiring very little or no damage, yet causing considerable damage to the receiver.

Head butting is an effective close range technique; you should use your forehead, which is quite strong, aiming at an attacker's nose, chin or jaw. The back of your head can also be used if attacked from behind to strike at the same points as before (fig.21). It is important to avoid using the side (temples) of your head because they are quite weak.

Your **shoulders** are well padded, being quite covered by deltoids and can be used effectively in a close combat situation, ideally pivoting on your axis, especially to fend off blows.

One of the hardest parts of your body is the elbow. **Elbows** are

fig.20 - Muscles are very elastic and provide good cushioning. Go to page 226 fig.298 for a more detailed muscles description.

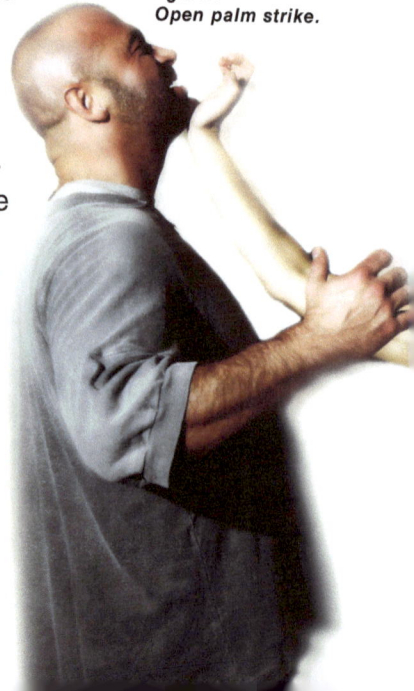

YOUR HANDS ARE THE WEAKEST PART OF YOUR BODY, BUT THE MOST VERSATILE.

tremendous weapons, very strong and extremely effective because of their pointy shape, especially at close range, and their position they are within our body (fig.14). **Forearms** are useful to deflect or block blows even from batons, since the bone is quite exposed and with very few superficial nerves.

The **hand** is a known weapon, especially when used as a fist, unfortunately, most people don't know how to punch correctly, and a badly landed punch can cause you severe pain and you might damage your wrist or even break your knuckles. In figure 22 we show you how to make a proper fist and several ways of how to use your hands to strike. Some of these will suit some people; some will not, it depends on the strength of your fingers and wrists; nevertheless it is important to know these are available to you.

It is equally important to remember that when throwing a punch, either a jab or a straight punch, your hips should twist to add more power to the blow, using the body as a loaded spring to unleash the punch.

To make sure your strike is effective always imagine 'punching through' your target (fig.22).

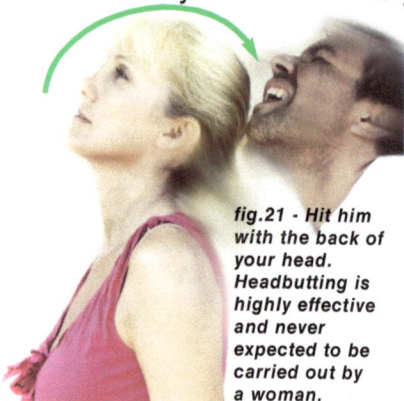

fig.21A
Open palm strike.

fig.21 - Hit him with the back of your head. Headbutting is highly effective and never expected to be carried out by a woman.

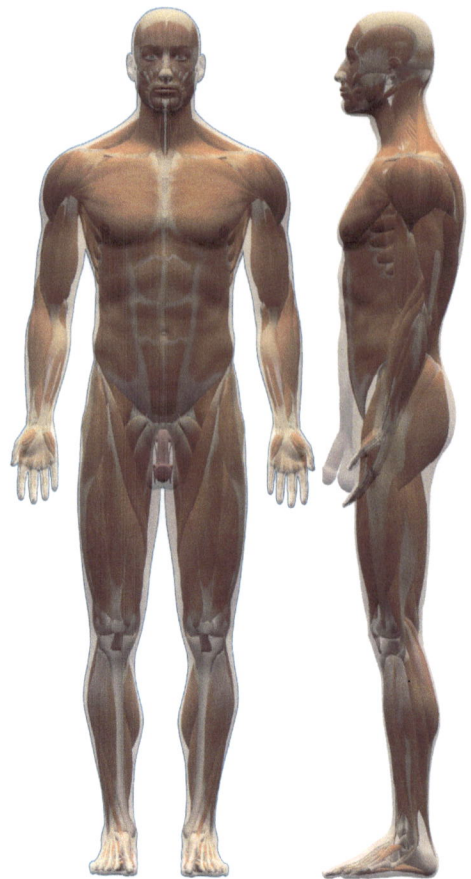

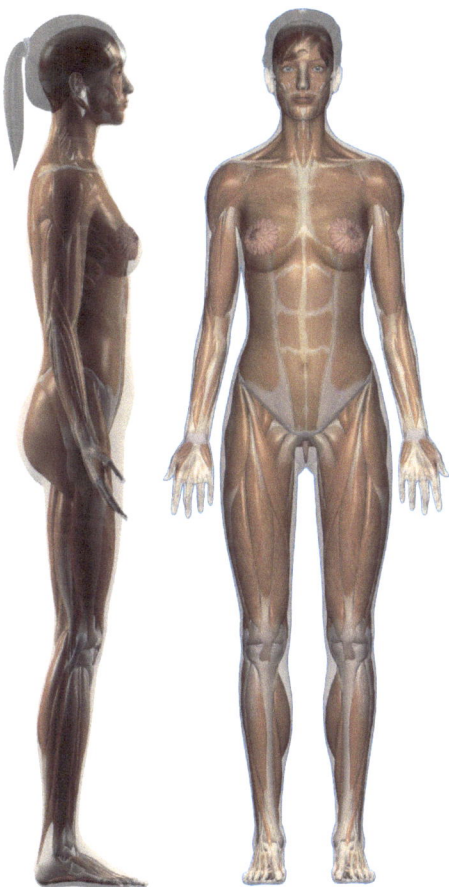

Another effective way of using your hand is an 'open palm' (fig.21A) strike. This type of technique has the advantage to hit a wide area of a target, for example if you are grabbed by the neck and you are facing your assailant, slapping an open palm on his ears will cause him some serious damage as well as great disorientation. The open-palm technique is also useful to disarm someone pointing a gun at you at close range, we'll see how to in detail in WEAPONS (page 102).

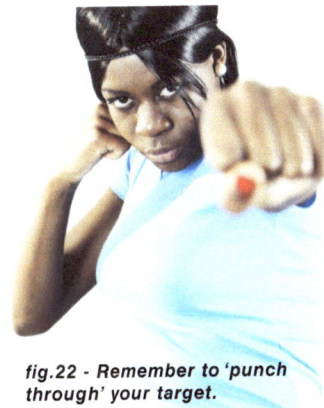

fig.22 - Remember to 'punch through' your target.

You can consider your **knees** almost as effective as your elbows, the thigh is a very strong muscle, and the knee is quite hard. Always remember that striking with your knee is good at close range, and can be more effective when projecting forward your hips as well.

fig. 23 - Pulling your opponent towards your knee as you strike.

Knee strikes are simple to perform, therefore easily learned, however the technique still requires a sharp and sudden move, not easy when adrenaline gives you a shaky leg and your clothes, trousers or tight skirt, won't help, therefore as we have said many times before, practicing under supervision is as usual highly recommended. What makes a knee strike extremely effective is the ability of pulling your opponent towards the knee as you shoot it up, grabbing him by his clothes (see fig. 23).

The knee strike should always be carried out in a sudden and explosive manner, not only because it will lack power otherwise but also because if you poorly perform it this will allow your opponent to grab your knee and throw you onto the ground in no time.

The knee can be very much used in a similar way as the foot when kicking: you can shoot your knee upward, forward and as a roundhouse move, aiming at the side of the thigh or the kneecap. Always thrust your hips forward as you strike and put your entire body weight into the action, it's not necessary that you aim high, a pointy knee to the side of his thigh striking with force will sure hurt him.

PRACTICE MAKES PERFECT. MORE PRACTICE MAKES IT EFFECTIVE.

fig.24 - How to make a fist correctly: fold your fingers tightly at the knuckles, making sure your thumb does not stick out, keep your wrist straight and in line with your forearm.

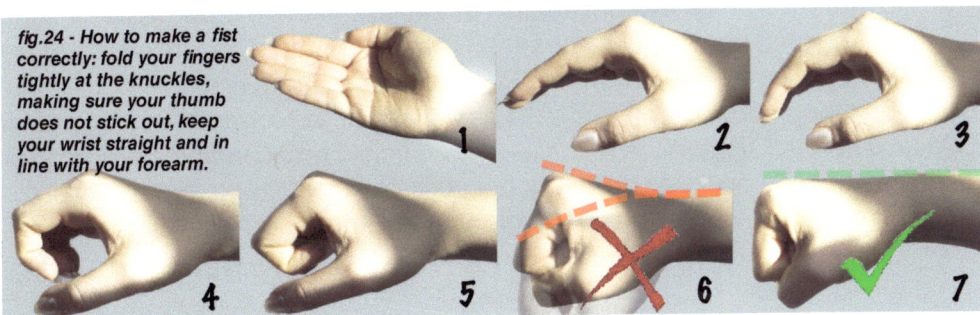

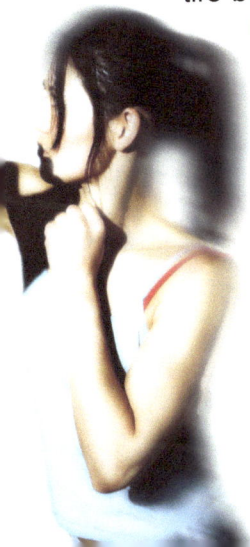

1

2

3

4

5

6

7

STRONG PARTS OF THE BODY

Your **foot**, especially if wearing shoes is a tremendously effective weapon.

It is quite important to learn how to use it properly, both to unbalance an opponent or to sweep as well as striking him from a safe distance and in fig.28 we show you the correct way to kick with your foot so as not to injure yourself.

Using your body as a weapon you should consider that obviously it's up to the individual to perfect striking techniques. In PREPARATION (page 36) as well as in the tables STRETCHING and FITNESS (page 224 and 228), you can see how to maximize your strength by perfecting your techniques, making every one count.

YOUR EYES ALLOW YOU TO BE AWARE, TO BE AWARE MEANS TO STAY ALIVE.

You will also discover through practice what can be used to expose your weaknesses, e.g. a side-kick can only be effective if carried out in a particular way, and practicing against a punch bag will reveal how good your technique is. The fundamental principles behind the Perfect Defence system are speed and simplicity: all techniques using the body as weapon are based on this, you will not see in here anything spectacular, you can go to a movie for that, but certainly you will find it extremely effective once you practice them to effect.

Your **eyesight** is another weapon: it's important to learn how to focus on an aggressor's actions and the environment, not using your eyes as an extra tool to fight back is a waste, you could find a possible escape route, spot an accomplice, find help, spot something you could use as a weapon, like a fire-extinguisher on the wall. Keeping eye contact if possible will help you read tell tale signs of your aggressor's intentions and as boxers know too well, a slight contraction of the

USE YOUR VOICE, DON'T BE SHY OR FEEL SILLY, IT'S SILLY NOT TO ACT.

muscles of the eye or variation in the size of the iris can indicate a change of action. You also have another powerful weapon at your disposal: your **voice**.

We will see in SWITCHING OFF (page 116), that a calm, firm tone can achieve great results even though obviously it is always best that you call for help, bearing in mind not to shout HELP but to shout "FIRE", this is because in our society most people are not too keen on running to rescue somebody being attacked but because of our heritage and a certain collective fear of fire we are more than keen to stop that threat in the shortest time.

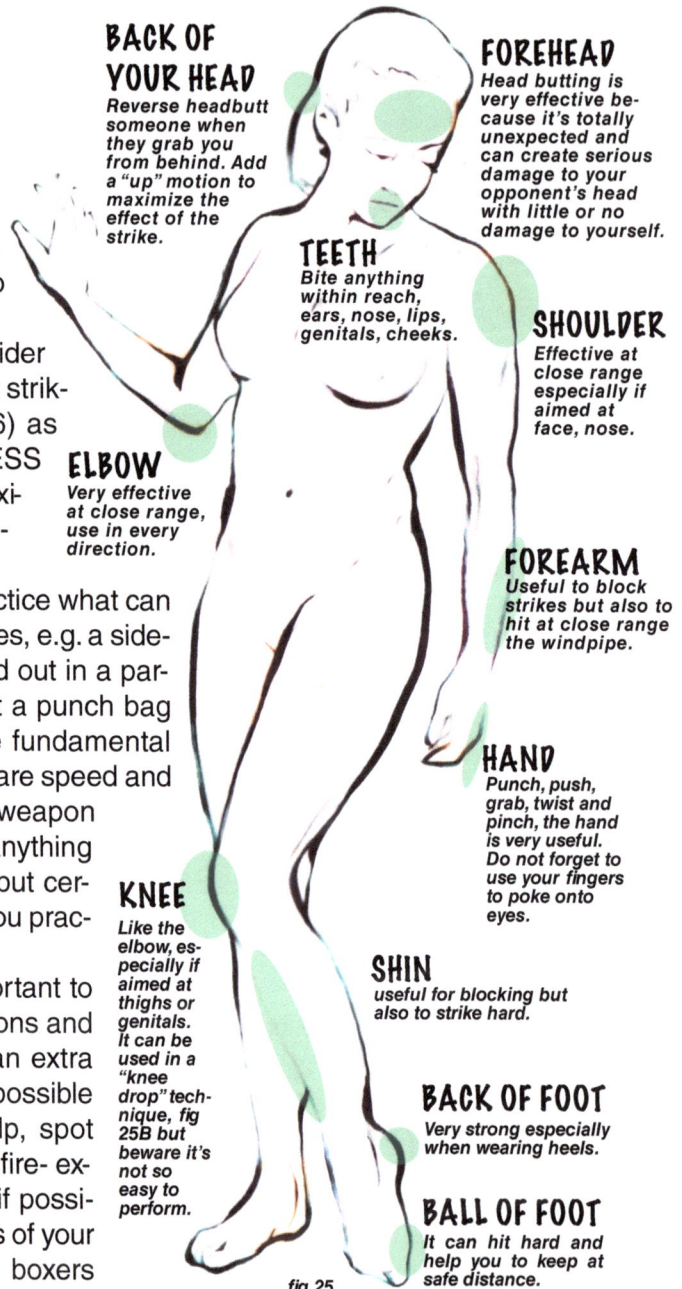

BACK OF YOUR HEAD
Reverse headbutt someone when they grab you from behind. Add a "up" motion to maximize the effect of the strike.

FOREHEAD
Head butting is very effective because it's totally unexpected and can create serious damage to your opponent's head with little or no damage to yourself.

TEETH
Bite anything within reach, ears, nose, lips, genitals, cheeks.

SHOULDER
Effective at close range especially if aimed at face, nose.

ELBOW
Very effective at close range, use in every direction.

FOREARM
Useful to block strikes but also to hit at close range the windpipe.

HAND
Punch, push, grab, twist and pinch, the hand is very useful. Do not forget to use your fingers to poke onto eyes.

KNEE
Like the elbow, especially if aimed at thighs or genitals. It can be used in a "knee drop" technique, fig 25B but beware it's not so easy to perform.

SHIN
useful for blocking but also to strike hard.

BACK OF FOOT
Very strong especially when wearing heels.

BALL OF FOOT
It can hit hard and help you to keep at safe distance.

fig.25

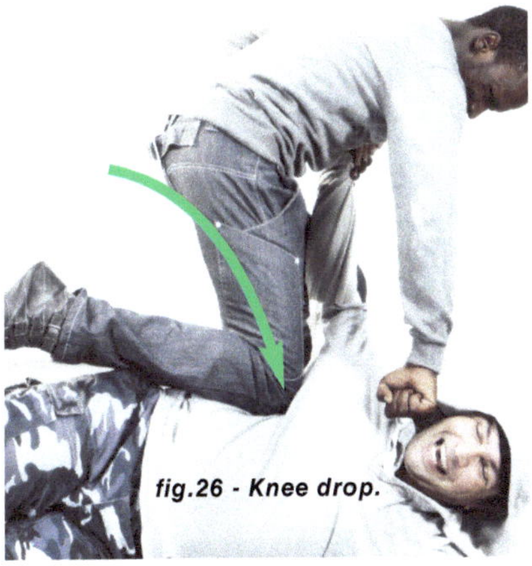

fig.26 - Knee drop.

People are more prone to come to the rescue in the event that something is burning down to avoid having their house following the same fate. It can also be helpful, in case of a sexual molester, just to shout something like "SHAME ON YOU!" or "YOU PIG!". Your tone and attitude may provoke a feeling of shame, especially if others are present, don't be shy.

Finally, especially when facing unruly teenagers, use a calm tone and appealing to their maturity, bearing in mind that often violent teenagers are only trying to establish contact with society, just in the wrong way and lack dialogue skills.

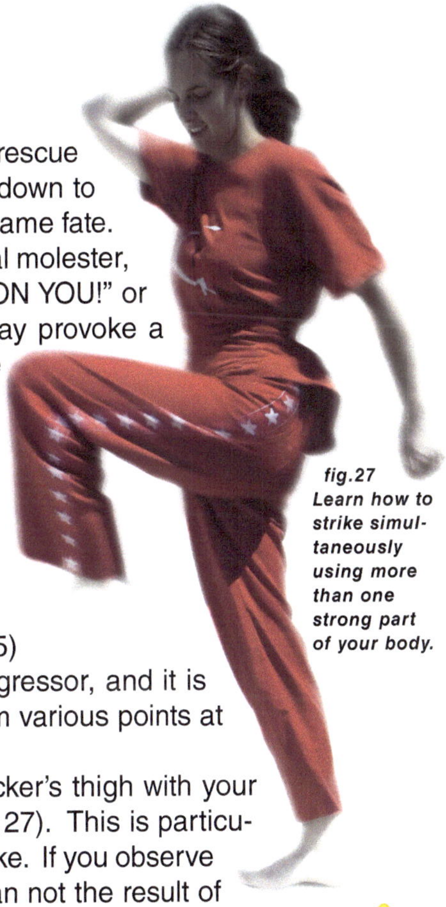

fig.27
Learn how to strike simultaneously using more than one strong part of your body.

As we have examined there are many parts of your body (fig. 25) that are strong and that can be used effectively to strike an aggressor, and it is equally important to remember that you can combine strikes from various points at various targets.

For instance it is more effective hitting simultaneously your attacker's thigh with your knee and his face with your elbow than just hitting his thigh (fig. 27). This is particularly useful in case you miss or he manages to avoid your first strike. If you observe a boxing match you will notice that knockouts are more often than not the result of a combination of different punches at different targets (right uppercut to the body and left hook to the jaw for instance (see more in HITTING page 44).

You should always practice a combination of different moves together. And lastly, remember that in a self-defence situation biting his face with your **teeth** can be devastating and especially effective, not to mention leaving a scar that can help with identifying him later on if suspects are caught.

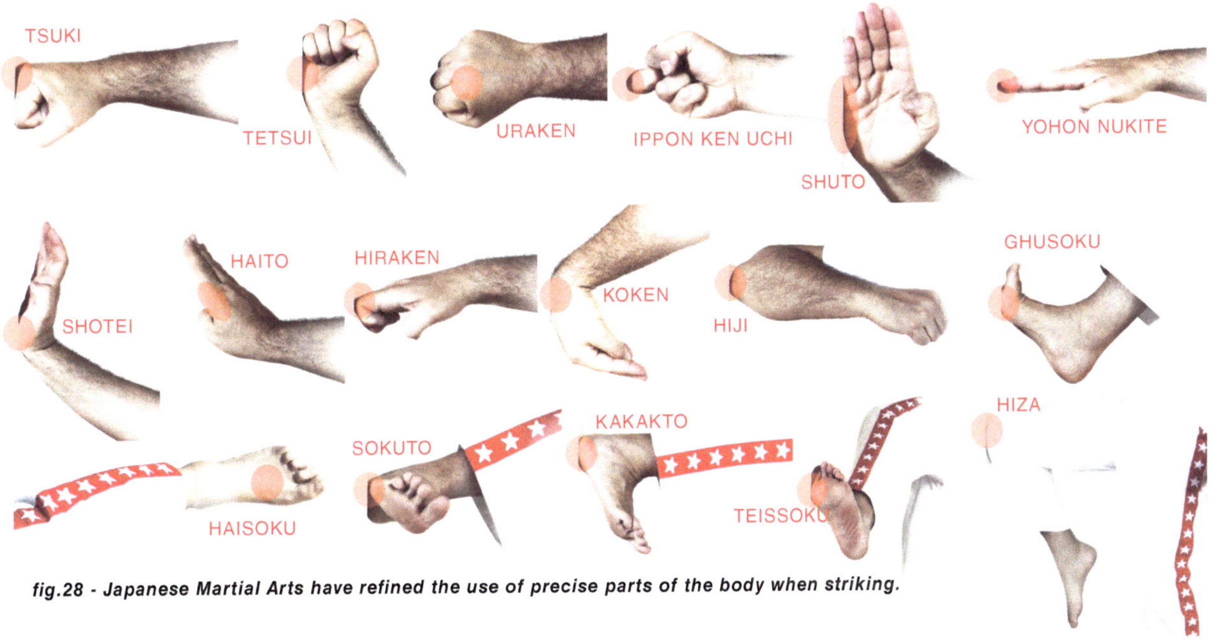

TSUKI
TETSUI
URAKEN
IPPON KEN UCHI
SHUTO
YOHON NUKITE
HAITO
HIRAKEN
KOKEN
HIJI
GHUSOKU
SHOTEI
HIZA
SOKUTO
KAKAKTO
TEISSOKU
HAISOKU

fig.28 - Japanese Martial Arts have refined the use of precise parts of the body when striking.

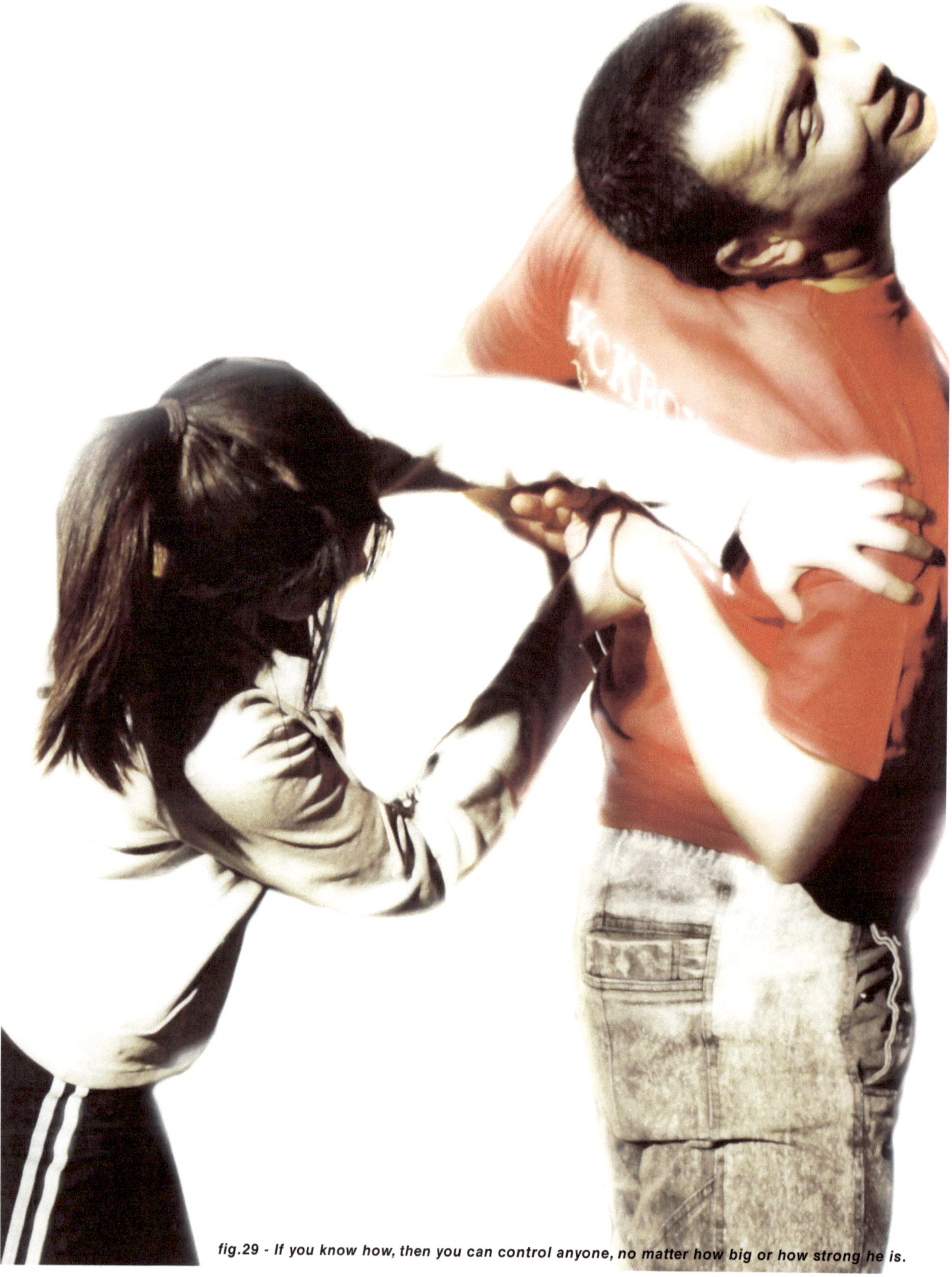

fig.29 - If you know how, then you can control anyone, no matter how big or how strong he is.

29

vulnerable

We have seen how strong some parts of your body can be, at the same time let's also examine how vulnerable you body is, if you know what to look for. You shouldn't be intimidated by somebody with lots of muscles, "pumped up" so to speak, for several reasons. The first one is that a big muscle is not necessarily a fast one, and often strength is not synonymous with mass, and mass can impede agility. On the contrary, speed is a great advantage, and professional boxers know too well that a fast punch can be as effective as a strong one. In our case, self-defence, speed will give you the advantage of surprising the assailant, and especially if hitting, irrelevant of mass, specific vulnerable points. Our body is made of hard and soft areas; some are more vulnerable than others. Nobody can really strengthen his own eardrums, testicles, throat, nose or eyeballs. In some points, nerves are just under the skin and knowing where (fig. 30) to strike can turn the odds against you even if facing a stronger and bigger attacker. It is also important to note the amazing capacity of our body, male or female doesn't matter, to take huge pain or strong blows if necessary.

ACHILLE'S HEEL, SUPERMAN'S KRYPTONITE: EVERYONE HAS A WEAKNESS.

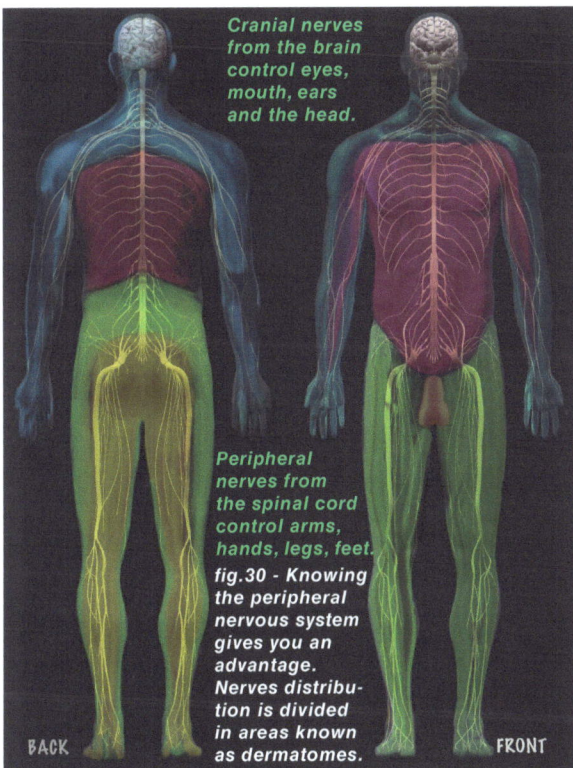

Cranial nerves from the brain control eyes, mouth, ears and the head.

Peripheral nerves from the spinal cord control arms, hands, legs, feet.

fig.30 - Knowing the peripheral nervous system gives you an advantage. Nerves distribution is divided in areas known as dermatomes.

BACK

FRONT

Adrenalin has an analgesic effect, and it is amazing what your mind can make your body do.

Our entire muscles envelope, sustains and protects our internal organs, and allows our skeleton to stand up or move.

This is why a fit well-toned body can take severe punishment better than the unfit one.

At the same time, there are areas that need to bend and move like the neck, wrists, knees and so forth, that are highly vulnerable, or the areas that have less protection, like your throat, or your head. Your entire body is surrounded by a network of nerves that if struck correctly can paralyse part of the system, causing permanent damage or even death. Knowing where and how to hit certain areas can give you an enormous advantage. In fact the more precisely you can strike these points the more effective you can be.

This is not quite that easy obviously but at the same time if we can focus on certain areas of your attacker's body we can give you an instant advantage.

fig.31 - Karate chop striking at the throat.

This knowledge as you can imagine carries great responsibility and by no means should you practice on anyone or strike these points unless you really want to cause some serious damage. This is a point that we will stress throughout many times, and safety in training should always come first. So what are the areas of the body that are the most vulnerable? Are they really as delicate as we are saying and so easy to damage irrelevant of the bulk of body mass?

Your first and easiest target should always be your attacker's face, eyes, throat, chin, all areas that if hit suffer pain easily, damage and quite importantly you can cause shock to the receiver giving you a strong and sudden advantage.

IF YOU CANNOT SEE YOU CANNOT ACT, ALL YOUR REFERENCES WILL FAIL YOU.

Any hit above the eyes, the forehead, is pointless since our cranium is designed to protect our brain and can take severe blows quite easily. Obviously, if you can strike to the head with a kick or your elbow, then do so, you can still cause serious damage.

fig.32 - If the fingers or the wrist are bent against their natural direction they can cause sudden sharp pain. See also fig.146 - page 91, LOCKS.

The classic uppercut to the **chin** or the **jaw**, causes immediate loss of consciousness because when hit at that point the head rotates and the brain crashes against the internal partial of your cranium producing local lesions. The jaw, especially in the middle section, is full of nerve endings which if hit properly cause instant loss of consciousness. It is the professional fighter's favourite target, but it needs to be hit with power and accuracy.

The **eyes** are also an easy target, and blinding your assailant in whatever way you can, including throwing dust or sand in that direction is extremely effective. Most Special Forces techniques to neutralise for example a hijacker, employ quick systems that blind the target (e.g. flash-bangs grenades, pepper sprays, a simple bag on top of the head). Pressure with your thumbs or a finger strike to the eyes can cause severe pain and serious damage. If you ever find yourself in a situation where you have to come to somebody's rescue, get on top of the attacker's head, achieving a superior advantage, making him a lot easier to control.

The **face** is the best target to hit with the back of your head, if attacked from behind.

The attacker's **nose** is an obvious target and when hitting that region you'll cause tears in his eyes that will impede his vision, and if hit precisely where the nose connects to the forehead, can fracture the bones and cause serious injury or death.

Because of the delicate situation that we are discussing, defending yourself against somebody who wants to seriously harm you, we will mention that if you find yourself in the right position, meaning extremely close to your attacker's face, don't hesitate to bite whatever comes at your teeth's reach, disgusting maybe, but very effective. Hold his head as you do it if you can to maximize your move, so he cannot move away at first contact.

Ears are designed to detect weak pressure waves in the air. The tympanic membrane will rupture at a pressure of 5-7 pounds per square inch (PSI) above atmospheric pressure, and that is very little. If both ears are slammed with your hands slightly cupped, this can be fatal or cause unconsciousness. Also biting the ears of your attacker causes horrendous pain. In the region just behind the ears, you can find a little bone called **mastoid process**: when hitting that area you can cause internal ear damage and consequentially immediate loss of consciousness.

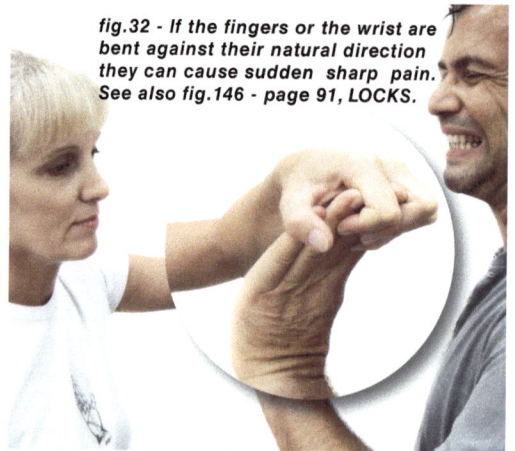

The **throat** is probably the most delicate and exposed part of our body, more delicate than the genitals.

A hit carried out in Karate chop-style (fig.31) can cause serious damage; hitting the Adam's apple can cause death, and it should never be rehearsed.

HIT FIRST AT WHATEVER IS WITHIN YOUR REACH.

If you are trapped underneath by someone and have one hand free, consider grabbing his throat, squeezing his windpipe hard (see figure 34), do the same if cornered frontally.

Striking the **side of the neck,** or the **back**, can cause serious damage and possible fractures, and especially on the side of the neck, 1 inch from the trachea, you'll find the vague nerves that reach all the vital internal organs from the cranium.

Hitting those nerves could interrupt breathing or cause cardiac arrest.

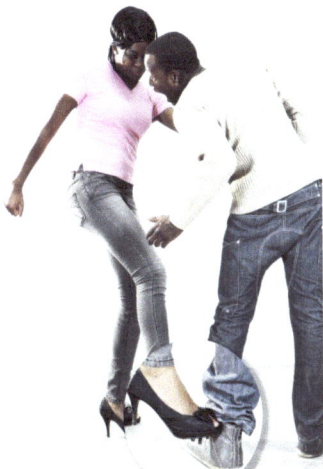

fig.33 - Hitting the malleus.

fig.34 - Grabbing the windpipe (larynx).

It is a technique that should never be practiced in training because it has caused quite few deaths, especially during Karate full contact competitions.

Alongside these nerves we also find important blood vessels that carry blood to the brain, and if hit accurately will cause immediate loss of consciousness, and is more effective than strangulation, however it needs to be precise and powerful.

All **articulations** are poorly protected by muscles, by definition; they have to articulate, meaning be free to move. That's why hitting articulations like the **knees** or the shoulder cause severe pain and damage. Even **fingers** if bent against their natural direction can cause severe pain (fig.32). We'll see more in LOCKS. (page 90) Hitting the **inside of the forearm**, e.g. with your elbow, can actually neutralise the use of the hand and weaken the assailant grasp. If attacked from behind you can also hit the side of your assailant's foot, the **malleus** and ideally you should try to hit it several times in a rapid sequence, causing severe pain and making your assailant lose control of his leg. (fig.33) All these points have been targets in several

KNOWING ALL VULNERABLE POINTS MAKES YOU LESS VULNERABLE.

martial arts, notoriously Ninjitsu and the famous Dim Mak (see GLOSSARY page 198) whose secret technique some people consider caused the death of Bruce Lee, and are just refined ways of hitting vulnerable points of our body with great accuracy.

A word of warning when thinking of hitting a man in the **genitals**: it is a very effective and often quite debilitating technique, causing severe damage, but the reaction to a blow to this area causes such an adrenaline boost that can produce a very violent retaliation attack for a few seconds. If you decide to hit the genital area, consider hitting other parts of the body in a sequence at the same time, in rapid succession with determination.

There really isn't much point trying to hit a fit man in the torso area or his back, even if inside there are vital organs, do keep in mind that they are

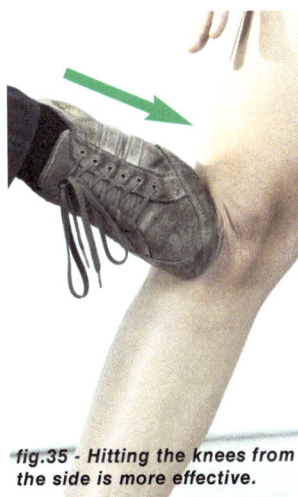

fig.35 - Hitting the knees from the side is more effective.

protected by a great muscular mass with a great deal of elasticity.

However the **lower part of the vertebral spine**, near the lumbar region and the kidneys are full of ganglions of nerves, very close to the surface and a precise hit in that region can do damage, and that's why it isn't allowed in boxing (fig.36).

If you have no other choice except for hitting the torso, consider that there is only one point of that area of your body that is not covered by muscles: the **solar plexus** (fig.36 and 40).

It causes tremendous pain, and literally takes your breath away for a few seconds. (fig.37) and that is enough to create a diversion or escaping.

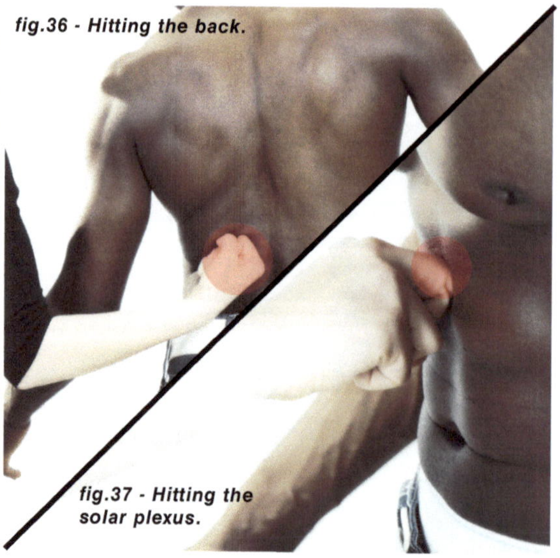

If positioned sideways or almost frontal to your attacker, kicking the **floating ribs**, (fig.38) the only two ribs at the bottom of your rib cage that are not connected to the sternum, can easily bend

fig.36 - Hitting the back.

fig.37 - Hitting the solar plexus.

them inside and potentially cause damage to the internal organs and loss of breathing.

There is one more very sensitive part of the human body that at close range, lying on the floor with somebody on top of you for instance, is still very vulnerable: if with your middle finger you push where the jaw bone inserts into the cranium and push towards the brain, you cause very sharp pain to the receiver (fig.39). If you push the jaw insertion to the cranium deeply enough it causes enough distress and pain to your attacker to let go for few precious seconds.

KNOWING WHERE TO HIT MEANS KNOWING WHERE TO PROTECT.

Now that you know what parts of our body are vulnerable, and represent a perfect target to disable an assailant, but you also know what areas you'll need to protect first. Also you should think that if you decide to strike these targets, you have to do it in the most rapid and powerful way you can, because if you miss your target or you are not effective, your assailant will react accordingly, with avid rage.

Deciding to react or not is entirely your choice, remember though that submission when it comes to sexual and violent assaults often results in the victim being killed.

The thought process "if I comply it will be over soon" does not really always equal surviving the situation, and the majority of threats carried out by dangerous attackers always start with " do exactly what I say or I'll kill you" or more cunningly " do as you are told and you will survive."

This is why we put so much emphasis on prevention trying to create the Perfect Defence, a state of alerted mind that can warn you when things might go wrong.

But when things are definitely going wrong, fast, it is up to you to respond, fast and explosive, using every part of your body to bite and strike, using everything within reach, such as keys, bag, shoes, anything that can inflict damage, and remember to hit first and foremost the face or throat.

Your first strike is the most important and it might be your only chance, do not waste it.

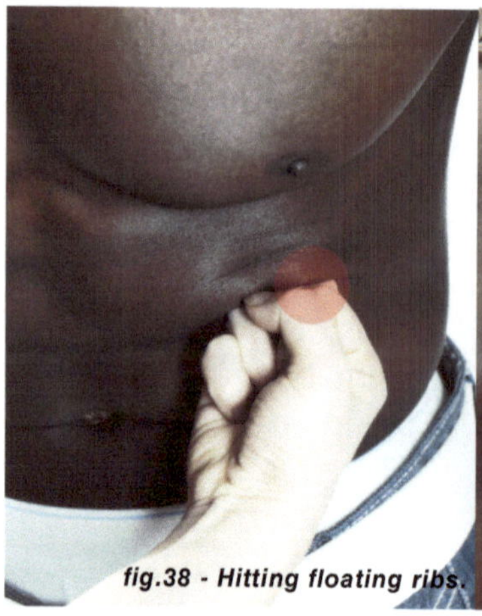

fig.38 - Hitting floating ribs. 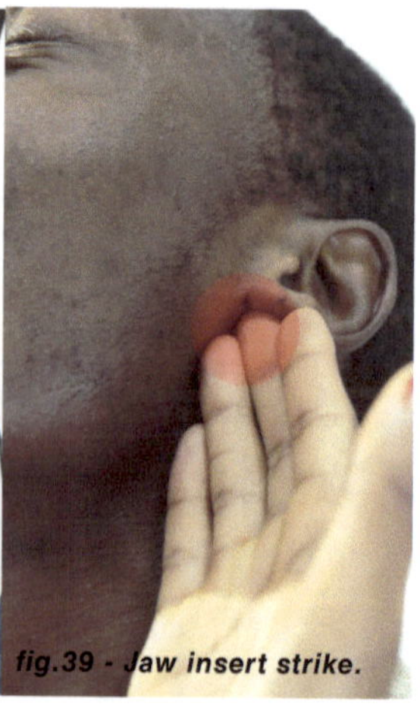 fig.39 - Jaw insert strike.

BODY's WEAK POINTS

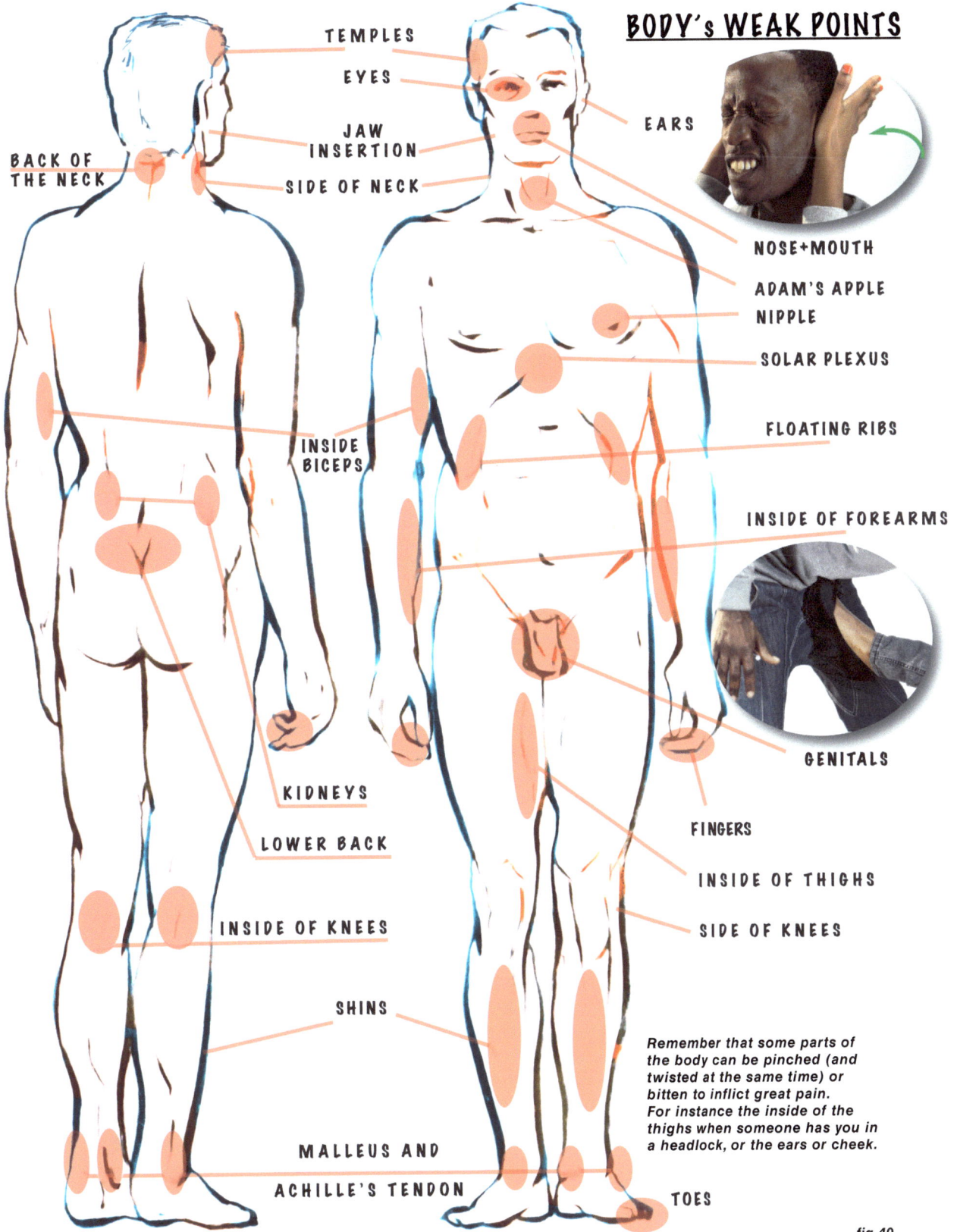

TEMPLES

EYES

JAW INSERTION

EARS

BACK OF THE NECK

SIDE OF NECK

NOSE+MOUTH

ADAM'S APPLE

NIPPLE

SOLAR PLEXUS

FLOATING RIBS

INSIDE BICEPS

INSIDE OF FOREARMS

KIDNEYS

LOWER BACK

GENITALS

FINGERS

INSIDE OF KNEES

INSIDE OF THIGHS

SIDE OF KNEES

SHINS

Remember that some parts of the body can be pinched (and twisted at the same time) or bitten to inflict great pain. For instance the inside of the thighs when someone has you in a headlock, or the ears or cheek.

MALLEUS AND ACHILLE'S TENDON

TOES

fig.40

34

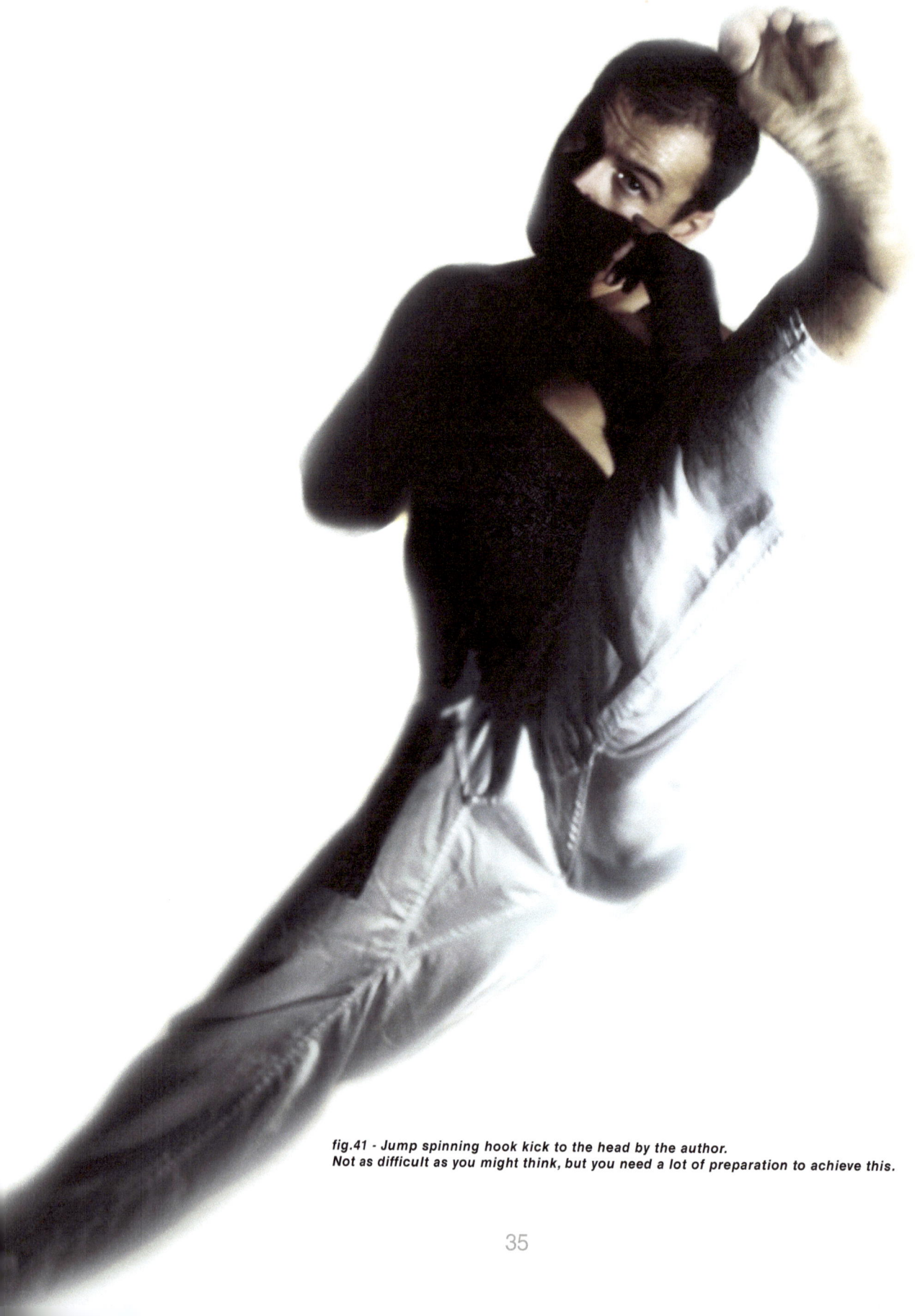

fig.41 - Jump spinning hook kick to the head by the author.
Not as difficult as you might think, but you need a lot of preparation to achieve this.

preparation

A big stumbling block in teaching anybody effective defence techniques, obviously involving hitting someone, is that most people have never taken part in a sport requiring physical contact. That's why before going into detailed striking or hitting methods we really should spend a little time discussing physical and mental preparation required to hit someone.

Popular sports such as jogging, tennis, swimming, even football do not really require physical contact with the opponent while obviously boxing, judo and rugby do.

It's not so much learning how to grab and throw somebody; it's more about coping with someone breaking that sphere around you, which is roughly as wide as the extension of your arm, that most people consider their own space.

Every animal, man included, has an area (fig.42) that ethologists (scientists who study animal behaviour) call "individual distance", if you enter this area the animal must attack or flee. With the PD system we have implemented a system that simplifies and maximises certain techniques adapting them to people who have little or no experience of contact sports. Over the years, we have taken all the best and simplest techniques from contact sports, like boxing and most martial arts for instance, bearing in mind most people wouldn't spend time hitting for hours a makiwara (see GLOSSARY page 198) or a punch bag for even longer, even though some training can do a great deal of good. Training means not only building stamina and increasing your power, it means perfecting technique through repetition as well as learning how it feels to hit something (see also fig.12). In the PD system course the participant is asked to hit the instructor hard wherever he/she likes for 15 seconds to learn how hitting a body feels, and how hard it can be. It is a bit extreme maybe, but it is always worth remembering that in a real life scenario, you will have no choice. When soldiers train in hand to hand combat for special operations, the focus is in hitting as hard as possible to break bones, causing maximum damage in the shortest of time or even to kill, but when teaching self defence, the focus should be kept on neutralizing the aggressor, trying to cause minimum damage.

This is more difficult because if requires a greater degree of control.

> SIMPLICITY IS OUR SECRET AND THAT IS DAMN COMPLICATED TO PUT INTO PRACTICE.

> REPETITIONS, REPETITIONS AND MORE REPETITIONS. ONCE FINISHED, REPEAT.

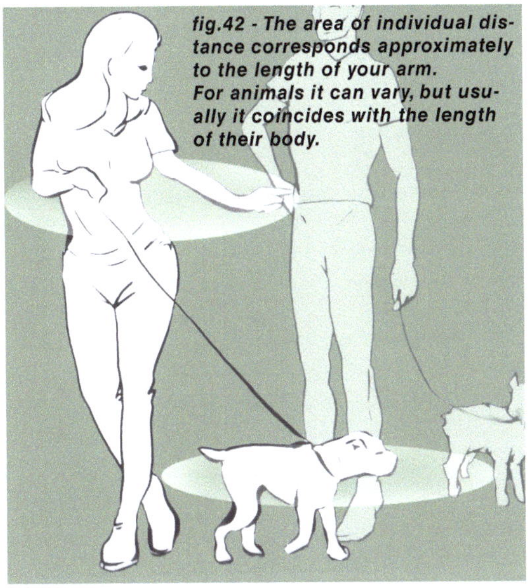

fig.42 - The area of individual distance corresponds approximately to the length of your arm.
For animals it can vary, but usually it coincides with the length of their body.

Normal training for paratroopers includes "milling", a one-minute fight where everything is allowed. This is a very important part of the training for anyone who will ever find himself fighting someone. Our emphasis with the PD system is speed, meaning speed of execution, fast reaction, lightning reflexes. That can be achieved through repetition. In FITNESS (page 228) you'll find tables with exercises to improve that.

We have made a specific selection of techniques that Special Forces operatives employ as part of their training. Often the commando operative is trained for a particular mission and the instructor concentrates just on those techniques.

FOCUS ON WHAT CAN APPLY TO YOUR LIFESTYLE. We'll do the same here, showing you what to do in case somebody traps you a lift, pins you against a wall, tries to get you out of your car and so on (see SCENARIOS page 214), obviously not to be applied if you find yourself surrounded by armed bandits in some remote region on earth.

If you do require specific training for war zones or a particular environment you can always contact us through our website (www.perfectdefence.com).

Training someone to become an effective fighter takes years and some serious commitment, let's not be unrealistic about that. However, we are confident that it is possible to train someone to effectively defend himself/herself in few sessions.

Effective self defence ability can be achieved by insisting on keeping the number of techniques to a minimum and making sure that you don't try to memorise specific techniques but that you learn how to react to a generic movement, e.g. the response to a roundhouse kick

YOU MUST LEARN TO REACT, NOT "HOW" TO REACT. can be the same if somebody tries to punch you with a "over head" (it looks like someone throwing a stone far away) or if being attacked by someone with a stick (fig.43).

This is why we have already mentioned that you would not find on this book too much emphasis on high-kicks and fanciful techniques, however you can still look here to see throws, kicks, and techniques common to a lot of martial arts for your general interest or as a reference to a particular technique applied to an attack.

Your initial training should include a good understanding on how to fall and roll on your back. We will show you how that is done further on (FALLING page 76) but then you should practice only under supervision. Absolutely essential in fighting is to understand balance, both your own and your opponent's.

It is easier to make a big man fall, offsetting his balance with a simple push–pull technique than punching him to the ground.

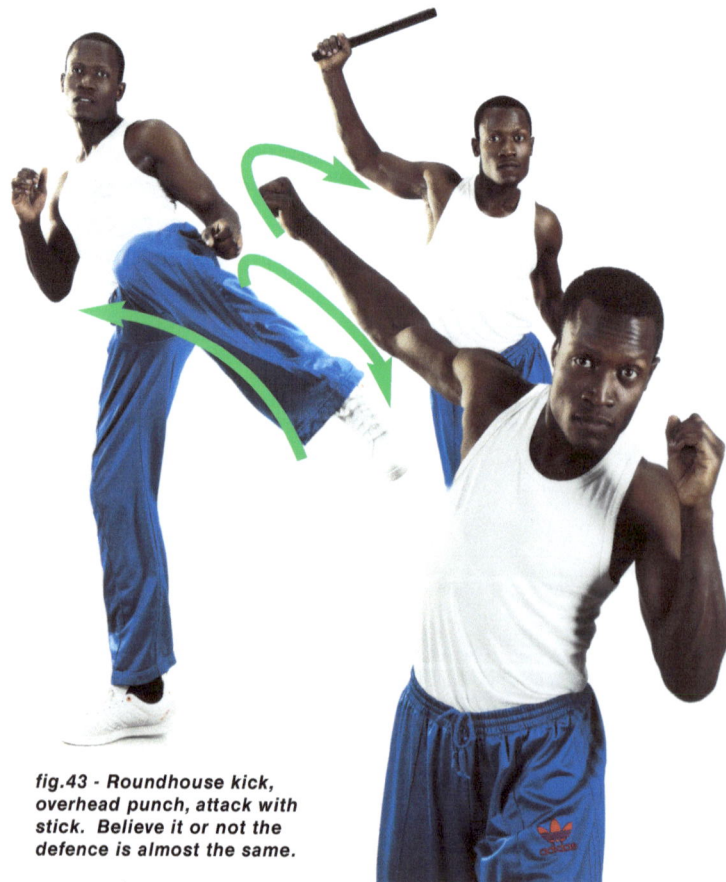

fig.43 - Roundhouse kick, overhead punch, attack with stick. Believe it or not the defence is almost the same.

fig.44A
Your chin should
be tucked in.

If you examine figure 44, you can see how to achieve a good stance if you have to prepare yourself to fight. Always remember that you shouldn't let your aggressor know that you are getting into a stance or similar position; otherwise you will spoil your advantage almost immediately. Let's see what really makes a good stance. Your knees should be slightly bent, and your feet slightly spread, roughly as wide as your shoulders.

One foot should be in front and one firmly behind; if you are right-handed your left foot should be in front and your right foot slightly back. Your feet should be at a slight 45º angle at the direction of the attack; your bodyweight should be spread equally on your legs. As you can see this is the classic boxing/kickboxing stance.

Furthermore, your arms should be bent 45 degrees and your forearms and your fist should cover your face without impeding vision, keeping your elbows close to your body to protect the ribs (see fig.44). We'll explore more what makes a good stance in TAKEDOWNS (page 52). It's not a good idea to close your fists at this time because the muscles of your forearm when clinching your fist are contracted, slowing down your arm and increasing your reaction time, the fist should be closed just before it lands on the target.

Finally your chin should be tucked down to your chest (fig.44A), using the natural protection of your shoulders, keeping your eyes fixed on your target.

We suggest you practice this basic stance in front of a mirror, and it is equally important that someone tells you if you are doing it correctly. In this posture when moving you should never lift your feet, just drag them, and you should never cross your legs.

Also you should never bend forwards or backwards, if you need to go low with your torso.

The best way to "go low" is to bend your knees, going down on your hips, because in doing so you can keep control of your balance more effectively (fig.46).

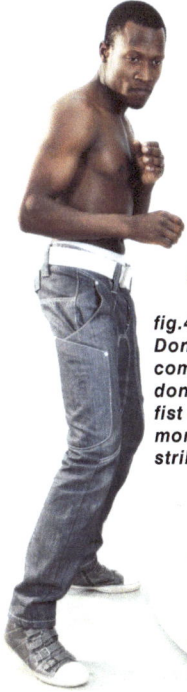

A GOOD STANCE ALLOWS YOU TO REACT EFFECTIVELY.

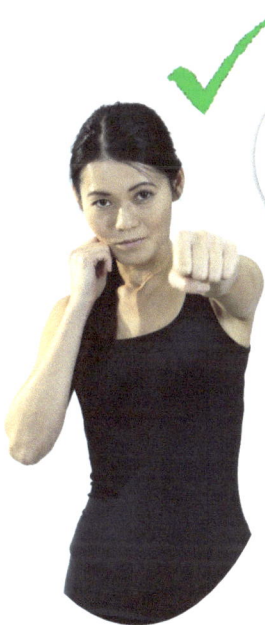

CAUTION

TAKE SMALL STEPS AND MAKE YOURSELF SMALL TO ACHIEVE BIG RESULTS.

fig.44 - The perfect stance: your arms should be bent 45° and your forearms and your fist should cover your face without impeding vision, keeping your elbows close to your body to protect your ribs. Keep your chin tucked in and your elbow in also when you punch.

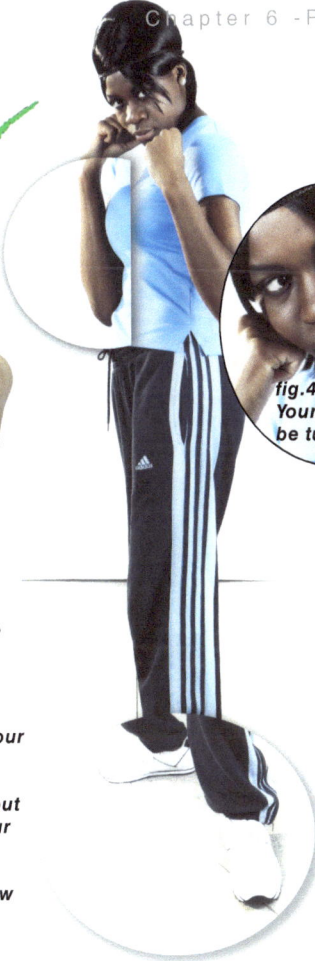

fig.45 - Small steps. Don't lift your foot completely and don't clinch your fist until the last moment before striking.

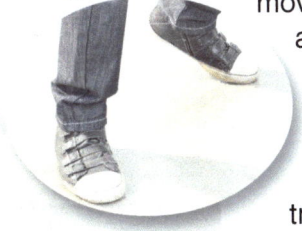

⚠ Your hips are your centre of gravity and ideally they should be at the right height to keep you stable.

Movements with your feet should be small and fast, it's better to have three half steps than one giant step, for different reasons: first because you can adjust your distance better, secondly you can retreat quicker without losing balance.

Watch a boxer moving around a ring, there is a lot to learn there. What we cannot do through a computer screen is to make you repeat the exercise or ⚠ check that you are consistent and accurate enough. Always remember to repeat at much as you can, to improve your speed.

Needless to say, before starting any kind of exercise you should always stretch and warm up properly (see STRETCHING page 224). What is very important for your training, so important that it would require an entire book dedicated to that argument, is your breathing.

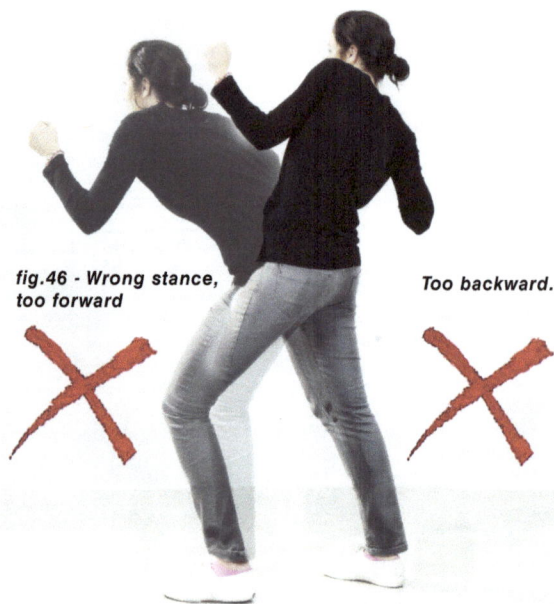

fig.46 - Wrong stance, too forward

Too backward.

If you ever assist training in a martial art dojo, or two boxers sparring, you will notice, they are making a lot of loud noises through their mouth, and the reason is because respiration is an essential part in generating power, explosive power. This concept translates into the "kiai", made famous by Bruce Lee, and is basically letting as much air out of your lungs as possible at the moment you are landing a hit, translating your breathing out into a yell.

BREATHE OUT AS YOU HIT, YOUR TENSIONING INCREASES THE POWER OF THE STRIKE. The purpose is that you'll increase muscular tension in your torso and abdomen, and that means your entire body follows with the impact. In any case, always remember to breath out as much as you can every time you hit something.

What you can't do by yourself in training is perfecting your hitting technique with an instructor who is using focus pads (see GLOSSARY page 224).

This is designed to improve your ability of hitting a moving target from different directions, at any moment, in every position, effectively and precisely, with power and speed. You will find out that as you hit a focus pad, the sound coming off it will tell instantly how precise your hit was (fig.48). On your own, you can practice on a speedball, ideally the ceiling to floor type that will dance around enough to make you adjust position and stance unless you want to get hit by the ball (fig.49). If properly set up the reaction of the ball to your strikes can simulate how an opponent would respond to your punch, and I promise, it will hit you back, hard and unexpectedly, eventually with proper training and supervision you can

IF YOU CAN CONTROL YOUR SPACE YOU CAN CONTROL YOUR AGGRESSOR. also practice kicks on it, but always wear a groin guard, and be careful not to hyperextend the kick and damage your ligament, quite possibly kicking the ball if not careful.

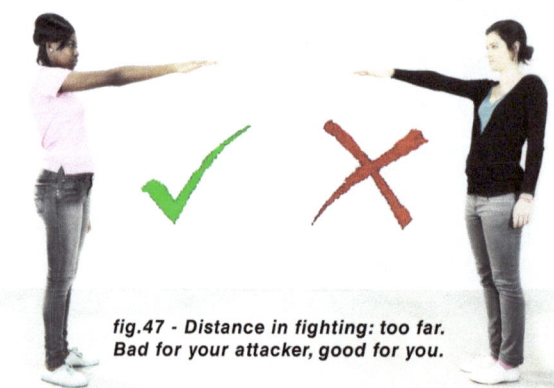

fig.47 - Distance in fighting: too far. Bad for your attacker, good for you.

fig.49 - Floor to ceiling speedball.

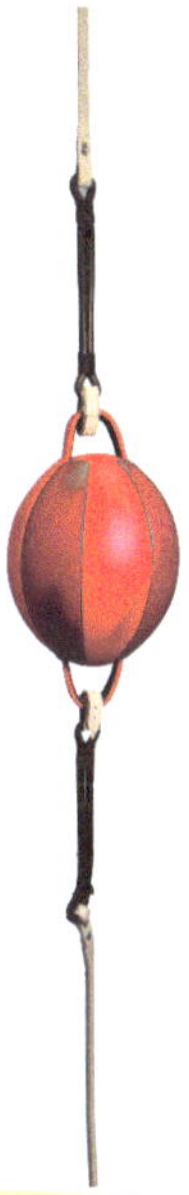

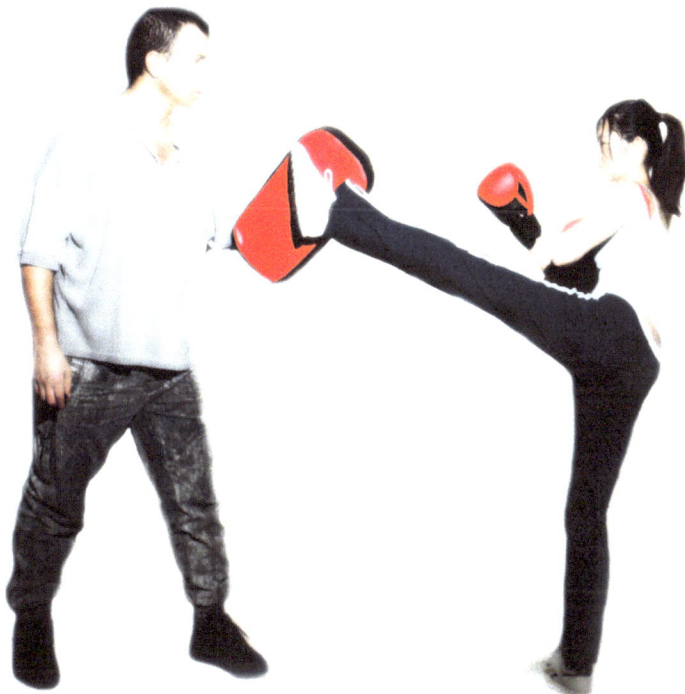

fig.48 - Hitting the focus pad increases your accuracy and speed.

If you have good preparation, learning how to achieve the correct stance and how to move properly, you will be able to control distance and strike fast and accurately.

Distance, seen as the space between you and an aggressor, is a fundamental element in personal defence. Doubling your arm's length from your aggressor makes your chances of being hit by an unarmed aggressor quite slim, or reduced consistently and shorter than that, let's say a couple of metres or less. You should already realise by now that it takes no time to receive a kick and then a punch, without forgetting that you can use distance to your advantage, e.g. shortening it

BEING AT CLOSE RANGE COULD BECOME AN ADVANTAGE.

and attacking first, could be a good form of defence but, needless to say, you really have to know what you are doing and have experienced in training.

You shouldn't consider close range as a disadvantage: for instance it's much easier, so to speak, to disarm someone who is pointing a gun holding you close than to tackle somebody pointing a weapon from a safe distance (see WEAPONS - page 102).

Preparing yourself to execute a punch or a kick, it is worth considering how important it is that once you start an action you should complete it. It is worth pointing out that women in particular have an innate fear of physical pain (quite amazing thinking that they can give birth) but also women are often much more concerned than men about causing pain to someone else.

Let's see now what makes a strike effective, causing damage through technique and not strength. We have all seen spectacular demonstrations of martial art techniques, when someone could hit the opponent many times in a space of a few seconds: well, it might look spectacular to you but believe me, unless your punch or kick penetrates at least 3 cm (approximately one and half inch) deep in your opponent skin it has no more effect that a caress (fig.51).

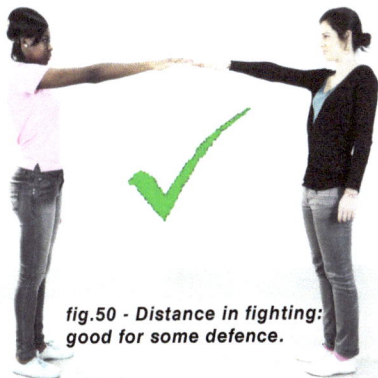

fig.50 - Distance in fighting: good for some defence.

During your preparation, it's fundamental to feel your hit landing and carry though the hit. Training in a gym environment or the comfort of your own home, presents obvious advantages but do consider though that you might have to defend yourself while you are wearing a tight suit, slippery shoes, high heels or a tight skirt, while you are tired or when you are having a good time, and fighting is the last thing on your mind (often a discotheque or club is fertile ground for unpleasant confrontations).

You might even have had a couple of drinks or a heavy meal, or have just woken up from a deep sleep, there is no technique that can help you with that, it's just the nature of things and you should try to be prepared for the unexpected.

YOU COULD BE FACING DANGER WEARING HIGH HEELS AND A TIGHT SKIRT ON AN ICY ROAD.

fig.51 - You must punch through at least 3 cm (1.1") to be effective.

What I can suggest is that every once in a while you practice a couple of simple techniques of your choice wearing normal clothes (away from view, so the occasional passer-by will not think you are a weirdo) and in different moments of your day.

While rehearsing, especially with a partner, you should wear protective gear specifically designed to avoid injuries to yourself and to your opponent.

Even if most certainly in a real life scenario, you'll probably be wearing every day clothing, often not suited (pardon the pun) for fighting, make sure that for training you wear a tracksuit and remove all jewellery (earrings, necklaces, rings, watch) and protect all your vulnerable parts (see fig. 40 - page 34) such as your head, breasts, shins, groin and so on, and on the opposite page (fig.54) you can see samples of clothing designed to protect you and your partner while training. It will be repeated many times throughout this book the importance to have an Instructor supervising your training, especially when physical contact is present, to make all activity safe and supervise your technique during practice.

In any case there are certain techniques that should be not rehearsed at all (a karate chop to the Adam's apple for instance) because they are just far too dangerous even to the trained professional. It is sufficient to know where to hit and how. There is a wide choice of protective clothing designed for sparring or practicing, and plenty of sellers, however remember though that the cheapest does not constitute the safest, and sometimes is not worth, for the sake of saving little money, to buy a poorly finished item that will fall apart when hit or won't stay in place. I wouldn't really recommend buying second hand, protective clothing because the chances that they contain bacteria or fungi that can give contaminate is quite high from the previous owner/s. If you train in a gym and borrow the equipment that is available make sure is regularly disinfected.

fig.52 - Kick through at least 3 cm (1.1").

Traditional training aids are always the most effective.

If you train mostly by yourself a good punch-bag is still no substitute to improve your striking power and practice combinations, available in different shapes and types, heavier or lighter. For simplicity lets say that the most commonly used are the classic (A) punch bag, normally cylindrical and suspended by a chain allowing to swing freely. (B) is similar but "torso" shaped and allows the practicing of uppercuts to the body, representing a more realistic target. In the past few years many "human" shaped bags (C) have flooded the market, some reproducing a realistic torso in silicone rubber, with a base that allows it to swing when hit. This type (C) also allows you to practice precise strikes to vital points (fig. 53).

A good ten minute workout on the punch-bag will make you stronger and improve your stamina. Don't forget to practice your knee strikes as well on the bag.

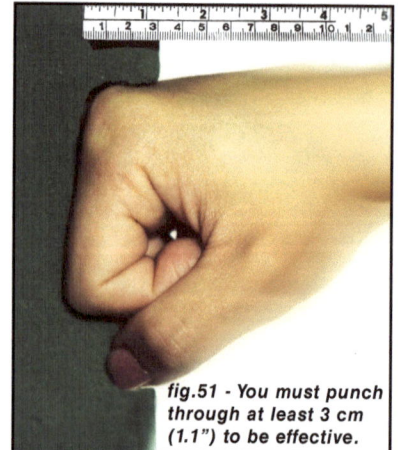

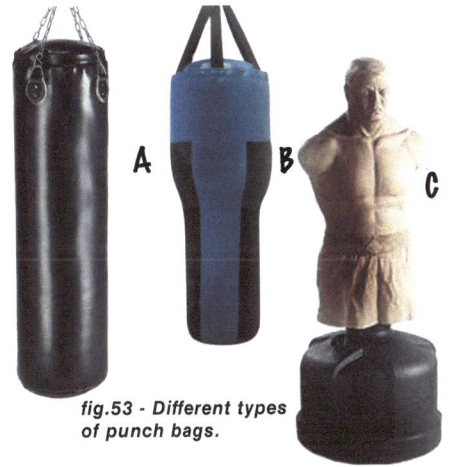

fig.53 - Different types of punch bags.

And lastly do not forget that the best way to prepare oneself for a physical confrontation is a simulated physical confrontation, either with an opponent using focus pads or with some sparring. If you have anyone who can help you with your striking technique using focus pads remember to ask for as many changes of directions as possible and to make it as difficult and varied as possible, varying the angle and height of the pads, moving onto performing combinations as son as comfortable with hitting the pads with single strikes.

Once you have completed the combinations (straight punch -left hook-right uppercut for instance) the person holding the pads should move away and offer the pads from a different angle, maybe even different height and more sudden. It is all well and good that you train your body and sculpt your muscles. By all means train against a punch-bag for hours on end but do not forget that albeit it does help to strengthen your body you should also strengthen your mind. This is the most difficult part, to toughen up your spirit and learn to overcome fear, to control the adrenaline rushing through your body, your legs turning to jelly and your mouth drying up.

Your body freezes and you have the feeling you are watching someone else, almost an out of body experience that lasts a few seconds but seems an eternity, then everything comes crashing down fast, the pain, the sweat, that cold feeling of impotence that will turn into shame and frustration afterwards because you did not react, you let it happen.

To toughen up to that takes more than a few sessions in a gym, even after fighting in the street many times it still happens to me, I still get scared.

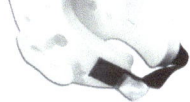

fig.54 - Protective gear.

Mouthguard

Head guard

Breast plate

Gloves (10oz)

Hand wraps

Groin protection

Shin and foot guards

fig.55 - Hand wraps are an essential part of the training equipment.
To learn how to wrap your hands go to KICKBOXING page 240.

HOW TO CHOOSE YOUR TRAINING EQUIPMENT

We all know that color and brand play a big part in everyone's choice, but in this case consider that safety comes first. Make sure that all protections cover what they are supposed to cover properly and with adequate padding, that all straps are holding in place what they are supposed to and that there is nothing protruding that can poke your partner or get caught as you perform a move. Comfort should also be considered: an ill fitting garment will restrict your movements or worse can cause sores where you least need them. Absolutely remove ALL jewellery when you train, including rings and earrings. If you end up doing a lot of bag workout you better invest in an extra dedicated pair of gloves, normally less cumbersome. Always wrap your hands. Make sure your groin protection or breast plate fits well and stays where it should as you move or kick, and that your headgear allows for good vision and fits quite snug. Always wear a mouthguard. Have fun.

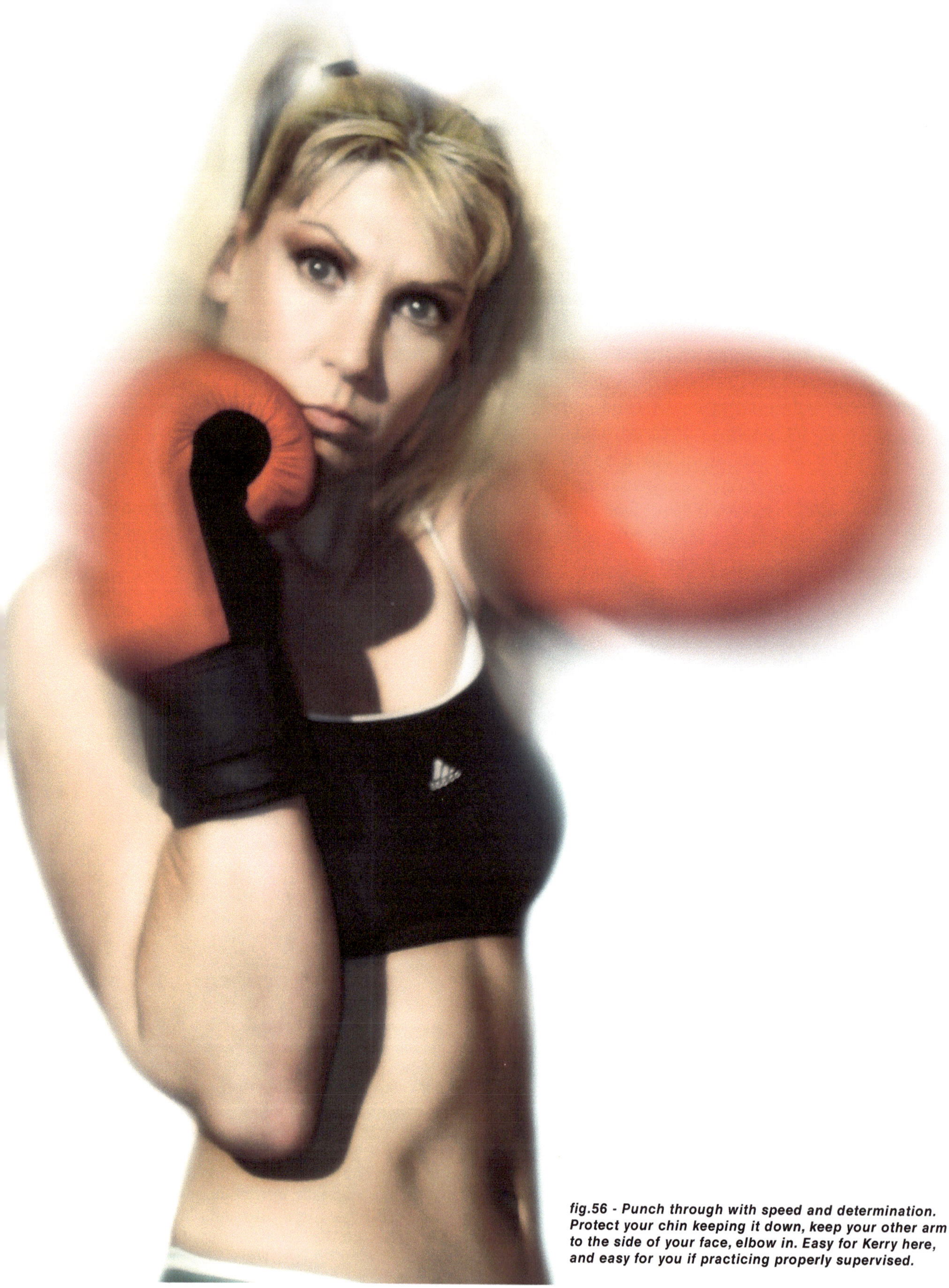

fig.56 - Punch through with speed and determination. Protect your chin keeping it down, keep your other arm to the side of your face, elbow in. Easy for Kerry here, and easy for you if practicing properly supervised.

hitting

   If you would ask me what is the perfect hitting technique, the perfect strike so to speak, I have no doubt answering "the powerful one"; hitting hard has no substitute, always wins.

However not many people can do that naturally or have the time to practice on achieving hard hitting in the gym and it's for this reason that we should go over what makes a good hitting technique. We have seen previously that one of the biggest muscles, if not the biggest, of your body, is your thigh muscle, being one of the strongest. If you do manage to keep your distance, and remember what we discussed on a proper "fence", your first resort should be a kick.

Like a punch a kick should be delivered using your entire body, to apply maximum power to the blow. In fig.58 you can see different types of kicks (see also KICKBOXING page 240).

The most effective kick is the front kick, especially when delivered to the knees of your opponent, to the groin or the chest. It's a fast kick and can be hidden easily.

It's worth saying that kicking with a good technique is not easy; it still requires good balance, good elasticity and good control. If improperly executed, a kick can do more damage to the giver than to the receiver, just for overextending the leg.

The reason why we will not bother with high kicks or spinning kicks is because unless you perfect the technique through serious training you'll never achieve a decent result not to mention that quite often you might find yourself wearing a skirt, suit or tight dress and you cannot raise your legs much, or fast enough.

DRESSED TO KILL DOES NOT GO WELL WITH DRESSED TO KICK.

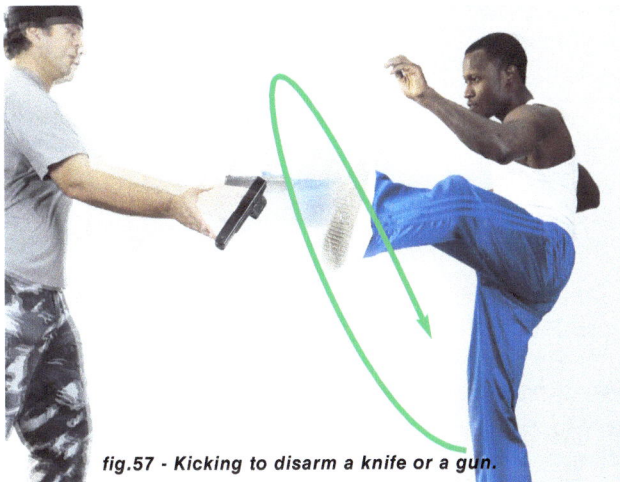

The other advantage of kicking is that often you are wearing shoes that offer both protection as well as adding extra sharpness to the blow, think of sharp heels.

 A kick can be used aiming at the hand holding the knife or the stomach as your attacker launches forward, or as part of a sequence of blows that started maybe with a punch or a feint (see fig.57). And never forget that even if wearing boots you should always try to have your foot positioned correctly as shown in fig.28.

An effective kick to the tibia or shin can provoke a dislocation of the knee and in any case tremendous pain, often the person being hit will fall to the ground in no time.

You should always remember to follow up with a second kick, as powerful as the first one, even if the opponent has fallen to the ground.

fig.57 - Kicking to disarm a knife or a gun.

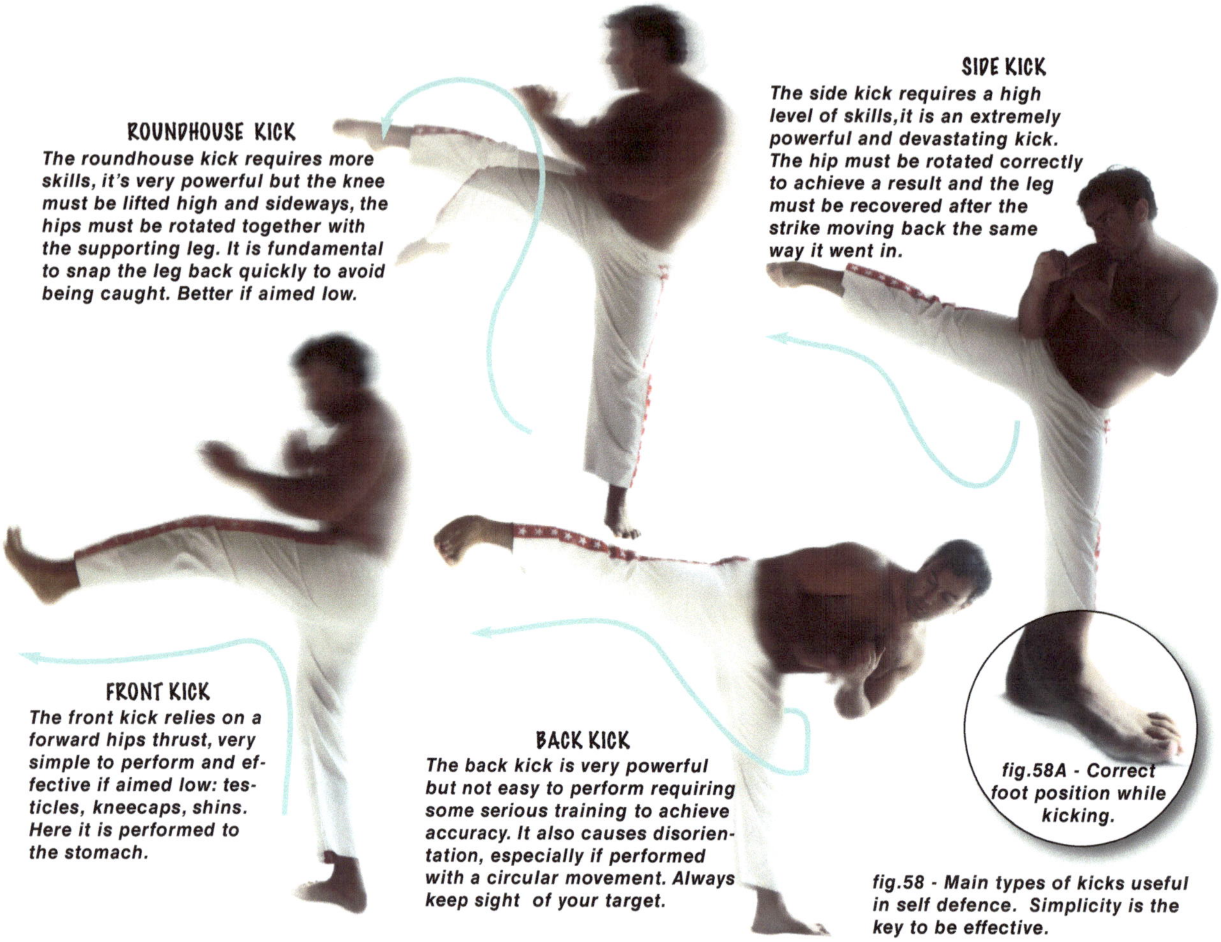

ROUNDHOUSE KICK

The roundhouse kick requires more skills, it's very powerful but the knee must be lifted high and sideways, the hips must be rotated together with the supporting leg. It is fundamental to snap the leg back quickly to avoid being caught. Better if aimed low.

SIDE KICK

The side kick requires a high level of skills, it is an extremely powerful and devastating kick. The hip must be rotated correctly to achieve a result and the leg must be recovered after the strike moving back the same way it went in.

FRONT KICK

The front kick relies on a forward hips thrust, very simple to perform and effective if aimed low: testicles, kneecaps, shins. Here it is performed to the stomach.

BACK KICK

The back kick is very powerful but not easy to perform requiring some serious training to achieve accuracy. It also causes disorientation, especially if performed with a circular movement. Always keep sight of your target.

fig.58A - Correct foot position while kicking.

fig.58 - Main types of kicks useful in self defence. Simplicity is the key to be effective.

In actual fact if you can you should follow up with a stamping kick (fig. 59) aimed at the face, neck, ribs or genitals. This because in this book we will always assume that life is at risk and you should not take chances, and always try to neutralise the assailant.

A second kick possibly to the head will definitely send him to sleep and give you enough time to run to safety. However if your first strike has achieved a good result, meaning he is on the ground and incapacitated, then run to safety. The risk of overdoing it after succeeding with a defending move is very high and I have seen people getting into trouble because they wanted the icing on the cake. The roundhouse kick, always directed to the torso (floating ribs or solar plexus) or below, has to be delivered with a good rotation of the hip, and once landed you should quickly snap back your leg, ready to strike again to avoid the opponent grabbing your foot.

KICKS ARE WOMEN'S BEST FRIENDS. Kicks are particularly well indicated for women's personal defence, the female cox femoral articulation (the hip) is suppler than the equivalent male even if you don't practice sports, and generally legs are often stronger than arms. Needless to say, women's shoes very often are pointy and quite sharp, making them an ideal weapon to use (see also OBJECTS - page 132). Don't forget if you are practicing any of the high kicks illustrated in fig.11 or fig.41 do stretch properly to warm up your joints and articulations before performing any of the above (see STRETCHING - page 224). Of course you cannot start stretching during an attack scenario, but why risk unnecessary injuries during training?

We have seen that in order to deliver a good kick, it is important to be able to control your balance effectively: it is always a good exercise to learn standing on one leg without holding onto anything and slowly raise the leg without touching the ground, in whatever way you feel like.

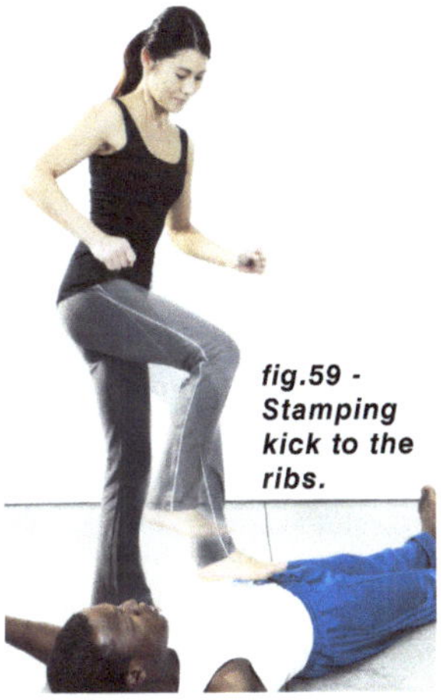

fig.59 - Stamping kick to the ribs.

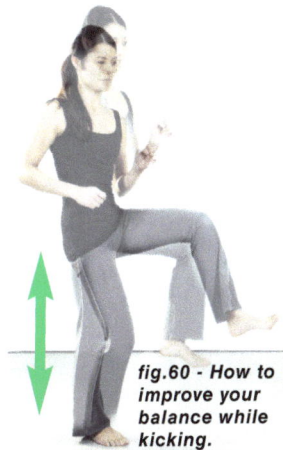

You can do this simple exercise whenever and wherever you are, and bending slightly the other leg, going up and down will also strengthen your other leg muscles (fig.60).

Always practice the moves slowly and consistently.

We can break down any kick in four fundamental movements that should be executed as one continuous movement: first is flexing your thigh, looking ahead of you, raising your knee towards your chest.

Second, you extend your leg away from you, third you snap back your foot and last you return your foot to the ground to your initial stance (fig.59). This is all performed obviously as one smooth movement.

To fully understand how a kick works you can do this very simple exercise (fig.61): position a chair in front of you and aiming at the seat, push it away from you, retaining muscular control of your movement only using either your right or your left foot. Repeat until you can push the chair away without making it topple, smoothly and evenly.

If you observe figure 58 carefully you will notice how important it is with all types of kicks to extend, also called "projecting" in technical terms, your hips with the kick to achieve maximum power; this helps to put all of your body's weight behind the kick, adding power.

One common mistake is closing your eyes when kicking, don't forget that you must keep your eyes open and never lose sight of your target; what you also have to remember is that a kick is effective when executed with a whip movement.

KICK AS IF YOU CRACK A WHIP, IF YOU DON'T WANT TO CRACK YOUR LEG.

fig.60 - How to improve your balance while kicking.

You should always kick out and snap back your leg immediately, as fast as possible. That as we've seen makes it stronger, less predictable, and makes it very difficult to grab hold of your leg. Training to kick is much more complicated that training yourself to punch, and do not forget that you have to practice against a target to understand how it feels when your foot hits something. At the beginning of your training session practice very slowly: it's very easy to hyperextend your leg, damaging your ligaments, especially your knees. The most common mistakes are closing your eyes or looking away, not breathing out, forgetting to keep your hands up or pushing your hips back instead of forward as well as being conservative with the speed of your kick.

As we've seen, a kick is very powerful and effective, it should be your first choice in most situations, and even if you fell to the ground you can still kick from that position (fig.62).

We'll see more of that in GROUNDWORK (page 82).

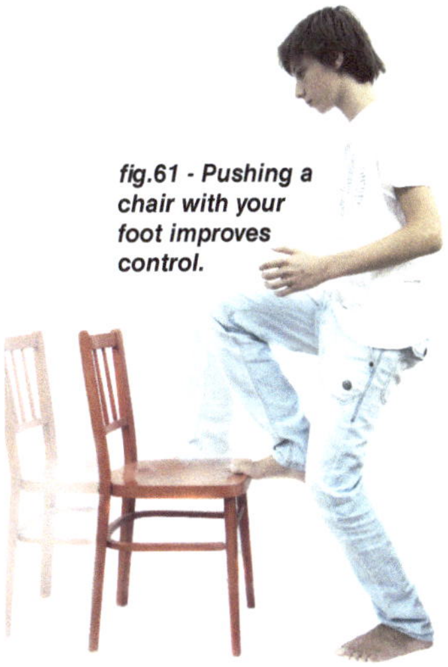

fig.61 - Pushing a chair with your foot improves control.

You can increase the power of the kick, especially in a close quarter's environment such as a lift, a phone box or even a small room, kicking your assailant and at the same time holding onto something or pushing yourself from a wall or an object (fig.63).

Finally, be mindful that you might be on the receiving end of a kick, and you should know how to deal with it.

You'll see more later on, but let's say that often the best defence against a kick is either to move out of the way or to grab the leg, ideally by the ankle, and twist or raise the leg to unbalance your opponent.

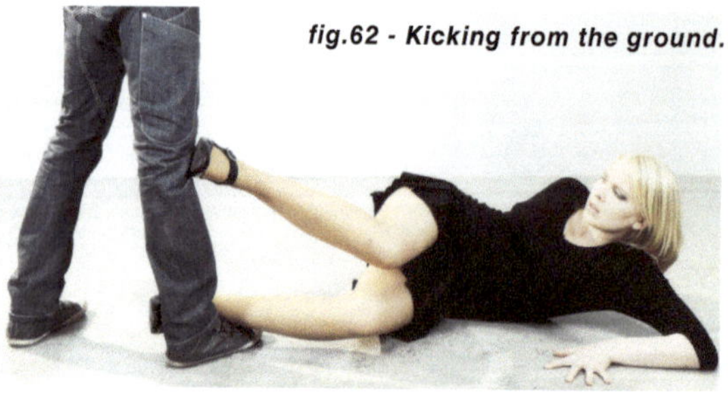

You should react with a fast and sharp movement with no hesitation, maybe even stepping closer to un-balance your attacker as you grab and twist his leg.

fig.62 - Kicking from the ground.

Punching, like kicking, requires a good technique, even more so because we are so used to seeing punches in films that we tend to assume that punching is dead easy, when in fact is much more difficult than you might think.

As you have seen already (fig.22) making your hand into a proper fist is important, you might land a fist incorrectly and easily break your wrist or knuckles. Contrary to most people's perception, the power of the punch has little to do with the size of your arm; in actual fact big biceps don't necessarily deliver strong punches.

I have trained fragile looking women who could punch twice as hard as a man with the arm the size of their thighs, all because their technique was great and you should never forget that a punch is delivered using all of your body behind it: as you throw the punch either straight or as a jab, you should rotate your hips to maximise the power of the strike (fig. 64).

This is also what you should do when kicking. Don't forget to snap your arm back to avoid the opponent catching your arm as well as protect the part of the body exposed to a counterattack.

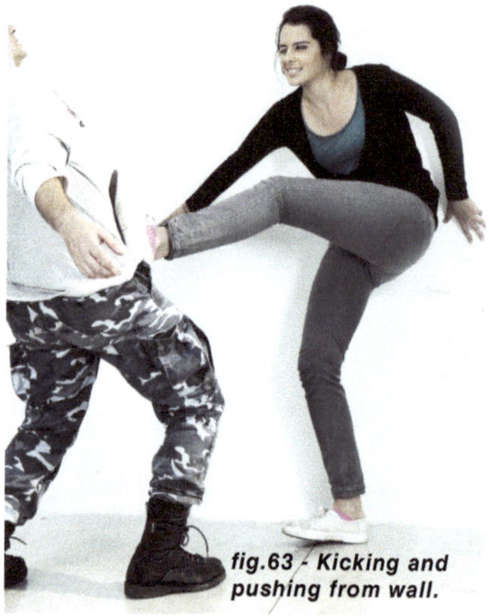

fig.63 - Kicking and pushing from wall.

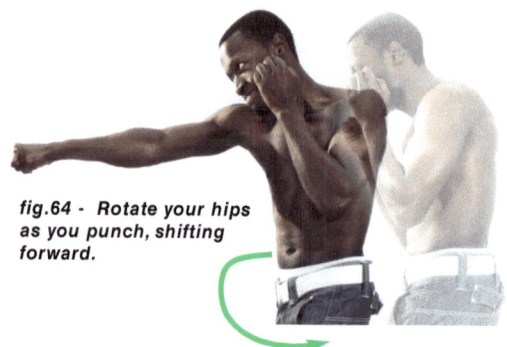

ALWAYS PUNCH THROUGH AN IMAGINARY PIPE OR TUNNEL.

You should imagine, as you throw a punch that you are travelling with your arm with a slight twisting movement anti-clockwise (right hand, rotating left) through an imaginary pipe or tunnel (fig. 67). We have already mentioned that we should close the fist as you punch, not before, to avoid contracting the forearm, slowing down your action.

The very moment you hit your target, tense up all your muscles, especially your torso's, to avoid absorbing the force of the impact.

Finally, learn how to breathe out deeply and fast as you punch to increase power.

Always practice very slowly, almost slow motion: this will allow you to see your mistakes more easily and it is better to practice facing a mirror or siding a wall, (fig. 66) to see if your elbow sticks out and becoming aware of what your body does and how to breathe properly while punching.

You can punch at close range or long range, and you can see in fig.72 types of punches and their use: you can strike using your hand "hammer style" (fig.65) and you should at least try once to have someone training you using hitting focus pads to learn how to punch at different range, angles, and positions (fig.48).

A punch can become very effective for women if done correctly because women often wear reasonably big rings that can cause serious damage (see OBJECTS - page 132).

We do consider part of punching techniques also striking with open fingers to the opponent's eyes (fig.68) or chop style to the side of the neck, (fig.70) as well as open-palm to the chin (fig.69).

fig.64 - Rotate your hips as you punch, shifting forward.

fig.65 - Punch hammer style.

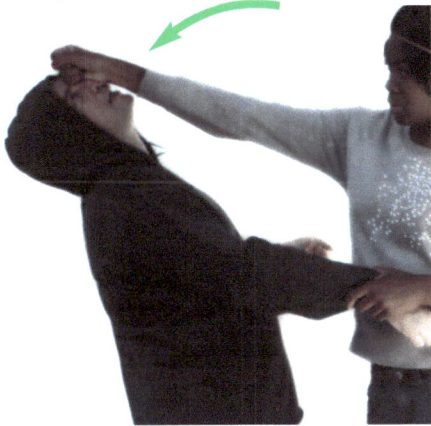

fig.66 - Punching siding a wall.

The latter has great advantages at close-range, and should be used with your full bodyweight behind it.

YOU CAN STRIKE WITH YOUR HAND IN MANY WAYS, BUT ALWAYS KNOW WHERE.

The advantage of this particular blow is that it doesn't require particular strength and can be very fast: your arm can be in any position, even relaxed down the front, and suddenly you can strike open-palm under your attacker's chin with great effect, especially when carried out at close-range.

You can maximise this effect, grabbing and pulling your opponent towards you, causing quite possibly a fracture of the neck. Furthermore, a punch can be followed up by a leg sweep: very effective and disorientating, especially if you didn't manage to land the punch properly.

Always remember that speed is more important than power, and don't forget you will not achieve a knockout with one punch, it should always be followed by another punch or kick or even a foot sweep (fig.71) straight away.

Hooks require good technique and a good rotation of your legs to maximise the power of the blow; a left-hook should be followed through with the rotation of your

ROTATE YOUR HIPS AS YOU PUNCH!

hips and a slight rotation of your left leg, a right-hook rotating your right hip in the same direction of your punch (fig.60).

Uppercuts are devastating punches but are difficult to carry out effectively because you should load the punch properly before you discharge its power. This is achieved bending your knees and lowering your body, and you must hit as you come up, releasing the punch. Remember to punch slightly away from you to avoid punching yourself in the face. See in fig. 72 the correct position of the fist in relation to the position of body. Hitting a target Karate-chop style allows great precision and considerable damage. It is a classic Karate strike

fig.67 - Punch through an imaginary pipe.

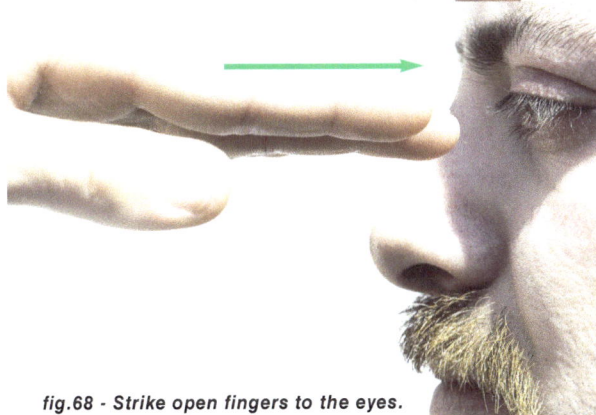

and inflicts considerable damage because it concentrates in a very small area, less than three centimetres, and all the energy of the strike. Imagine hitting something with a bar and hitting the same object with a sharp blade and you understand why it makes a difference.

It is very important to practice this strike supervised, you can easily break your wrists or your fingers, and it's easy to hit with your wrists instead of hitting with the edge of your hand.

Also equally important is to snap back your hand before the impact is absorbed by your body through your arm.

fig.68 - Strike open fingers to the eyes.

A PUNCH IS EFFECTIVE IF YOUR TECHNIQUE IS AS TIGHT AS YOUR FIST.

It can be used with both hands at the same time, coming from high, from low, from the side, from any direction, always bearing in mind that this type of action needs precision in hitting the designated target.

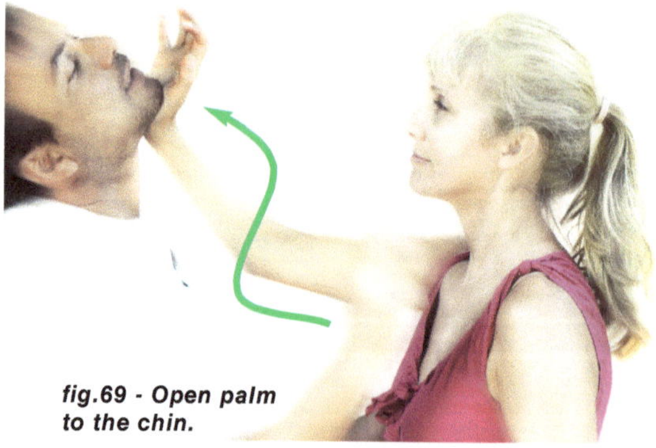

The main principle when using punches is to always follow a punch with another blow to a different target, not necessarily with another punch, it can be a kick or elbow/knee strike, but in any case very rarely an isolated punch can produce the desired effect, unless it comes as a complete surprise, such as in the case of a sucker punch (see SWITCHING OFF - page 123).

fig.69 - Open palm to the chin.

Learning how to hit someone effectively will help you to overcome fear.

If you become more proficient and less shy about physical "hard" contact you will be able to use actions to overcome fear. If you talk to fighters, boxers, kick boxers or wrestlers, they will almost all agree on one thing: the moment they initiate the action the fear is gone.

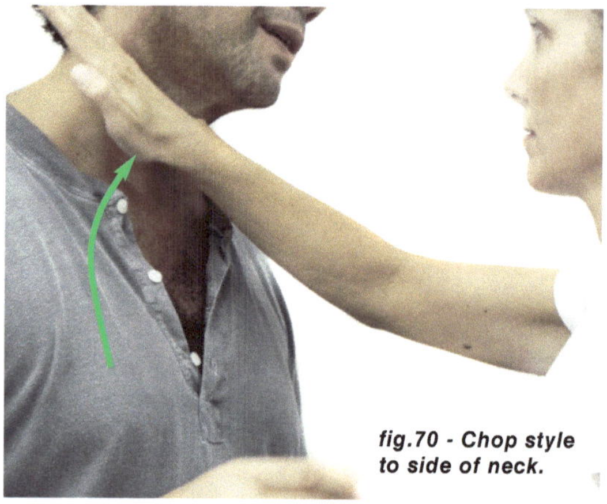

Until the moment they are stepping onto the ring or taking place onto the mat all the fear is controlling their movement but after the first initial contact of gloves the training and hard work in the gym done when sparring takes over: action is what channels adrenaline to a positive force.

Knowing how to effectively act, the knowledge of what that action can cause can put our mind at rest.

The worse type of fear is the fear of fear itself, an incontrollable sensation of panic fearing what we do not know or understand.

fig.70 - Chop style to side of neck.

The concept alone of being hit or having to hit someone scares most people, especially women. The majority of people prefer to avoid confrontation, staying away from trouble, and thank God for that. Speaking to people when they start training in martial arts I always hear the same reasoning over and over "I am happy to hit the bag but I don't want to spar or hit anyone" as if that will cause irreparable damage or you might kill someone or get badly hurt. It does not happen like that. In any sensible gym or dojo you will pair up with people who have your level of experience and gradually build up your skills and it's very important that you do that. The majority of men believe in their mind that they can fight anyone, only because they can hit a bag hard, unfortunately I have been right next to people with impressive physique and a big mouth that went with it yet at first contact or the thought of getting into a fight they would make excuses or just end up paralysed with fear. Why? Because they are fearing fear, they are building up in their own mind a picture of the consequences of fighting that makes the fighting itself more daunting that it really is, they fought and lost in their mind already.

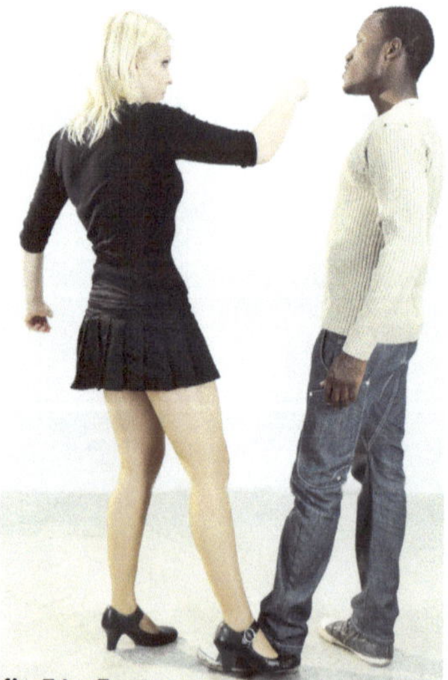

fig 71 - Foot sweep following punch.

I once had a man, who looked like a real beast, in a bar who kept staring at me.

I was with a friend who is very "camp" and "the beast" clearly disliked us... you get the picture. Anyway, after the classic verbal shower of abusive epithets this man asked me if I wanted to go outside. Staring at him I hissed "sure, can my friend come and watch as I beat you to a pulp?" And I moved closer. He quickly retreated and muffling something made a quick exit.

You might wonder why I said that, since I always believed in avoiding confrontation and try to diffuse a situation. Well, I knew he wanted to fight, he clearly did.

But I did not want to be intimidated by the thought of been beaten, I was ready to be beaten and put up with it. I had nothing to lose except a broken nose. I had my nose broken before and I know I can take it. But obviously my opponent couldn't.

Was I bluffing? No, I just handled my own fear. I just thought to myself, fine I'll get a black eye, no big deal. You can beat fear with action, not with the thought of action, real action such as hitting your attacker with speed and precision and more than once.

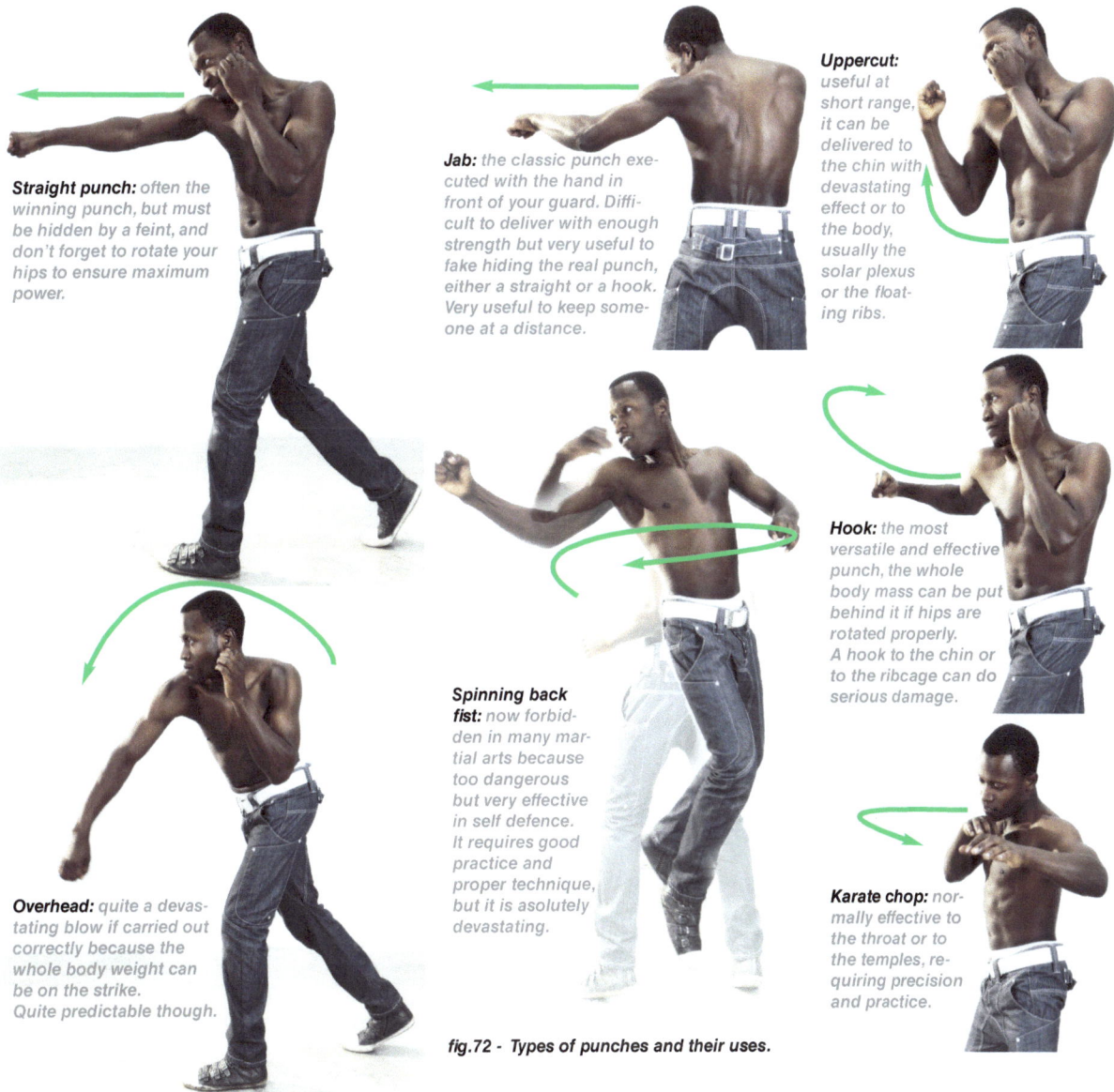

Straight punch: *often the winning punch, but must be hidden by a feint, and don't forget to rotate your hips to ensure maximum power.*

Jab: *the classic punch executed with the hand in front of your guard. Difficult to deliver with enough strength but very useful to fake hiding the real punch, either a straight or a hook. Very useful to keep someone at a distance.*

Uppercut: *useful at short range, it can be delivered to the chin with devastating effect or to the body, usually the solar plexus or the floating ribs.*

Hook: *the most versatile and effective punch, the whole body mass can be put behind it if hips are rotated properly. A hook to the chin or to the ribcage can do serious damage.*

Overhead: *quite a devastating blow if carried out correctly because the whole body weight can be on the strike. Quite predictable though.*

Spinning back fist: *now forbidden in many martial arts because too dangerous but very effective in self defence. It requires good practice and proper technique, but it is asolutely devastating.*

Karate chop: *normally effective to the throat or to the temples, requiring precision and practice.*

fig.72 - Types of punches and their uses.

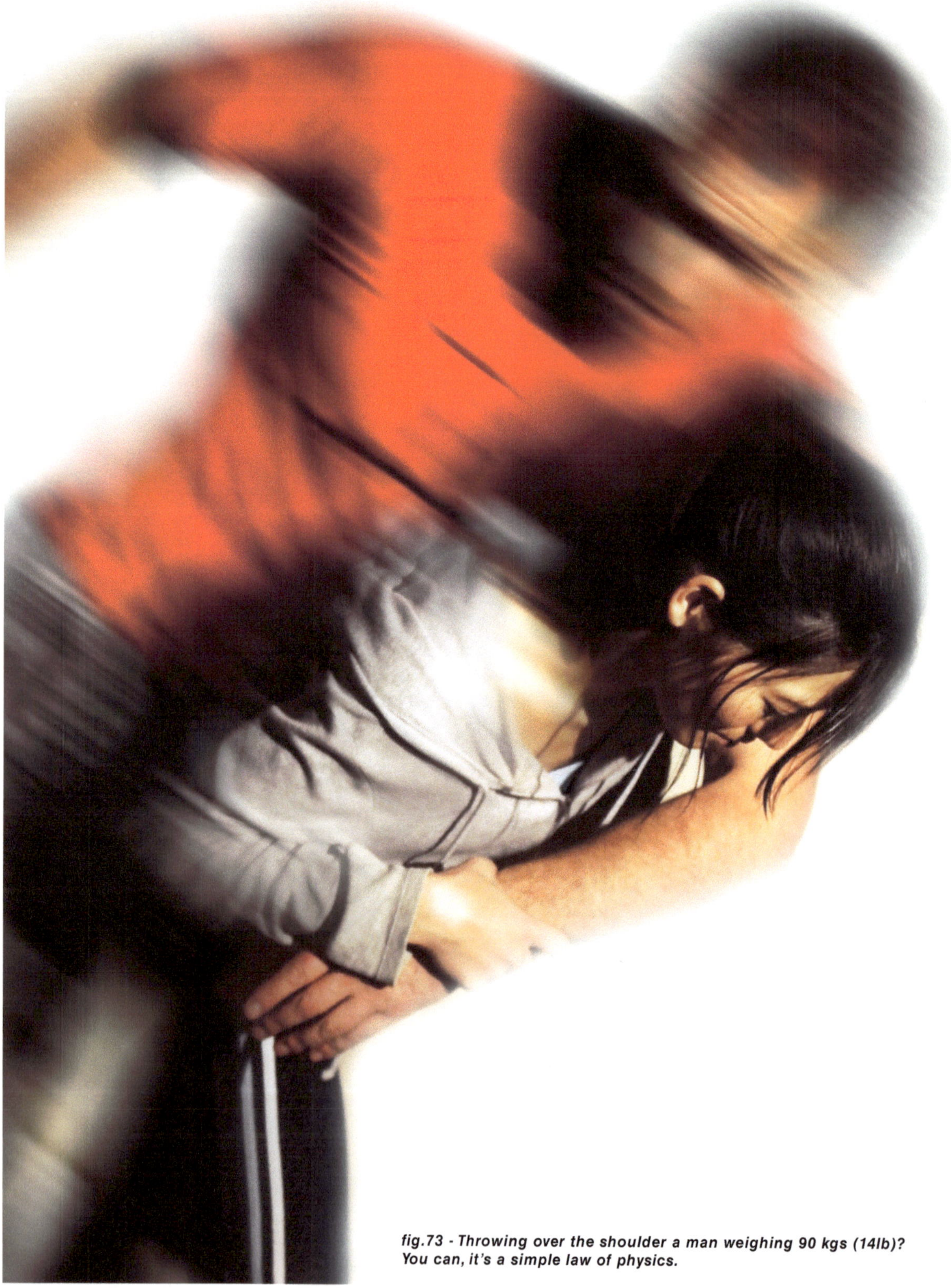

fig.73 - Throwing over the shoulder a man weighing 90 kgs (14lb)?
You can, it's a simple law of physics.

takedowns or throws

A takedown means getting your attacker to the ground without going down as well.
You can achieve this by making him lose his balance, and this creates a very disorienting feeling that can give you a huge advantage or a chance to run to safety: the moment your opponent hits the ground you basically can decide if you should immobilise him or run to safety, in any case you do have more control over the fight, at least for a few precious moments.
To understand how a takedown works, you have to understand the principle of balance, the most important notion when it comes to self defence. Balance is provided by the position of the centre of gravity, if you manage to disturb this centre of gravity in a way that no longer falls above the area of its foundation, your assailant will lose balance regardless of how big, strong or aggressive he is. At the same time we have seen how fundamental it is to have good balance yourself while kicking or punching, to maximise

ANY MASS CAN BE UNBALANCED BY MOVING THE CENTRE OF GRAVITY.

the effect of your strike or readjust yourself quickly if you miss.
Manipulating the centre of gravity requires practice and a good understanding of how the body moves and finds its balance.
Normally we can consider that the centre of gravity is located at the centre of your upper body, but your stance and body structure can change that (fig.74). The principle to remember is that the lower the centre of gravity, the more stable you are. It's easier to unbalance your opponent when he raises his centre of gravity but if you think that going very low with your stance will give you a very strong advantage, think again because it might do that but at the same time going too low stops you from moving quickly. If you observe two boxers fighting you will notice that they never lean back to avoid a punch, always sideways or ducking when necessary. This happens because

IF ATTACKED, MOVE SIDEWAYS TO GET INTO A BETTER POSITION.

leaning back or flinching to the rear, spoils the chance to counterattack, not to mention that a very simple push or punch can actually send you to the ground in no time.

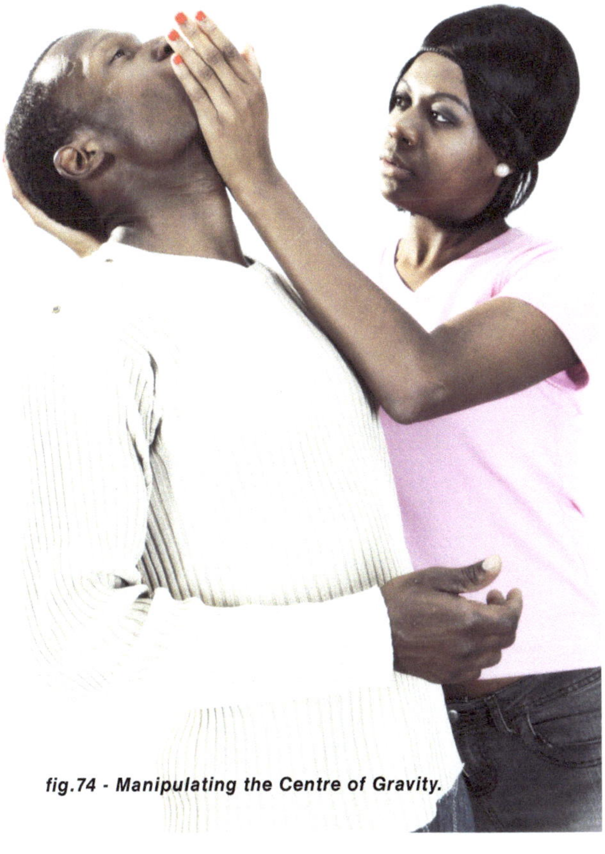

fig.74 - Manipulating the Centre of Gravity.

So the best first action if somebody moves towards you in a threatening manner, shouldn't really be to flinch back but to lower your centre of gravity and tuck your chin towards your chest. In training is so important to correct your stance and to be aware of your stance because your natural reaction as somebody attacks you is to lean back, and that puts you in a very difficult position to initiate any kind of self-defence move. This means you have to reset forwards your centre of gravity, your body's balance, before you can initiate a kick or a counterpunch effectively and quickly.

By all means, move back to avoid a strike, but be aware that it would be best to move sideways in a circular movement to get yourself into a better position to counterattack and to keep your balance. When we walk, we cross our legs, which makes us very vulnerable and any of the sweeping techniques in Judo take advantage of this or in any case it can provoke the opponent into taking steps.

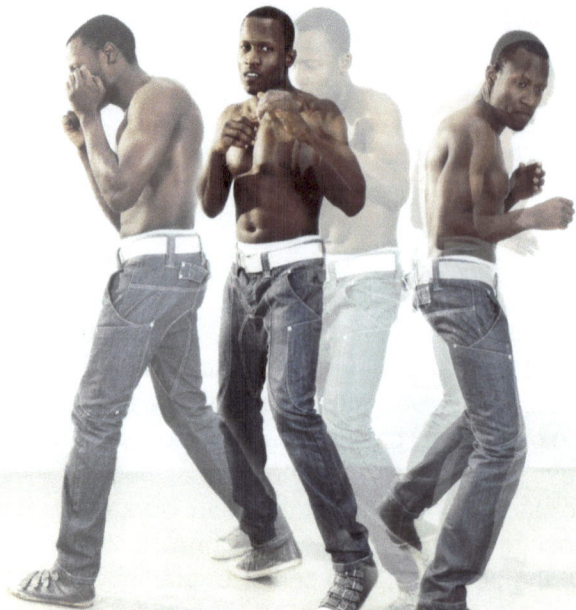

fig.75 - The right stance is a fluid ever changing position, that adapts to the opponent's moves allowing to defend yourself and counterattack in every direction.

In fig.75 we show you how your correct stance should be.

You should think of your stance as something fluid, you shouldn't be rigid but flexible, if you keep a stiff and rigid posture you can be unbalanced easily, not to mention that being flexible and supple will help you stay fit as well as have a better posture, and it will also help you to avoid joints problems getting older (see STRETCHING - page 224).

KNOWING GOOD TECHNIQUE ALLOWS YOU TO EVALUATE YOUR ATTACKER.

Knowing what makes a good stance also allows you to be able to judge your attacker's position and take full advantage of his bad positioning, e.g. somebody holding a knife quite often positions himself in a "wide-horse mount" stance (fig.75A), and this is quite an easy stance to unbalance, a simple push to the upper body will send him flying onto the ground.

You can easily try by yourself pushing somebody in the wide horse stance gently forwards or backwards, to see how easily you can unbalance someone in that stance.

A good understanding of what makes good balance will help you to know where to kick your attacker in order to achieve his falling to the ground: a kick in the middle of the chest will almost certainly make him fall backwards, but a well given hand push can be equally effective. Understanding balance will give you the opportunity to know when to strike, including a simple push, finding the best possible moment.

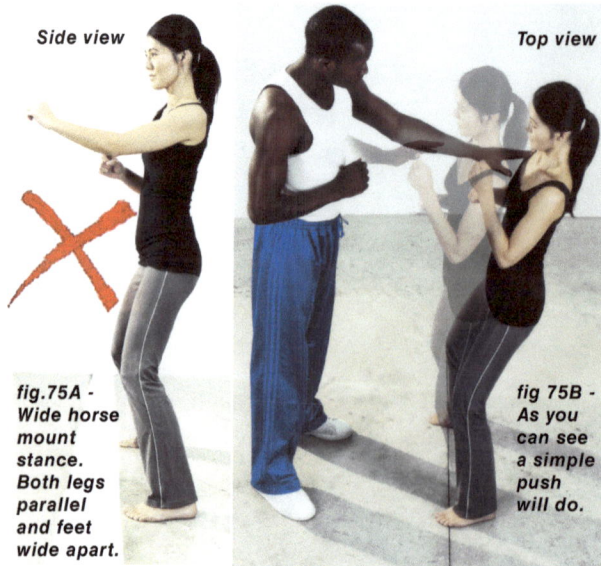

Side view

Top view

fig.75A - Wide horse mount stance. Both legs parallel and feet wide apart.

fig 75B - As you can see a simple push will do.

fig.76 - Grab one of his legs, pull him towards you and push with your other hand against his upper body.

For instance, if he's taken a step towards you, the moment his foot is in mid air, is your window of opportunity (see DE ASHI BARAI technique in JUDO - page 236).
We have seen that you can kick somebody to make him lose his balance but once again if he made you lose your balance or he's trying to get you to the ground, you can shift his centre of gravity and get him on the floor. You can grab one of his legs and as you pull him towards you push at the same time with your other hand against his upper body to unbalance him easily (fig.76).

The same can be done if you are coming to somebody's rescue, basically attacking the assailant from behind: you can kick the back of his knee, so as to unbalance him to the rear, remember it is easier to unbalance rearwards than forwards, because our body is not designed to bend back, at the same time grab his shoulder or around his neck (ideally you want him in a choke), to pull him down (fig.77), don't forget though all these moves should be done sharply and with a continuous movement until you get your opponent to the ground, without stopping or breaking the action at any time, one continuous move. A common mistake is to keep your elbows out as you pull for the takedown: don't do that but instead keep them closer to your body to have more power and more control in your pull.

GOING TO THE RESCUE MEANS TAKING THE ATTACKER TO THE GROUND IN A CHOKE.

fig.77- When coming to someone rescue grab the atacker's shoulder or around his neck (ideally you want him in a choke), to pull him down to the ground.

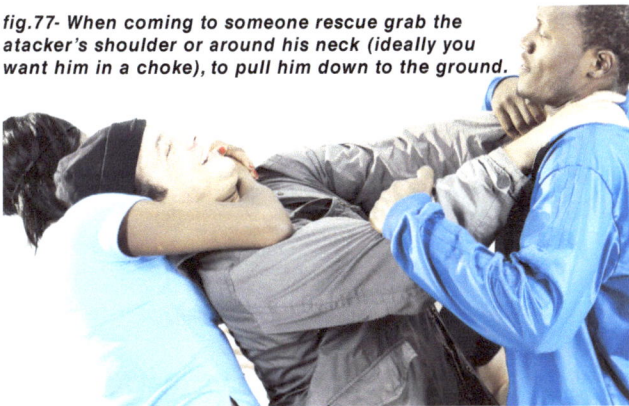

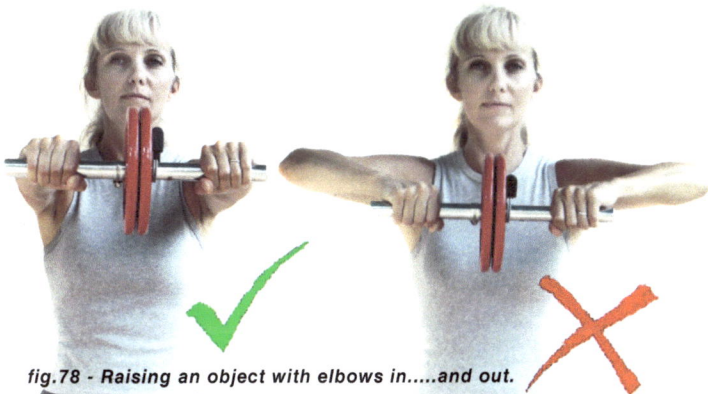

Raising an object with your elbow close to your side and raising the same object with your elbow sticking out can easily demonstrate why this is important (fig.78).
You should remember that once you have understood the principle behind a good stance, you'll be able to find or to create your window of opportunity as well as to position yourself ready for a takedown or a throw as we will examine further on.
The first thing to do is to shift your attacker's centre of gravity, moving his upper body to the rear, using momentum (mass by velocity) to pull your attacker off balance, ideally with a circular movement to increase his disorientation, acting fast to surprise him, because once you start with a takedown you can't stop for any reason.
You can also facilitate your capacity to shift his centre of gravity over his foundation using barriers to stop him from stepping back and regain his balance.

fig.78 - Raising an object with elbows in.....and out.

Using your foot behind his for instance (like O-SOTO GARI in JUDO - page 236), or a box, a chair, even the edge of the pavement, anything appropriate to make him trip over.

MOVING CLOSER WILL SURPRISE YOUR ATTACKER AND GIVE YOU MORE CONTROL. Also to be effective with a takedown, you have to close the distance so don't forget you cannot step backwards, instead you should crouch slightly forwards to get into a good position for your takedown.

You can go for a takedown when you find your window of opportunity, normally when the assailant is momentarily distracted either by something you say or do, or by something he does. This ability to move forwards and crouch, that boxers learn in the ring is not something you can learn by yourself, you must get someone to help you do that.

You will notice that sometimes in boxing when one of the boxers starts receiving a series of blows, instead of stepping away, he moves closer: this is a known technique to break the opponent's punches, making them ineffective at

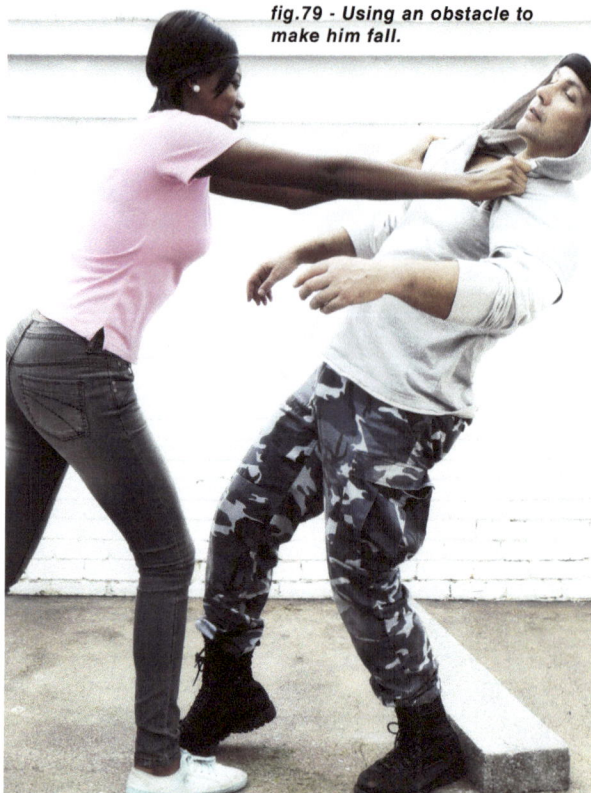
fig.79 - Using an obstacle to make him fall.

short range and clearly in this circumstance safety is in proximity, and not in distance.

The secret of a takedown is positioning in relation to your opponent.

DON'T SQUARE YOUR ATTACKER, MOVE TOWARDS HIS BACK OR SIDE INSTEAD. If you observe two Judokas fighting you will see that all they try to do is to unbalance the opponent and to get their body in the best position for their throws.

So how do we get into a good position? In a fist fight, squaring your opponent is asking for trouble, and what you should try is to move towards his back and this is why boxers in the ring move constantly in a circle.

If your opponent follows your movement, step suddenly in the opposite direction, closing the distance and try for a takedown, using his momentum to make the most of the technique.

What happens if your attacker has managed to grab hold of you?

Our natural reaction is to fight or grab the arm that is grabbing us. If attacked around the neck, your hands will instantly try to free yourself, grasping your attacker's arm around your neck.

If grabbed by the waist your immediate reaction will be using your hands to try to free the area. This should be avoided because you are fighting your attacker's focus of energy, he's putting all his strength into that arm lock, and you will fail against a stronger attacker.

What your attacker is not paying attention to at that moment is his balance and his stance.

The secret of any takedown really has to do with the laws of physics, that is why it is important that while practicing unbalancing techniques you understand how these work.

As we've seen, getting into the right position is as important, allowing you to either be the perfect fulcrum to be able to throw him to the ground or to unbalance him effectively.

You also should be careful not to step into your attacker's line of attack, and using a parry or block can delay him for a second, allowing you to get close for your takedown position.

fig.80 - If grabbed by your waist from behind you should push back, adding a head butt if you can.

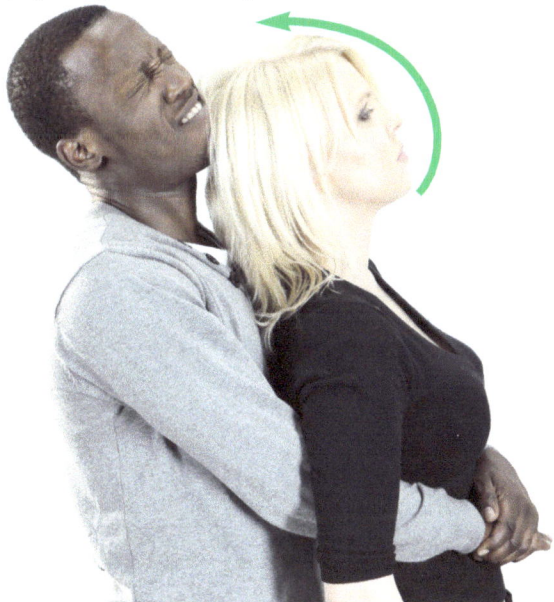

All this might sound quite complicated, and you might think "hang on; you said earlier that simplicity is the principle". It still is.

> **WORK AGAINST THE NATURAL MOVEMENT OF YOUR ATTACKER'S JOINTS.**

As a general rule, remember that your attacker's joints, like neck, knees, elbows, can only bend in one direction, and if you push him in the opposite direction he has to follow your action, or sustain pain or worse getting injured if resisting.

If you are going for a hand grab or lever, because arms bend forward, you have to position yourself behind or to the side of the elbow.

Regarding the legs, because they bend backwards your best position is in front or to the side of your attacker, working against the natural movement of the knee.

The neck can bend and rotate in every direction but being attached to the torso, that

> **THE BODY GOES WHERE THE HEAD GOES.**

naturally bends forward, positioning yourself behind the body will allow you to control the body just manipulating his head (fig.80,77,88).

A very important principle is that if you control the head of your attacker, you also control his body because the body goes where the head goes.

Let's examine closer how to reach the best position for a takedown: we have seen that fighting your natural reaction you should close your distance but you should remember that by doing so your attacker will want to grab you. It is important consequentially to be aware of any part of your body or even part of your clothing that can offer a chance to an attacker to get hold you.

If grabbed you should immediately try to either push or pull, make him lose his grip or balance, you can also make him lose his grip, striking e.g. the interior side of the forearm that as we can see in VULNERABLE (page 30) can momentarily paralyse his hand movement.

> **ALWAYS CONTROL THE HEAD OF YOUR ATTACKER, EVEN WHEN IT GOES DOWN.**

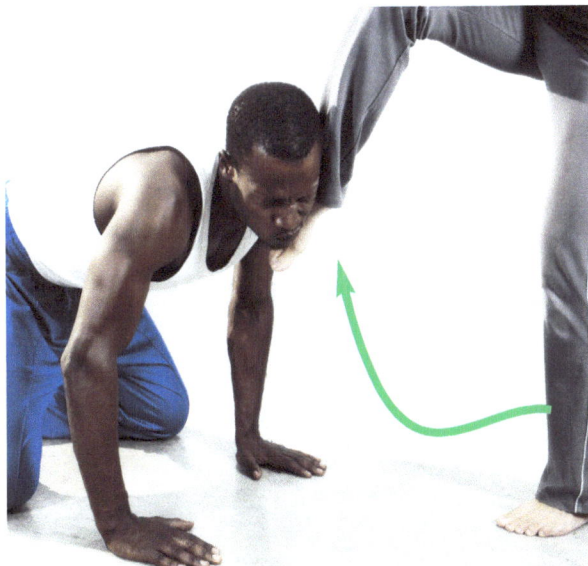

This book cannot make you experience how it feels, pushing, pulling or being pushed or being pulled, this can only be done with an experienced partner, but at least now you know the fundamental principles. It is also important to understand, and we have seen already that this is a difficult element in teaching self-defence, that practicing any techniques against an opponent who is helping us performing them is much easier than executing them against someone who's sole intention is to hurt us.

fig.81 - Kick his head once he is down or if he tries to get up.

56

Assuming that you have managed to take your assailant down, you have to decide what to do next, obviously run to safety if possible should be your first line of action, but this is not always practically achievable.

If you have to step over him always do it over his head, because if he manages to grab you, you'll find it easier to control him by his head than by his feet, don't forget.

An ideal line of action would be kicking him to the head, chest or throat to make him lose consciousness, but we are not expecting most

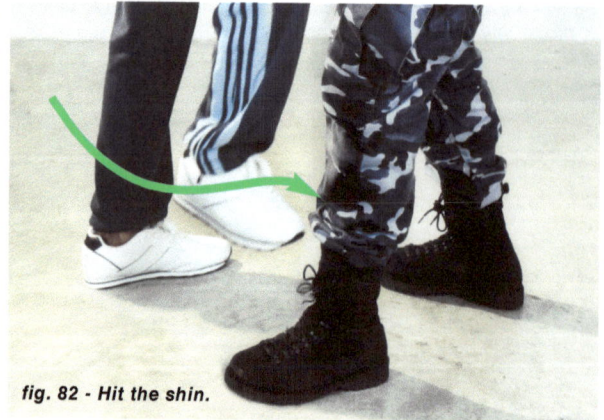
fig. 82 - Hit the shin.

people to do so, but nevertheless at least avoid hanging around complacently (fig.81).

What I have seen during a fight is people standing watching the result of their takedown, and waiting for the attacker to get back to his feet: big mistake. He's going to be angrier, and he knows you are somewhat experienced. He'll be more careful and at the same time more violent.

In other words, don't wait to see what results you have achieved just run to safety

All unbalancing moves rely on disturbing your attacker's technique, if we can call it such, in any case, you have to take control. Your primary aim when under attack is to break your attacker's focus and that should be done in the initial part of his action before he reaches its effect.

When we examined kicking techniques we purposely left out high kicks.

That is because assuming you do have enough flexibility of your joints you probably won't be fast enough to kick effectively but especially to stop him grabbing your leg.

A low kick to the shin, knee or mid torso can reach a better effect and split his focus more effectively and you can call this technique unbalancing your attacker through pain.

IF YOUR STRIKE IS ONLY SUPERFICIAL IT IS ONLY AS GOOD AS PILLOW FIGHTING.

You've also seen in HITTING (page 44) that a kick or a punch is only effective if it can penetrate 2/3cm past the skin and again you can only achieve that only getting close enough and being in a good position. This is important because if you decide to kick you should not kick waiting for your opponent to move, you should kick before he is in the middle of his action. It would be ideal that you could experience for real a bit of sparring, and that's why we keep suggesting that at some point you do take some practical lessons.

Practicing closing the gap following a strike effectively, deflecting a punch, kicking properly and getting into the right position are all moves that cannot be achieved against an unresponsive punch bag or by just looking at some images but only through supervised practice. Nevertheless, it's also important that you understand the principles to be able to put them into practice.

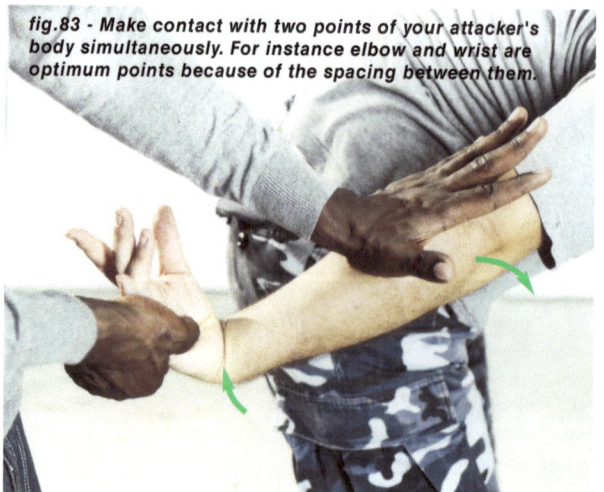
fig.83 - Make contact with two points of your attacker's body simultaneously. For instance elbow and wrist are optimum points because of the spacing between them.

IN A SELF DEFENCE SITUATION THERE IS ONLY ONE RULE: SURVIVE!

In self-defence unfortunately we cannot expect sportsmanship and fairness, in a street attack situation these are principles that find no place.

If you decide to defend yourself, think offensively, bearing in mind that thinking twice is not an option and that your window of opportunity, meaning the best moment to strike your attacker, is found through an understanding of timing, probably the most important concept in defence. Timing is the ability of taking advantage of your attacker's position, hesitation, distraction or a pause in his actions. It is a very difficult ability to achieve, your mind might feel and spot these gaps in your attacker's action but your body will either be too slow in reacting or reacting in the wrong way, the only way to achieve a good timed response is through supervised practice.

Believe us when we say it's pointless, like some other manuals do, giving you lots of scenarios and telling you when and how to react, scenarios should be kept to a minimum and should mostly sum up a general action-reaction, not indulge in specific techniques and its infinite variations.

If under attack you should not try to remember the sequence of moves you have seen in a book, you should react with an action that your brain has assimilated through practice following a easy to remember principle. To break down some simple principles to better understand timing, bear in mind that somebody launching at you using an overhead punch (a mix between a hook and a punch coming from high, very common in street fighting, (resembling someone throwing a stone fig.72) can easily be thrown to the ground if you move to the side and pull his arm using a circular movement.

UNDERSTAND TIMING TO BE ABLE TO REACT EFFECTIVELY!

At the same time, moving in when somebody kicks you frontally (front kick) is asking for trouble because you are doubling the power of his kick towards you, unless you can move in close so quickly that you make his kick useless, in that case it's fine to step back, and move in as he's flexing his leg back to regain balance.

An experienced kick boxer can defeat a kick, moving in at the slightest sign of his opponent initiating a kick, or moving to the side of his opponent the moment he throws a kick, striking him back when he's on one leg.

This, needless to say, requires experience and good timing, achieved through plenty of practice and all these techniques, getting into the right position and so on, relying on the main principle of the Perfect Defence system: speed.

To get into the right position for your takedown or for your kick, your movement has to be of absolute lightning speed, almost explosive. It is also a good idea to maximise

TIMING IS EVERYTHING IN SELF DEFENCE.. SPEED IS THE ANSWER.

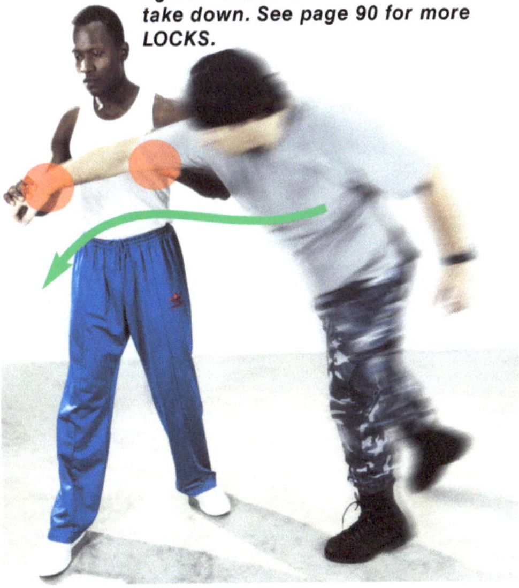

fig.84 - Elbow and wrist lever for take down. See page 90 for more LOCKS.

your results, to get into position as you throw a series of punches to his torso or kicks to his shin, this will achieve a distracting effect and causing pain and it will break the tension of your opponent's body. If you've ever watched two boxers fighting, you will have noticed that when one of them initiates a rapid sequence of blows, let's say five or six in a rapid firing sequence, the other can only cover and wait for him to stop.

The aim is to overwhelm your attacker raining blows mercilessly and then go for the takedown.

Unfortunately, you are not trading blows as De Coubertin preached, with fairness; instead you must be unsympathetic and furious, as your life might be at stake.

These fundamental principles in unbalancing your attacker apply in every other way also to leverage (see also LOCKS - page 90).

Leverage relies on torque, expressed in physics as lever = arm x force (fig.84).
The longer the lever's arm the smaller the force you need to apply to produce torque, meaning moving a mass or lifting a weight.

(!) Leverage is based on the push-pull main principle through two points of balance; this means that to be effective, you must make contact with two points of your attacker's body simultaneously. For example elbow and wrist are optimum points because of the spacing between them (fig.16 and fig.84).

The same can be said if you apply leverage to the neck; even if the distance is shorter the neck is quite weak and will suffer.

Applying a circular momentum in your pushing and pulling action will greatly increase the effectiveness of leverage, beyond your best expectations with great result.

Anyone can only resist one action in one direction at one given time, for example if you grab someone by his shoulders and push back, he can quickly regain balance by stepping back, but if you push him back and at the same time rotate his shoulders on his axis you'll achieve greater effect (fig.85).

ONE CAN ONLY RESIST ONE ACTION AT THE TIME. ALWAYS COMBINE TECHNIQUES.

(!) If you are of small build and not particularly strong, bear in mind that you should distance these two points of leverage as much as you can, making the lever arm as long as possible, for example if you grab his foot, try to push with your hand his upper body approximately at chest height, as you lift his leg.

You will throw him to the ground in no time with little effort (fig.86) and if you add a slight rotation to the move your technique is as perfect as it can be.

KEEP YOUR ACTIONS FLUID AND TOGETHER: DON'T BREAK MOMENTUM.

All of these actions should never be broken down because breaking your movements means stopping momentum, intended as your ability to continue motion, moving your bodyweight in the same direction as your attack's direction is the way to go.

To sum it all up, any action to redirect your opponent's momentum should be done following your attacker's momentum shifting its direction in a fluid movement. Imagine two American football players running towards each other at speed, going against each others momentum, translating into a clash of momentum (fig. 87).

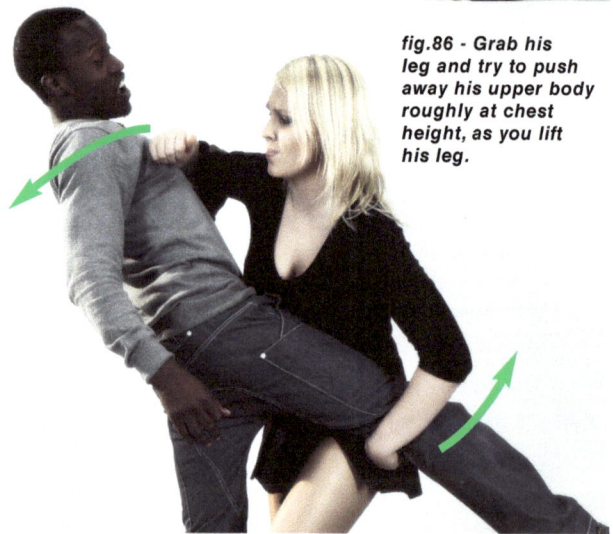

fig.85 - If you rotate his shoulders whilst you push him back you'll achieve greater effect.

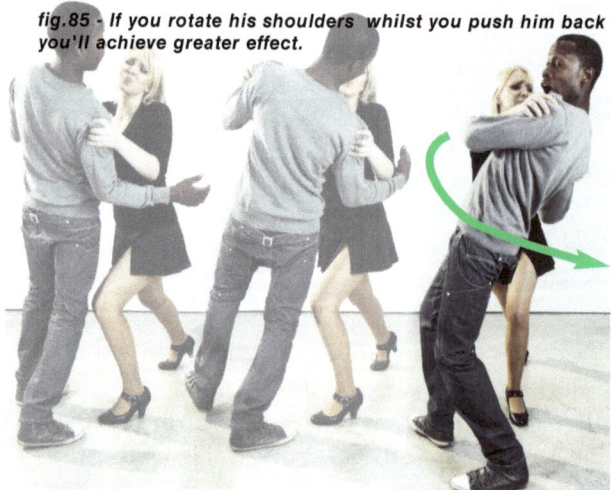

fig.86 - Grab his leg and try to push away his upper body roughly at chest height, as you lift his leg.

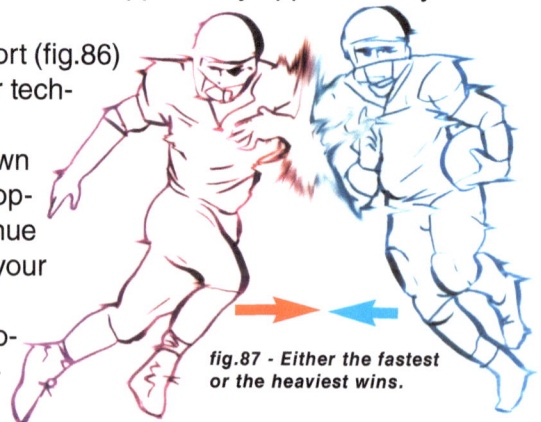

fig.87 - Either the fastest or the heaviest wins.

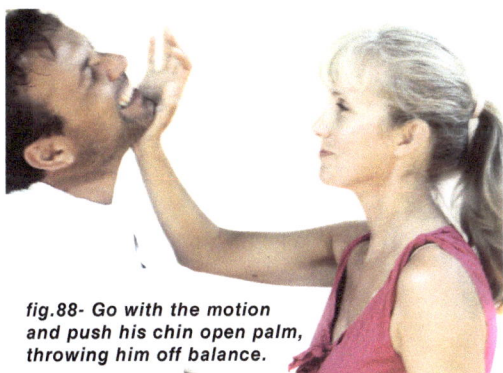

fig.88- Go with the motion and push his chin open palm, throwing him off balance.

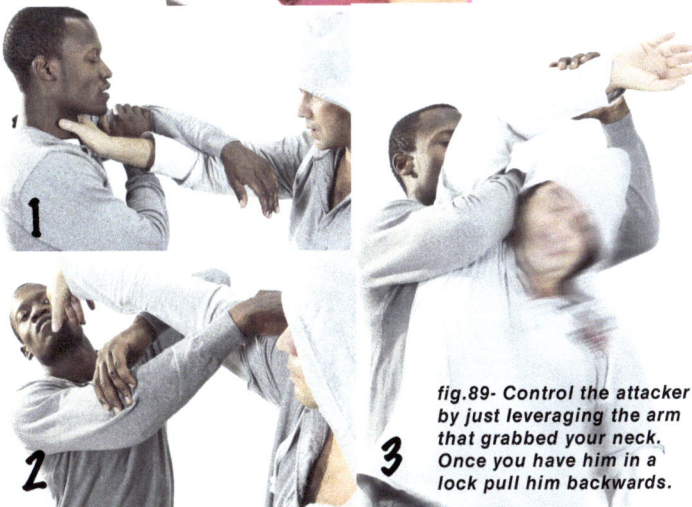

fig.89- Control the attacker by just leveraging the arm that grabbed your neck. Once you have him in a lock pull him backwards.

fig.90 - Push up your partner's chin open-palm, at the same time, put your leg just behind his (see also O-SOTO-GARI in JUDO TABLES page 236).

The result in this case will be that either the lighter person will succumb, or possibly the person with less speed: the basic principle is that you should step into your attacker's centre of gravity and joining momentum knock him off balance to your advantage.

You can also change the direction of your attacker's momentum, making a move or a strike to make him shy away, allowing you to join momentum in the direction that he has taken in his action. If for example somebody grabs your wrist naturally your reaction is to pull away, when in actual fact you should move forward, joining his momentum (he's obviously pulling you towards him) and that will allow you to go with the motion and push open-palm up his chin, throwing him off balance (fig.88).

We have seen that to achieve an effective takedown you should use a combined movement not just pushing him back but also down or pushing him down as well as circling.

In other words, always combine a straight move with a circular one.

This applies to all takedowns: the push-pull-principle combined with the circular move will allow you to control the attacker by just leveraging the arm that grabbed your neck (fig.77).

The principle is really simple.

Of all techniques to control and unbalance an attacker the best one and most effective is the one controlling his head.

Remember: where the head goes the body goes, but controlling the head doesn't mean pulling his hair: remember to always use two points, one high and one low, for example grabbing his chin and the top back of his head, to manipulate accordingly.

Manipulating the head means controlling the entire spine, and this can produce serious spinal injuries if your attacker resists your motion. It is important to understand that you should not practice these techniques unsupervised or with somebody inexperienced, the risk of causing a serious injury is very high.

Lets start with a very simple technique that shows how powerful head manipulation can be to unbalance an opponent even one much larger than you.

THE BODY FOLLOWS WHERE THE HEAD GOES. NO EXCEPTION, JUST SIMPLE LAWS OF PHYSICS.

(!) Put your hand open-palm up your partner's chin, and at the same time, put your leg just behind his. Ask your partner to try to maintain his balance as much as possible and perform the push accompanying it with a slight circular movement as illustrated in fig.90.

Even moving dead slow, he will not be able to maintain his balance. It is important to hold your hand in position all the way through it.

The two points of balance are your hand on his chin and your foot behind his.

The same can be applied approaching the opponent from the side and applying a circular movement to your push-and -pull action (see fig.91).

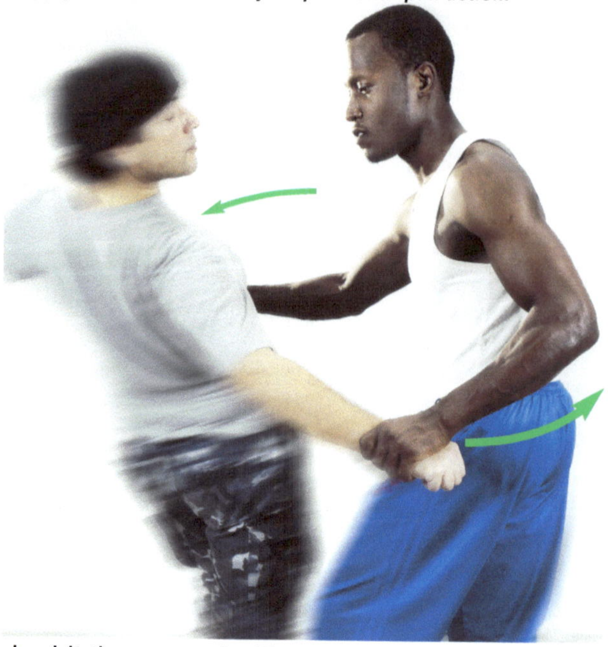

Finally, consider that if somebody grabs you bear-hug-style, lifting you off your feet, you can still manipulate his head just pushing up his chin (that he naturally will have away from you to avoid you hitting him) but you'll notice that a simple push will make him lose balance and maybe hit the ground with you on top.

fig.91- *When your opponent is attacking from the side, apply a circular move to your push-and -pull action.*

It is worth remembering that when somebody lifts you off the ground with a bear-hug technique, he cannot really harm you in other ways because both his hands are used, and he cannot strike you. Now you know why it is important that you assess quickly why he is using this technique: is he trying to drag you somewhere, a secluded spot or a car.

In this case, the moment you should consider to initiate a takedown is the moment he lets go or you touch the ground. The moment you have one hand free, or one leg on the ground, that's the moment you can join his momentum and steal his balance going for your takedown.

WHEN YOU HAVE BEEN LIFTED IN THE AIR JUST WAIT TILL YOU HAVE ONE POINT TOUCHING THE GROUND.

We cannot emphasize enough how important it is to always join momentum with your attacker and initiate a circular movement, in a spiral way at the same time.

This will work regardless of the way he is attempting to strike you.

What you will find most difficult is to close the gap, and physically grab your attacker.

As he throws a punch for instance, you evade his strike and should grab his arm stepping behind him or onto his side, and using circular momentum go in for your take down.

(!) So how exactly you decide when to go for your motions?

Any self-defence move is only effective if you surprise your attacker, if you hit his nose, eyes, if you strike his throat or kick his knee, all these reactions should be immediate, as soon as the threat is perceived: a moment later could be too late.

That's why takedowns are quite effective, it is more difficult to decide to kick first or strike first, and most people do not have that state of mind.

YOU MUST INITIATE YOUR ACTION THE MOMENT HE TOUCHES YOU.

However, you'll find it reasonably easier to react to someone trying to hit you or grab you, therefore, you should initiate your action the moment your attacker leans towards you, either to strike or to grab you.

If somebody who is threatening you for whatever reason, steps towards you, you can be sure, it is to harm you, or in any case to control you.

fig.92 - Ideal leg takedown: grab both legs of your attacker to avoid having him stepping back to regain his balance.
Best if you push with your shoulders against his thighs, and pull his knees together to narrow his foundation.

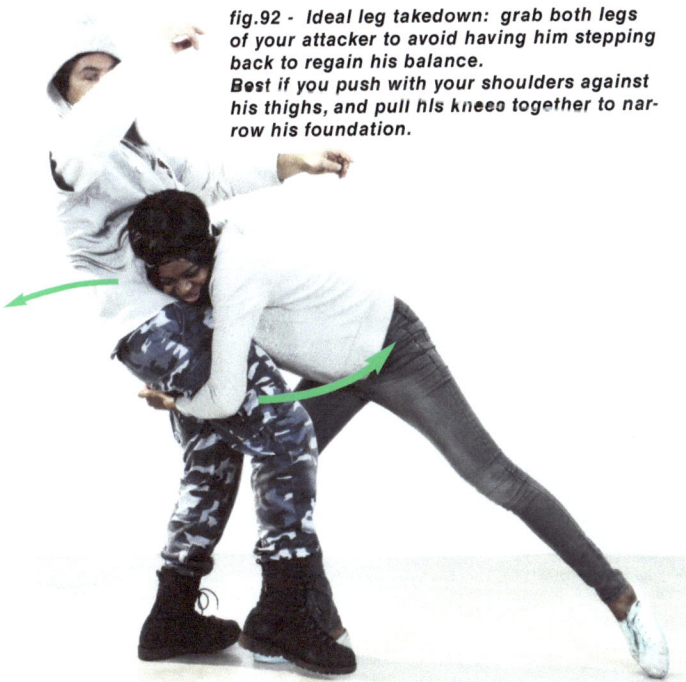

Doing so, he's in a temporary weaker position for the following reasons: he's stepping, meaning unbalanced, he's distracted because probably looking around checking if somebody is watching, and he's also confident of his actions, counting on this surprise factor.

This is the moment that you can par the strike and grab his wrist or arm, and pulling him along his line of attack, his momentum, you can get him in a circular movement for the takedown.

READING A BOOK IS NO SUBSTITUTE FOR READING REAL BODY LANGUAGE.

All this should be done in one continuous movement, no hesitation, almost in an explosive manner.

It is naive to think that just reading this book you can perfect these techniques; you should remember that practice is essential especially when done with experienced people. Do not forget that even in a training environment, you will find that your opponent is cooperating; making things too easy for you, and that obviously you are not applying an explosive action for fear of hurting your partner or injuring yourself even.

Nevertheless, as we said many times before, remember the principles and practice in a safe and controlled manner, (possibly supervised by an instructor.)

YOU MUST REACT THE MOMENT HE MAKES A MOVE. NO LATER NO EARLIER, RIGHT THEN.

The principle to remember is that the moment to initiate your push-pull-technique with a circular movement joining your attacker's momentum is the moment he touches you in any way. It takes lots of practice to get into that frame of mind, as well as forcing yourself not to react, as your instinct would tell you, leaning backwards or just covering your face closing your eyes and it's also important that you try positioning yourself for a takedown with your opponent attacking from different angles and directions.

We have seen so far how applying takedowns you can control your attacker's arm or head: in all takedowns you should always remember one simple principle: the focus of your takedown are the two points of balance, for example the wrist and the shoulder, the arm and the head, the foot and the head, but always two points.

THE FOCUS OF ALL TAKEDOWNS IS TWO POINTS OF BALANCE.

You can also manipulate just the legs of your attacker, with great effect.

The principle is to shift his upper body, the centre of gravity, and changing the relationship between centre of gravity and foundation, to then get him to the ground in no time.

In this case, moving or removing the foundation (the legs) will make your attacker fall.

The ideal leg takedown (fig.92) should consider grabbing both legs of your attacker, so to avoid having him stepping back to regain his balance.

Pushing against his knees with your shoulders, rugby-style, will achieve a faster, greater result if you also manage to pull his knees together, narrowing his foundation, shifting his centre of gravity.

If halfway through the attacker manages to bend over to resist your action, switch your momentum into a circular movement to make him lose balance to one side.

The result of the takedown is ideally your attacker onto the ground in as little time as possible with maximum impact.

Once you have achieved this, your next action is to run to safety, and unless you are really good or extremely well trained we suggest you don't try to control him any further.

If you cannot run anywhere drop with your forearm with all your weight on his throat, going for a choking maneuver, or if you have managed to stay up, or you managed to get up before he does, kick his head.

If for whatever reason, you can only manage to grab one leg, maybe because his stance is quite wide, keep your head onto one side of his body and as you pull up his leg make sure that you push with your shoulder, as high as you can, onto his thigh or his waist (two points of balance, remember? (fig.93).

fig.93 - Grab one leg if his stance is quite wide, and keeping your head on one side, pull up his leg and push him with your shoulder in an upward movement.

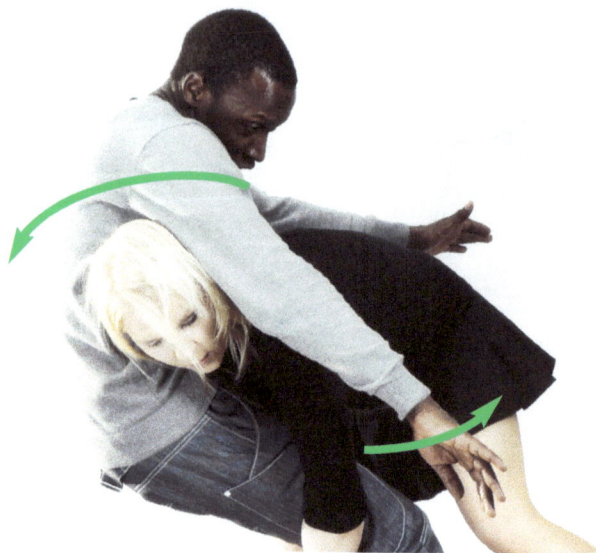

What you should absolutely avoid is going onto your knees, because it will become quite impossible to push him off balance, and you also have to be quite precise, aiming at knee level, not higher because obviously you decrease the length of the lever arm.

As always one explosive action without hesitation will achieve a perfect result.

As we pointed out before, make sure if you only managed to catch one leg, to keep your head tucked on the side to protect yourself being kicked or hit in the other leg and don't forget that, twisting his leg as you throw him to the ground, will quite surely help you achieve maximum result.

Another situation where you might be able to grab someone's one leg is when you managed to catch a kicking leg: this obviously requires perfect timing and good distance closure: ideally, you should close the gap the very moment his leg leaves the ground to kick.

A common mistake once you grabbed his leg is to rely on him for support: this should be avoided at all costs because if he manages to suddenly pull his leg away from you, he will throw you off balance quite easily.

Obviously, if we perceive that a kick is coming towards us, the natural reaction is to move away, normally backwards: force yourself to move closer to 'break' the kick, moving backwards as many kick boxers know, could actually put you on the receiving end anyway.

The most difficult kick to catch is the front kick and you should bear this in mind if you decide to kick first for whatever reason, while the roundhouse kick (see KICKBOXING - page 240) is normally the easiest to catch or intercept, especially when directed to the head.

fig.94 - The rotation of the leg, if done correctly, maybe even sidestepping him, might cause the attacker to fall forwards.

fig.95 - Side-step him and push his chin with your open palm whilst pushing his back with your other hand (always remember 2 points!) By simultaneously pushing and pulling, you'll get him to the ground).

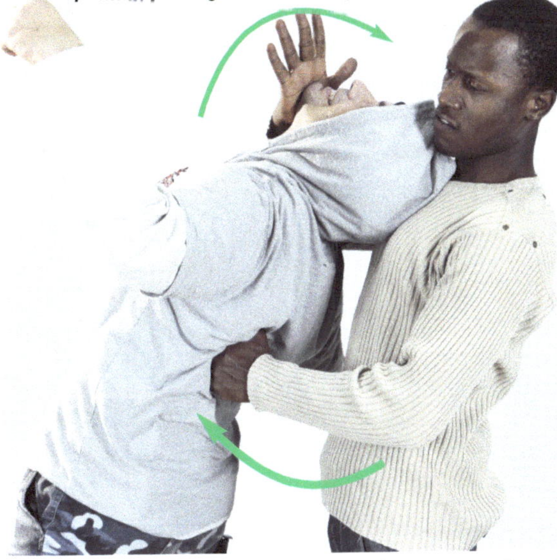

You can only achieve a 'feel' for kicks by practicing with a partner, also to see what part of the body will 'telegraph' your kick.

Normally, espccially when preparing to kick, someone will get into a particular stance or switch feet or lower himself, or in any case narrow his eyes to focus.

These are all telltale signs that can help you to prepare yourself to move closer to him the moment he initiates the kick. You will also notice, that if you perfect your timing and you are quick enough, you might be able to sweep the foot left on the ground, the moment he is kicking with the other leg.

Do no expect though, if moving closer, that you will be totally safe from receiving any impact from his kick, you certainly will, but at the same time, it

MOVE CLOSER, UNLESS YOU WANT TO BE AT THE RECEIVING END.

won't be as bad as it could be if you remain where the foot lands receiving the full force of the blow. As you grab his foot, raise his leg and step even closer, don't just simply push back.

Our emphasis is on executing these techniques in an explosive manner, fast, decisive and with all your strength, tensing your body. You can increase your chances adding a push with your free hand to the top of his torso, or stepping with your leg behind his on the ground, and adding a circular move. Do all this, and he stands no chance at all.

The rotation of the leg, if done correctly, maybe even sidestepping him, might cause the attacker to fall forwards (see fig. 94). Falling forward causes more damage than falling backwards because it is more difficult to cushion your fall considering your joints bend in the opposite direction (see FALLING - page 76).

The successful forward takedown relies on a good rotation of your attacker's leg and in the accuracy of your positioning and you should always remember not to allow his leg to bend, keeping his leg in contact with your own body, pulling him in a spiral movement.

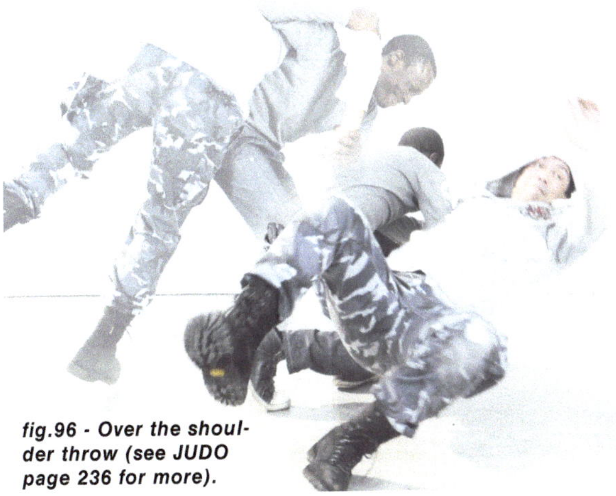

fig.96 - Over the shoulder throw (see JUDO page 236 for more).

On all these takedowns, you can use your free hand to hit or push open-palm his chin as well as confusing him, this will cause more pain and allows you to have even more control over his centre of gravity.

You can also apply takedown techniques to your attacker's body or arm but this normally presumes that you should initiate the action, not wait for him to act first.

Body takedowns require that you get as close as possible to your attacker, this is because you can apply the two-points-of -balance-principle easier at close range.

GETTING CLOSER IS THE SECRET. YOU WILL HAVE THE ADVANTAGE.

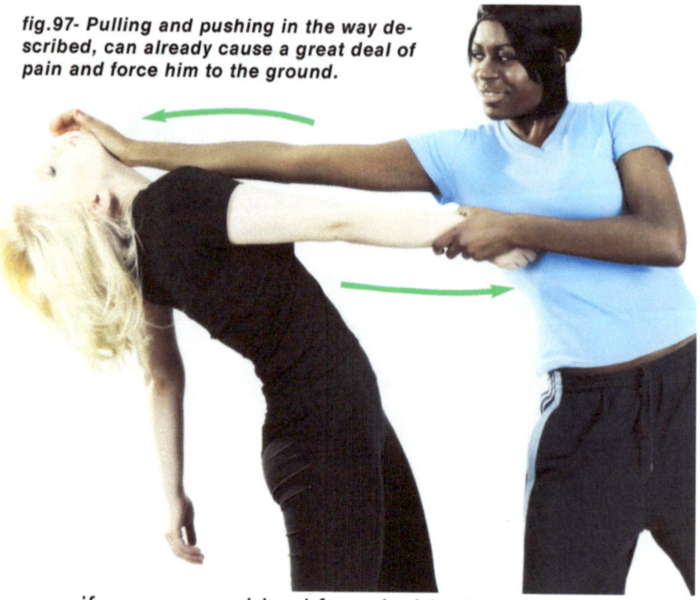

Obviously a body takedown is more difficult if your size is much smaller than your attacker's, but believe me if you are confident and explosive in your action you will achieve the results, this is the simple law of physics.

() For instance, you can side-step him and grab his chin and push on his back with the other hand (always remember two points!) and push and pull simultaneously, you'll get him to the ground (see fig.95).

If you join hips with your attacker and apply a circular movement you will achieve a throw in no time. It is much easier if you differ in size to achieve a takedown, controlling your attacker's arm even if you are grabbed from behind.

fig.97- Pulling and pushing in the way described, can already cause a great deal of pain and force him to the ground.

The moment he wraps his arm across your body, you should grab his wrist and elbow and using his own momentum you will successfully throw him over your shoulder (see fig.96 and IPPON SEOI NAGE in JUDO - page 236).

() Grabbing your attacker's arm is complicated enough, and you should refrain from using complicated techniques that require precision and training.

For instance, in fig.97 you can see that pulling and pushing in the way described, you can already cause a great deal of pain and force him to the ground.

IF YOU PUSH AND PULL, DON'T FORGET TO ADD A ROTATION AS WELL. There are several variations on techniques applying levers to the arm, all equally effective, and all exist because the angle of the attack changes.

For more see LOCKS (page 90), but for now just remember a very simple principle: applying a push-and-pull technique you should always add a rotation, to maximize the momentum and follow the line of attack, independently from the angle.

(!) As seen before, you can also combine manipulating the arm with manipulating the neck.

It is worth remembering that just twisting the wrist and pushing on the elbow doesn't necessarily resolve in a takedown. Obviously always use his arm as a lever against the natural movement of the elbow, that way you'll turn him with his back towards you and once you have him in this position, grab the chin and go for a takedown (see fig. 98).

Never forget to always apply a circular, spiral move in a down-direction with a quick turn of your body to unbalance your attacker. Needless to say, you must always try to keep the lever as long as possible to make it more effective, the longer the lever the more the torque, that's why you should always try to grab the wrist. You might also find yourself attacked by surprise by someone who grabs you with one or both hands around your neck, maybe to pull you to the ground or to direct your face towards his knee.

ALWAYS WORK AGAINST YOUR ATTACKER'S ARTICULATIONS NATURAL MOVEMENT. If you just oppose strength to his move, you only are going to win if you're stronger or bigger. In this case, you can't just free yourself either going backwards or stepping forwards, as he has the advantage of the grip. You can however, take advantage of the arm's natural weakness when pushing against the natural movement of his arm.

fig.98 - Grab the chin and go for a takedown.

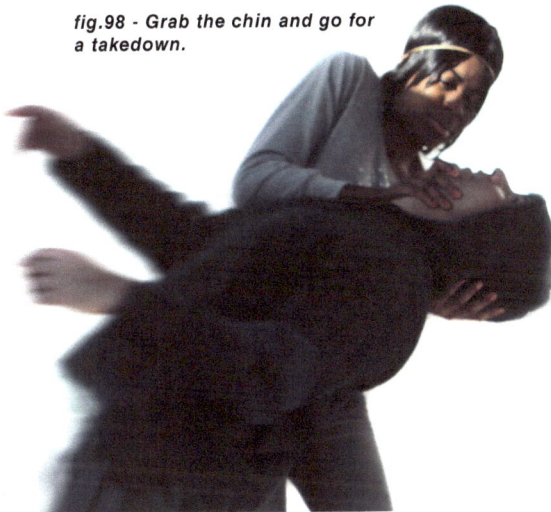

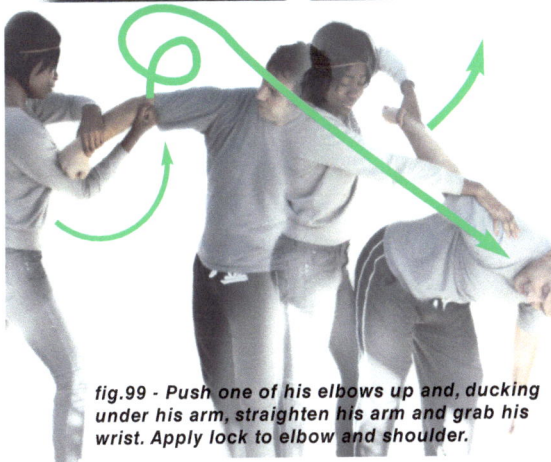

In this case, push one of his elbows up and, ducking under his arm, straighten his arm and grab his wrist (fig.99).

As you've seen in fig.90 as you hold his arm close to your chest, pull his chin in the opposite direction, arching his body back and keep pushing the chin until you achieve the takedown (see fig.100 for the whole action).

fig.101- If you can squeeze your hands between his arms, grab his chin, now bend his head back and down.

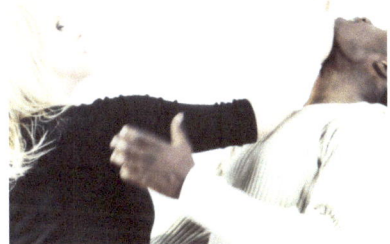

If you can squeeze your hands between his arms, grab his chin with one hand, and the back of his head with the other one (always two points, remember?) and then now bend his head back and down, applying pressure with your thumb under his chin to cause pain and to distract him (fig.101), even though it is a less favourite technique because it does not put you behind your attacker, that is a superior position for the takedown (fig.98).

However, it might seem more natural as a line of defence because your natural instinct is to grab the arms that attack you and also he wouldn't expect an attack to his neck.

fig.99 - Push one of his elbows up and, ducking under his arm, straighten his arm and grab his wrist. Apply lock to elbow and shoulder.

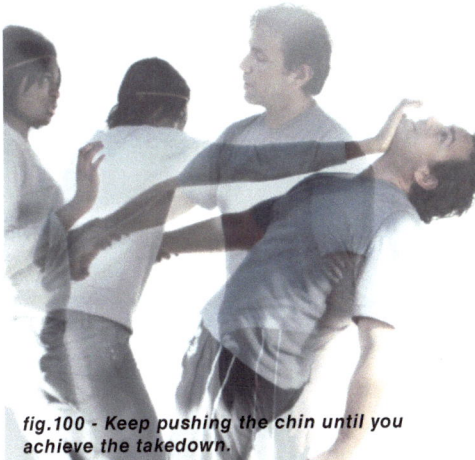

The principle is that you should always manipulate at least two points at the same time, the only way to achieve a takedown because you move his centre of gravity.

A very successful way to control your attacker's arms is a classic 'Figure Four', so called because the position of the arms resembles the number 4 (fig.102).

It is a technique ideal if someone grabs your shoulder or the top of your torso, a controlling technique against the joints.

It can also be used if somebody is attempting to strike you with a baton: starting with the opposite arm to his (if your are facing him), if he attacks you with the right, you react with your right, and quickly grab his wrist or forearm and at the same time bring your other arm around grabbing your own wrist (fig.104).

fig.100 - Keep pushing the chin until you achieve the takedown.

Let's now go back to the situation when your attacker has grabbed you around your neck: to get him to bend his arm and for you to achieve the "figure four" technique just grab his little finger and twist it hard against its natural movement and once you bend his elbow, proceed as we have seen before.The whole reaction is performed fast and in an explosive manner.

It is worth constantly reminding you that unless you can act decisively and precisely, you don't really have a second chance, so if you start fumbling just forget it and strike him open-palm to his chin the moment he grabs you.

KEEP YOUR ELBOWS IN TO JOIN THE TWO MOMENTUM.

If you do manage to him into the "figure four" lock, all you have to do now is step with your foot behind his body and go for a takedown and don't forget, to keep elbows together so that you can join momentum.

This takedown, using a "figure four" lock can also result, if you position yourself correctly, in a powerful throw (fig.102).

The difference between a takedown and a throw is that, in the takedown, your centre of weight is not one with your attacker, they are joined and very close, in fact as joint as possible, but they can't be one (fig.103).

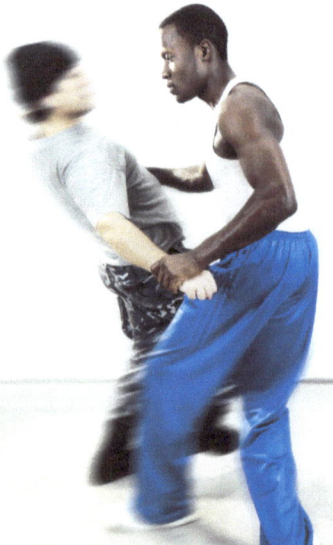

In a throw you join centre of gravity and as you pivot your body, you shift his centre of gravity away from his foundation.

It is worth remembering that the natural positioning of the centre of weight in a man is about eight centimetres below his hips.

So what is more effective, a takedown or a throw?

It depends: it's easier for most people to achieve a successful takedown than to achieve a decent throw an at the end of the day, they both achieve stunning your attacker and make him hit the ground even though a throw most probably will disorient him more and will make him hit the ground harder.

fig.102- Figure-of-Four throw.

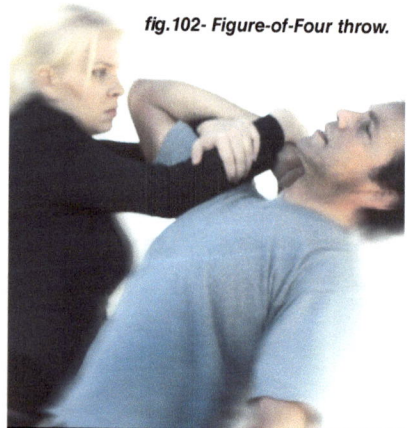

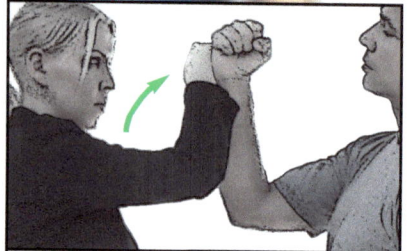

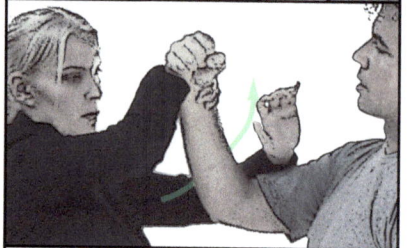

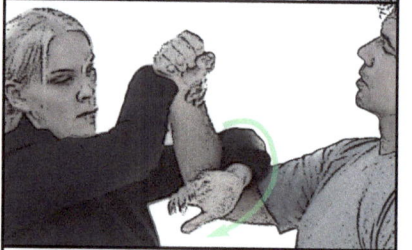

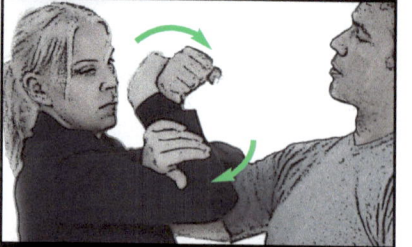

fig.103 - In a takedown the centre of weight is not joint.

Before we move to discuss throws, let's see what to do if a takedown fails.

If you fail the takedown, it is because you either failed to shift the centre of gravity of your opponent past his foundation or because you executed your moves in a broken manner, and hesitated: remember that your action should always be explosive and fluid at the same time, one continuous uninterrupted action. There is no point, continuing or trying to repeat a failed technique, you have to switch quickly to plan B without thinking, without hesitation at all.

fig.104 - Figure-of-Four explained: if he attacks you with the right, you react with your right, and quickly grab his wrist or forearm and at the same time bring your other arm around grabbing your own wrist.

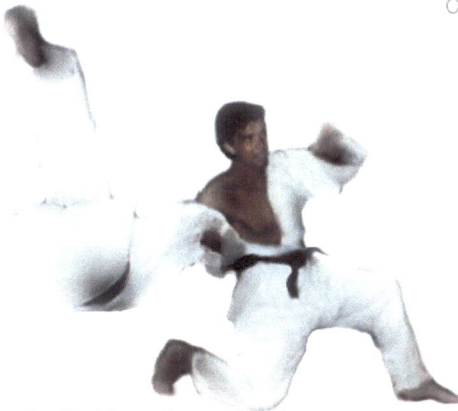

fig.105 - The author performing
a spectacular throw (KATA GURUMA kneeling).

Because you already moved closer to your attacker, you would be better off using an open-palm push or jab to your attacker's chin , maybe grabbing his leg at the same time, applying your action always on two distant points on his body (fig.88 and fig.92).

One last technique discussing takedowns is called FULL NELSON (fig.106), a technique used mostly standing and facing an opponent: all it takes is bringing your arms underneath his armpits and capping his face with your hands, covering his eyes. As you force his head back, he's going to lose balance and won't be able to see. Applying pressure to his eyeballs will make the technique more effective (fig.106A). A throw is certainly more violent than a takedown, and without a doubt is much more spectacular. However, because of inherent problems like resistance from the opponent, difficulty in getting into the right position, timing and so on, throws are very difficult to achieve. The classic movie scene, in which a very small person throws a big guy a few feet away, using just one hand movement is most of the time Hollywood fiction and more realistically it requires for someone to achieve easily only after many years of hard training (fig. 105).

Throws utilise the same concept as takedowns, joining momentum, but they differ because while takedowns allow you a certain gap between you and the other person, throws require very tight contact, really close. Throws require a small circular motion over your body while takedowns are performed with a wider circular move around it.

Once more the principle is the same because torque (an applied lever) is applied on both: a takedown could be transformed into a throw if your opponent tries to counter-

THROWS
REQUIRE A
SMALLER ARCH
THAN
TAKEDOWNS.

act in any way. The same can be said for the other way round. The most common throws utilise your hip as the pivoting point and that means joining hip with your opponent as you apply downward leverage.

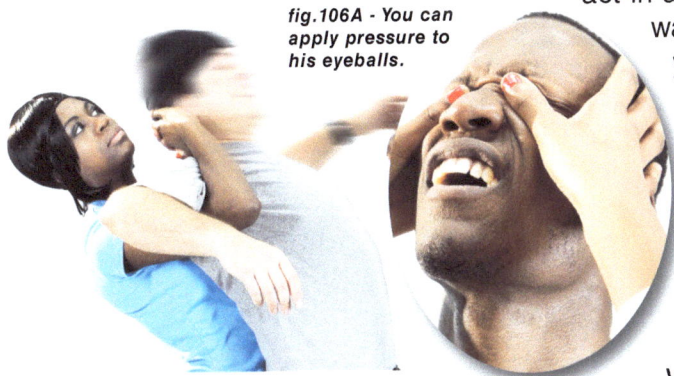

fig.106A - You can
apply pressure to
his eyeballs.

If you go too deep with your position you are basically carrying his weight, if you are slightly off centre, almost certainly, there comes a takedown if you still manage a successful circular movement as we have explained earlier.

Watching two Judokas fighting you will notice all they are trying is to join centres of gravity meaning closing the gap between the bodies.

But this is only part of the secret, you must be able to centre your opponent's weight, finding the balance point not to mention that you should never start a throw lifting your opponent with your hip or, worse even, on your back, but always try to position his body to combine your centre of gravity (fig.107).

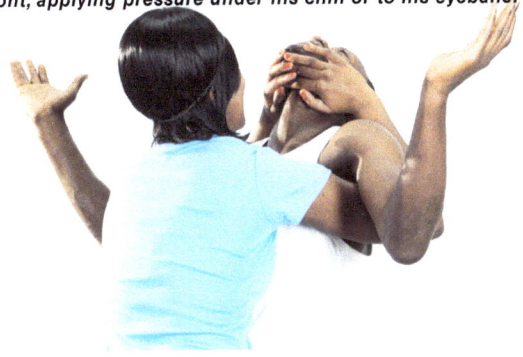

fig.106 - FULL NELSON takedown from the back and from the
front, applying pressure under his chin or to his eyeballs.

This means thinking his body is as yours is, moving as one: you shouldn't move faster because you will end up dragging his mass with you, and at the same time you shouldn't allow your body mass to be slower than his because you may lose balance. It is a question of joining momentums, or even better, synchronising them, always finding opportunity or creating it.

Similarly to the preparation for the takedown, you should also slightly unbalance your opponent before executing your throw.

For instance, you can throw him effortlessly if you can shift his centre of weight or narrow his foundation.

ou can use the same unbalancing technique for the takedown, using your forearm or striking with your palm to his chin, or any other way of shifting his weight.

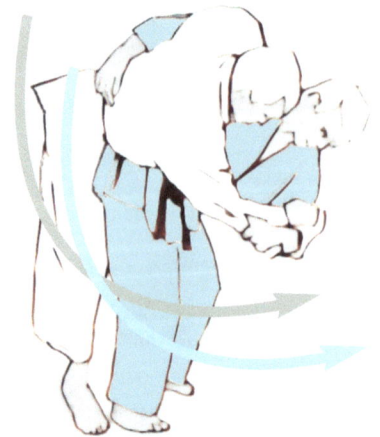
fig.107 - Join your opponent's momentum to succeed in your throw. (OGOSHI)

We show you in FALLING (page 76) how to hit the ground without hurting yourself and this is important because you might end up, as you practice, falling onto the ground. What is important is to avoid absorbing all the impact of the fall with your body, so as you can see in fig.108 you should round your back and roll with it, trying to spread the shock gradually over a wider part of your body.

As you do so it's very important that you tuck your chin towards your chest to avoid banging your head on the ground.

FALLING REQUIRES SUPERVISION AND CONSTANT PRACTICE. Like all techniques, falling requires practice and someone with experience and who is also qualified to follow you, pointing out possible mistakes but especially guiding you physically through the movements, especially at the beginning.

Takedown and throws work very well if combined with other techniques. When we examined earlier the "figure four" arm lock we noticed how it is useful to control your attacker, especially when he's trying to hit you with his arm with a downward motion (see more in LOCKS - page 90).

As we have seen, use the opposite arm to block his strike, grab his wrist with the same arm and quickly bring your other arm around his and grab your other wrist (see fig.90).

This can be achieved even if he attempts to grab your neck, as we have already seen, lifting his arm and grabbing his little finger and bending it backwards.

We remind you about this over again because manipulating small body articulations can be very effective. Because of the great control that "figure four" gives you, you'll find it very easy to simple step with one foot behind your attacker to throw him onto the ground.

It is important that you keep pressing your forearm against your attacker's shoulder while in "figure four" to help your unbalancing move to succeed, staying close to his body to join centre of gravity: now you just throw him diagonally over your hip, spiralling your body downwards (fig.102).

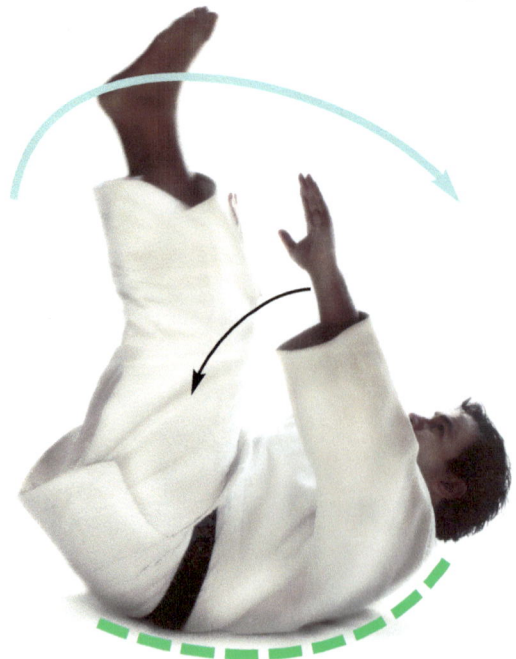
fig.108- Curve your back and roll with it.

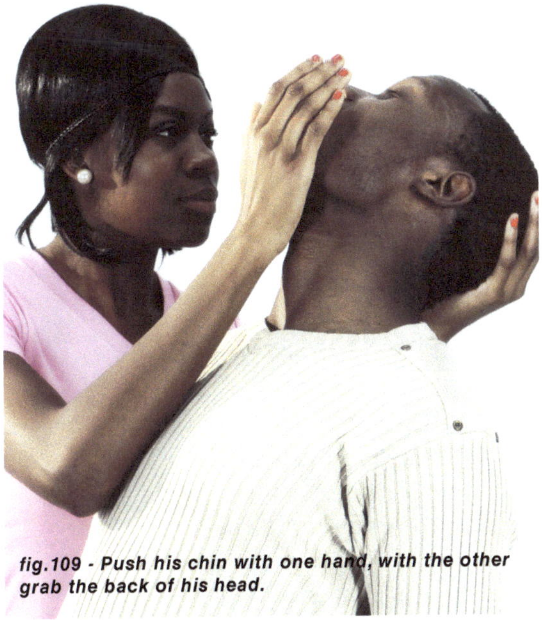

You can always resolve to a takedown starting in the same way, but obviously without stepping behind your attacker, you just pull him rotating his body downwards and remember that combining the "figure four" with a throw is much more effective, quicker and certainly more violent.

We have established that controlling the head of your attacker will let you control his body, this is even more evident when you apply throws manipulating his neck with both hands.

BE EXPLOSIVE AND DECISIVE WITH YOUR ACTION IF YOU WANT RESULTS.

To find your window of opportunity you can take advantage of the following approaches from the attacker: as he approaches you from the front, grabbing you around the neck with one or two hands, as he swings at you with a punch, or if he pushes your upper body backwards with both hands. If any of these actions happen just close your distance

fig.109 - Push his chin with one hand, with the other grab the back of his head.

(he definitely won't expect that) and put your hands between his arms or one hand between his arms and one hand outside of his arm, in other words get inside his arms.

With your hand in between his arms, grab his chin, with the other grab the back of his head (fig.109) and as you can see, we still apply the same principles of two points of balance, and always remember to start your move as soon as he touches you, without letting him finish his action.

ALWAYS ACT ON TWO DISTANT POINTS OR YOUR OPPONENT'S BODY.

The same applies if he takes a swing at you, the moment that you block or avoid his punch, and just before he can regain his balance, go with your move.

Obviously, you'll find it difficult to move closer if somebody is throwing a punch at you, but as you will remember we said many times in previous pages, sometimes safety is in closeness, even more so here.

With a push to your upper body, you probably won't be able to react at his first touch, often these pushes are often explosives accompanied by a loud "WHAT?" or with an insult, and your window of opportunity is the second push, that's going to come next, be prepared for that and close in.

IF YOU GO FOR A THROW, YOU MUST JOIN HIPS WITH YOUR ATTACKER.

You might also find that you want to prevent his action and go for a throw or takedown before waiting for his first move, if you are sure that there is nothing left to diffuse the situation (see also SWITCHING OFF page 116) then go for it, better to strike first, always. In this case add a distracting move, like a kick for instance, to hide your real target, his head (fig.110).

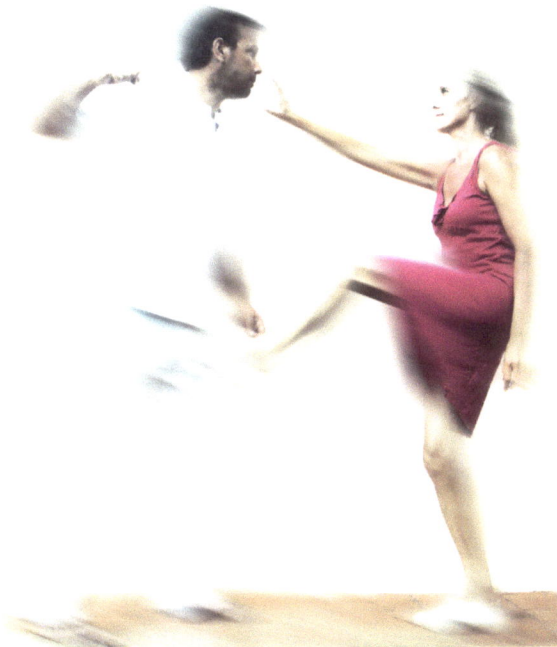

fig.110 - Hide your real target, the head, with a kick. Or hide a kick to the groin with a hand strike .

Once you have grabbed his head, step behind him, on the same side of the hand you have on his chin, the back of your leg touches the back of his leg, pushing up and back his chin, tilting his head back, all carried out at top speed. Do this decisively and without any hesitation, turning fully his head to the side and throwing him backwards over your hip in the usual downwards spiral.

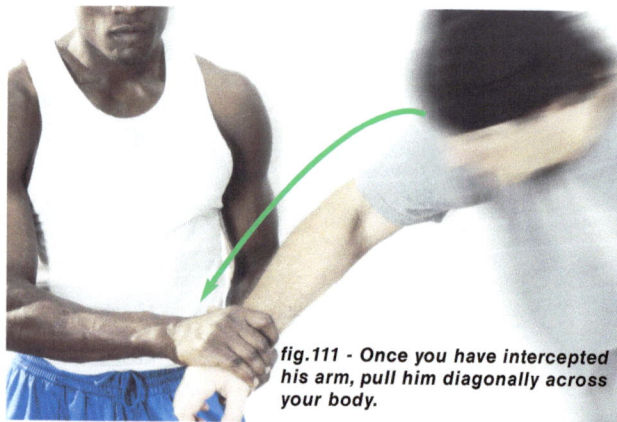

fig.111 - Once you have intercepted his arm, pull him diagonally across your body.

Now you can flee, or you can pin him to the ground with your knee, but is important to remember that as he starts to lose his balance, his first instinct is to grab you wherever he can, to avoid going to the ground. Carry on regardless, if anything, increase the speed.

The same principle applies if you have managed to grab your opponent's wrist for whatever reason, intercepting a blow or, maybe you are grabbing it first to prevent a blow and probably he would step forward and then try to reach for you.

Once you have intercepted his arm, pull him diagonally across your body. This is obviously if he grabs the opposite arm, or you have grabbed his opposite arm, such as right arm grabbing right arm for instance (fig.111).

It is fully natural that you'll find it difficult to grab somebody's wrist or arm, as he tries to punch you, or worse, knife you, but you should remember, it's actually quite easy, if you don't think of it as "grabbing" but just to par or block first and then grab, as shown in fig.111, and you will already be in a good position, slightly behind him, ready now to grab his chin with your free arm and stepping behind him at the same time without hesitation.

As quickly as possible, switch hands and throw him off balance using the hand on his chin that was originally holding his wrist (fig.112).

Always remember that every time you go for a takedown or a throw using a grip on somebody else's wrist, head or arm, you should be forceful and grip tightly, this will also give you a strong psychological advantage over your attacker, selling yourself as very strong and determined.

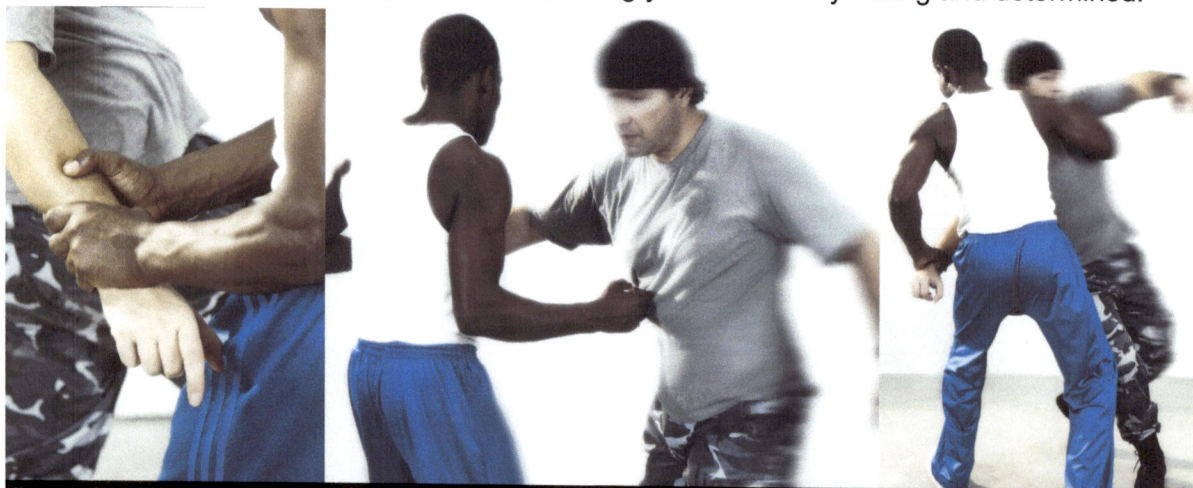

fig.112 - Switch your hands, using the hand that was holding his wrist to push his chin. Keep pulling with your other arm down and in a circular move. If you have positioned yourself towards his back he cannot resist the takedown.

Of course in reality, your hands might be cold, his clothing might not allow you a good grip, and his neck might be sweaty and slippery but in any case, go for it, always in an explosive and decisive manner, without second thoughts or interrupting mid action, even when successful.

Another point seen more than once already is that sometimes you have to make your own window of opportunity, normally with a some distraction.

Unfortunately we cannot show you how to fake convincingly and properly with a book, this can only be done through practice.

PULL, PUSH AND ROTATE ALWAYS!

You can try with your partner in training, practicing a few distractions and see how often you can succeed with your intent and make your partner react to your distraction in the way you plan.

Throws work in the same way independently of direction, the principles behind a reverse or forward throw are the same: you should still use a straight or circular momentum, at the same time apply torque and always use two points of balance (for example your hip and another part of your opponent's upper body).

It is absolutely fundamental to always join your attacker's centre of gravity, and that means leaving no gap between your body and his, a principle well observed in JUDO (page 236).

We will explore possible scenarios INSERT LINK, but do remember the general principle, instead of trying to remember a specific technique, most important of all is finding your window of opportunity in response to your attacker's aggressive action, most of the time the very moment his action commences, not one second late.

As for takedowns if you manage to intercept your attacker's wrist as he's launching at you with or without weapons, you can still apply a throw as in fig.113.

As for takedowns it is important to keep your movements fluid and avoid a stepping motion, in this case you swirl as you turn to join the centre of gravity and position your arms, locking his wrist and his upper arm going for the throw and don't forget most forward throws work best pulling diagonally across your body (see O-GOSHI in JUDO- page 236).

DO NOT REVEAL YOUR INTENTION, SURPRISE YOUR ATTACKER.

Of course, your timing and the way you join the momentum of his attack has to be spot on, otherwise the throw will not work but just end up a tug of war scenario where you pull and he pulls and the strongest wins.

Another danger to avoid is to "telegraph" your intention to the attacker, so as we have seen for takedowns, to reveal in advance your action, always hide your true intention, in this case grabbing his wrist, with some distraction.

To make most hip throws 100% effective make sure that you don't just pull your attacker by the arms but you also push with your hips in a backwards movement to maximize the effect (fig.113).

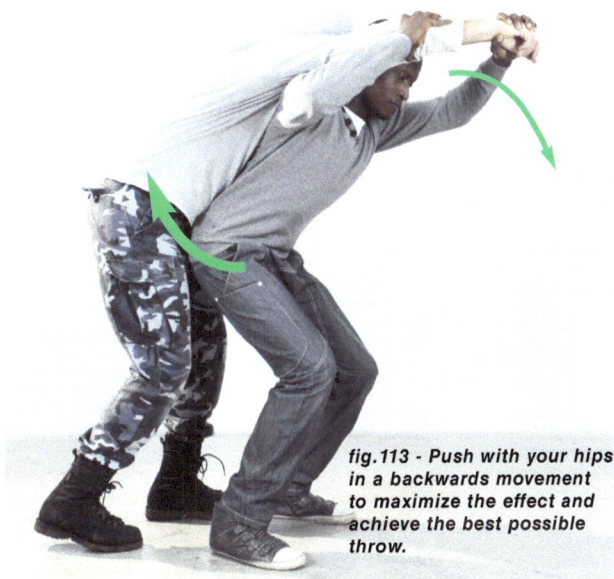

fig.113 - Push with your hips in a backwards movement to maximize the effect and achieve the best possible throw.

Once on the ground, you can kick his head, drop with your knee onto his head (see the knee drop technique on fig.26) or twist his arm (you should still be holding his wrist) and turn him on his back, face down.

As we have mentioned before, we always suggest running away without looking at the consequence of your throw or takedown, because restraining techniques require some serious training and they might put you in danger.

So once you have successfully thrown your attacker to the ground, you have quite a few moments for your attacker to recover from his shock, and that should give you enough time to flee and look for help.

A forward throw should be your number one choice if attacked from behind, and you have been grabbed by the neck in an attempt to choke you.

At the first feeling of contact, you should already been grabbing his arm (fig.114) with both hands and as you twist diagonally again, project your attacker's body onto the ground.

SAFETY IS IN CLOSENESS.

The reason why this is an ideal technique is because you start with your centre of gravity already joined to your attacker thanks to his initial action and since he is probably trying to pull you backwards to maximise his choking technique.

To get him forward, that is how you want him to be to execute your throw, push back trying to unbalance him to the rear.

In reaction to that he will be instinctively pushing forwards, giving you the perfect momentum for the throw and even if by sheer chance, you actually totally unbalance him, and make him fall backwards, hit him with the back of your head on his nose as you both fall to the ground, in any case, he'll hit the back of his head violently onto the ground.

With all throws, you have to remember the following: join your centre of gravity at the very earliest opportunity with your attacker's, bend shaping your back in a curve, not flat, twist diagonally as you pull his body across yours, push your hips into his to maximise your pull-movement (remember: pull-push-move, always.).

REMEMBER: PULL, PUSH... LIKE ARROW AND BOW.

Like most of the techniques shown on this book, you cannot expect that only mentally executing them will give you good results, everybody is brilliant in their own mind, remember that practice makes perfect, and it's important that you get a feel for throwing somebody to the ground for real as well as equally you experiencing being thrown.

fig.114- Grabbing his arm with both hands and twisting diagonally, project your attacker's body onto the ground.

fig.115 - A classic technique is called SASAE TSURI KOMI-ASHI (foot stop-pulling and lifting). To perform it successfully you must pull the opponent towards you and rotate his shoulders as seen in the sequence, then use your foot to stop his ankle to side step to maintain posture. Keep pulling and you will get him on the ground with one decisive and explosive move.

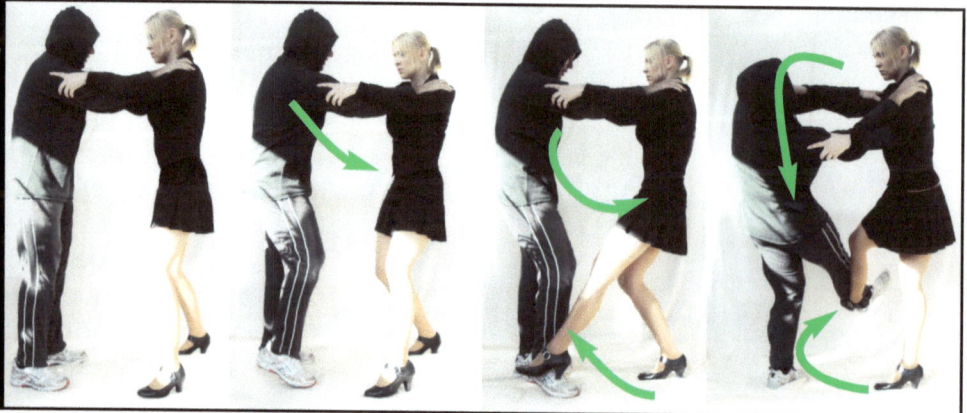

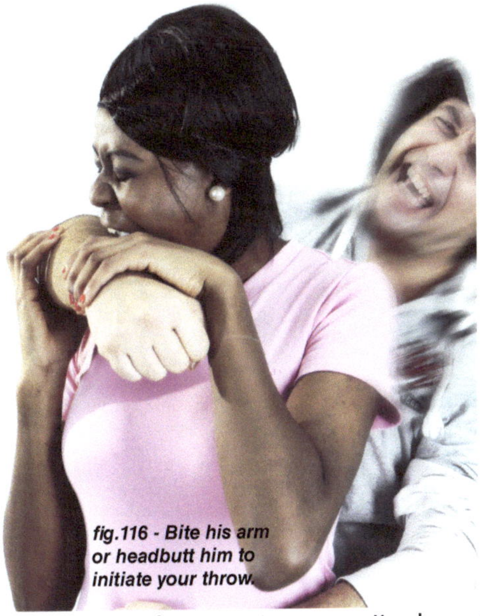

Like all techniques, you should only try this if properly supervised and in a suitable environment.

You must have mats on the floor to avoid injuring your partner with the throw or hurting yourself falling with him.

In other words, don't try this at home.

All throws can only be achieved by closing your distance. In order to avoid being thrown all you have to do, even if you are grabbed, is to keep a gap between the two bodies.

It is always worth remembering that all throws work at their best, applying some distraction or a different technique before initiating the throw, for example a kick or head butting, this is to interrupt the tension that adrenaline gives to the body as soon as somebody grabs you, and even biting his arm could be a good distracting technique (fig.116). Always be aware of your surroundings, it's more effective if you can execute a throw or a takedown against a chair or the edge of a pavement, or anything that can in-

fig.116 - Bite his arm or headbutt him to initiate your throw.

crease the damage to your attacker. Also, keep in mind that what you are wearing might impede some of the throws or takedowns, and you shouldn't employ techniques that require lots of movement when you are wearing tight clothes.

We have to think of throws and takedowns as kicks and punches, they have to be carried out ideally preceded by another action, be a kick, a punch or head butting, and then executed in an explosive and decisive manner, leaving your attacker no chance. Sweeps are also good especially at close range, and very effective especially in an initial confrontation where for instance you have been grabbed frontally by your clothing or pushed several times by your shoulders.

USE THE ENVIRONMENT TO MAKE THE MOST OF YOUR THROW.

A classic technique, as shown in fig.115 is called SASAE TSURI KOMI-ASHI (foot stop-pulling and lifting, see JUDO - page 236), and similarly there are many sweeping techniques that can be used effectively and they are based on the same principle as takedowns and throws, pushing and pulling, two points of balance, adding a twisting movement spiralling downwards. Timing and perfect understanding of momentum is very important to achieve good sweeps, you should always sweep the foot that is bearing most of the weight of your opponent, and the unbalancing technique is the same as the one we have seen for the takedown, either creating that opportunity or seizing it as he moves. Quite often it's good to push-pull your attacker in the same way as you would pull

SWEEP THE FOOT THAT BEARS MOST OF THE WEIGHT.

an arrow with a bow, an action that produces great results.

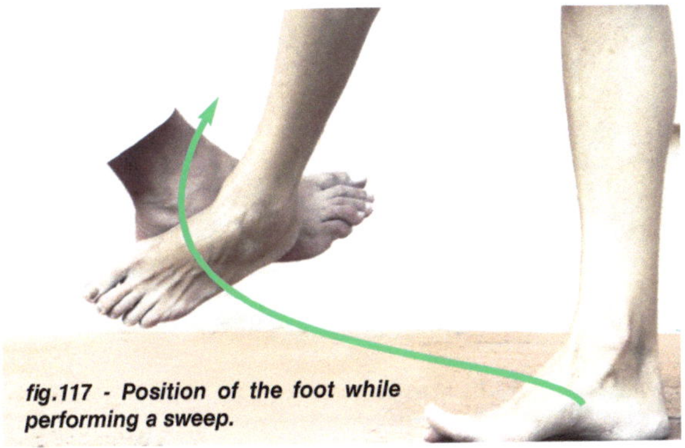

It is always a good thing to apply a distracting technique to soften up your attacker's tension and distract him from your real intentions; you must create your window of opportunity. Sweeping must be done without hesitation, in an explosive manner and with perfect timing; it's all about grabbing the opportunity or creating it.

For more details on foot sweeping techniques go to the JUDO table (page 236).

fig.117 - Position of the foot while performing a sweep.

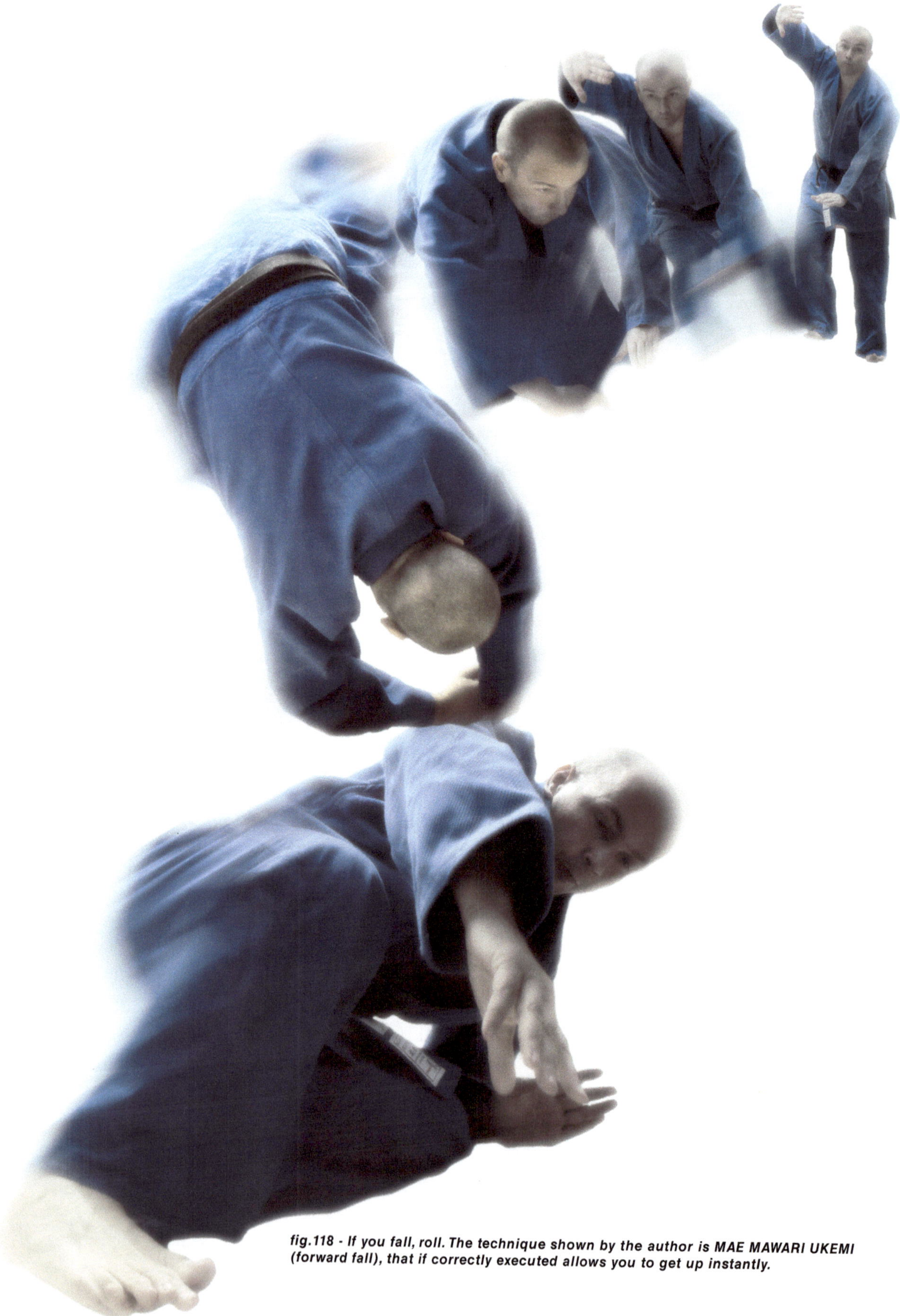

fig.118 - If you fall, roll. The technique shown by the author is *MAE MAWARI UKEMI* (forward fall), that if correctly executed allows you to get up instantly.

falling

In TAKEDOWNS (page 52) we have seen different techniques used to throw your attacker to the ground. You should also consider the possibility that he might take you down with him or that he'll be the one making you fall, in any case you might end up having to fight low on the ground. We will see GROUNDWORK techniques next (page 82) but first let's see how you should minimise damage to your body if, for whatever reason, you end up falling to the ground.

FALLING FORWARD HURTS MORE THAN FALLING BACKWARDS.

Fundamentally, this could happen for two reasons: you lose your balance due to your own fault or your attacker makes you fall to the ground.

Normally, if you lose your balance, quite often you will fall face first, and we say normally because in throwing a punch you miss your target or in throwing a kick you missed and couldn't recover quickly enough. Falling forwards is potentially extremely dangerous, because you have a lot of parts of your body that are not cushioned properly to rely on as when falling backwards (your buttocks or your back). Your knees are fragile, your wrists (as you try to absorb the impact) are delicate, and obviously, as you will probably remember from childhood, your chin and nose seem always prone at finding tarmac the hard way. So, if you find yourself falling forwards, you can help to soften the impact using your arm slightly bent and your hand cupped and not wide open: it is important not to hit the ground with your elbows and keep your legs straight to avoid hitting the patella of your knee (fig.118).

As you touch the ground, roll on your shoulder to break the impact, and keep rolling until you come to a stop, that also gets you out of your attacker's reach. Being able to roll effectively out of his reach could actually help if in a street situation: you can roll under a parked car and yell to attract attention.

IF YOU FALL, ROLL!

Your attacker will find it very difficult to pull you out (there are plenty of parts under the chassis that you can't hold onto) and you'll be difficult to reach, bear that in mind.

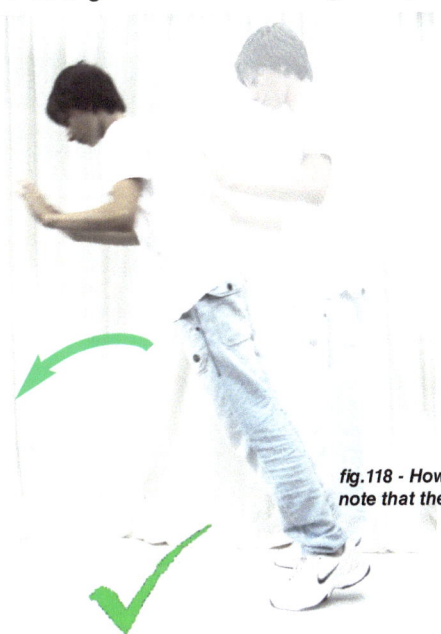

fig.118 - How to soften impact falling forward, note that the knees are straight.

A simple way to learn to fall forward is the classic forward roll that so many children enjoy, given the chance, on a muddy field.

Falling forward is slightly more complicated, since the majority of people are inclined to use their knees to break the fall.

You should avoid that at any cost. Instead of this, keep your knees straight and use your arms to absorb the impact. If you find all this particularly difficult you can start practicing standing against a wall few feet away and letting yourself go towards the wall, using your hand at the last minute to absorb the impact (see fig.121).

Eventually you will be practicing kneeling and increasing your height. In any case always keep your face looking sideways to protect your nose and chin in and add a roll to dissipate the energy once you are on the ground. Falling is easy, falling without hurting yourself is an art, requiring lots of practice, ideally on a mat, and a good understanding of how your body reacts, especially in mid-fall.

FALLING IN A CONTROLLED WAY IS A REAL SKILL, PERFECTLY ACHIEVABLE

Let's see now specifically the best techniques to fall in any direction without hurting yourself.

To avoid hitting the back of your neck, as you fall backwards, always tuck your chin to your chest, and if you are thrown back particularly violently, add a roll after you hit the ground (fig.119). Often we get hurt because we have an innate fear of falling when: we are comfortable in our natural position, that is standing, and as soon as we fear that we are losing our balance our confidence is threatened and we tend to react in a panic manner.

Judo has made an art and a science out of falling; there are few techniques and throws that utilise a fall on your back to throw your opponent (fig. 120) and this makes it a very effective martial art to learn how to fall properly and how to throw someone effectively even using your own fall.

MOST FIGHTS END UP CLOSE RANGE: LEARN HOW TO THROW AND FALL.

Our experience is that most fights always end up at close range with your attacker grabbing you at any one point, so learning how to throw him at this range is fundamental, but at the same time you must take into account that you might end up on the floor, and you must know how to do it safely.

You could find yourself falling sideways, for example trying to avoid being grabbed as you walk, from somebody hiding in an alley or doorway, but remember the principle is still the same, just directed in a different line. Arch your body and break your fall using the arm closest to the ground, keeping your head tucked to your shoulder or chest, away from the ground (this is called YOKO UKEMI, see fig.125 and see JUDO - page 236). Falling sideways is relatively easier and it should be your preferred choice if you find yourself losing balance, you should always try offering the least possible area of your body to the impact, to minimise shock and damage (fig.121A).

fig.119 - Add a roll after you have hit the ground.

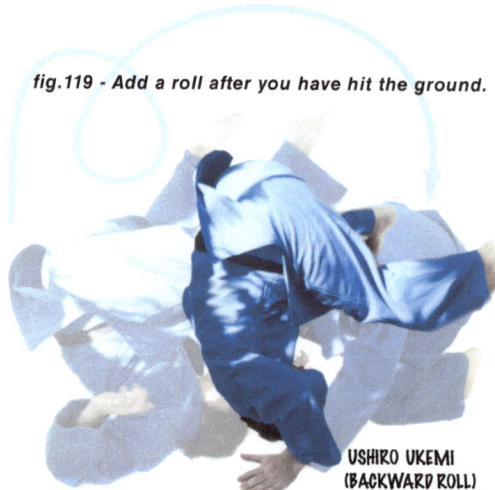

USHIRO UKEMI (BACKWARD ROLL)

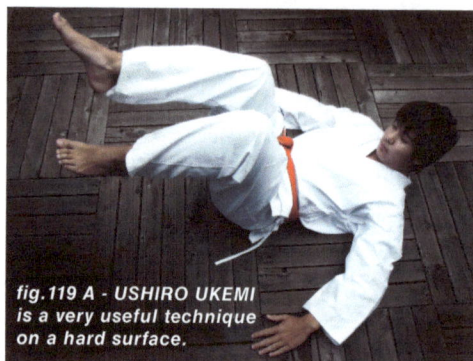

fig.119 A - USHIRO UKEMI is a very useful technique on a hard surface.

fig.120 - Throwing someone as you fall (TOMOE NAGE).

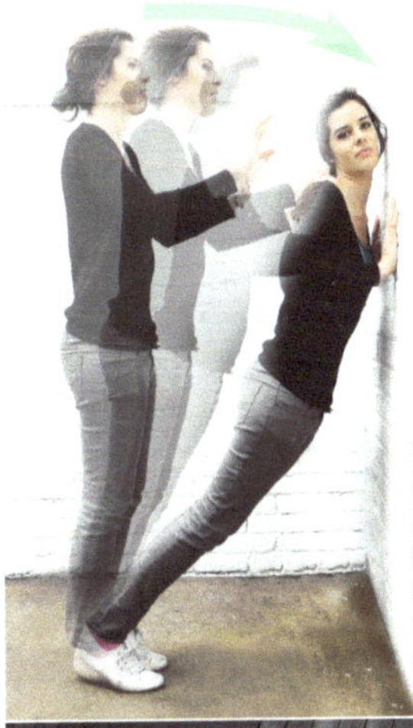

fig.121 Learn how to fall, starting with a wall.

Practicing falling techniques without proper supervision can be dangerous because if you hit hard with your lumber region, you could do serious damage to your spine, or in any case, damage your elbows or knees quite seriously.

Lets go over once more all the fundamentals of falling techniques, this is something that has saved me many times.

The best way to learn how to fall is starting in a crouching position; tuck your chin into your chest (so to avoid hitting the ground with the back of your head), breaking your fall spreading your weight on your forearms if falling forward, on your buttocks if backward.

CURVE YOUR BACK AND TUCK IN YOUR CHIN.

Remember that you should always curve your spine to ease the impact to the ground (rolling on your back).

To learn how to fall efficiently and safely is very important: falling is often a cause of injury and normally this is caused by making simple mistakes in an instinctive reaction but often enough it is the wrong reaction.

For example putting your arm out to stop the fall will almost surely result in breaking your wrists or arm, in any case suffering a serious bruise.

Falling forwards presents more danger because the knees tend to hit the ground first and because our natural reaction is to bend them to meet the ground first.

fig.121 A - YOKO UKEMI if properly executed works on any surface.

If you practice you should always try to do so on a soft surface such as grass or a reasonably bouncy mat. The most delicate part of the body as we impact a hard surface is the neck: in fact it only takes 10 pounds (4.5 Kilograms) of force to fracture your neck and this is why you should try and protect your neck at all times, tucking your chin into your chest (that should be well etched in your mind by now).

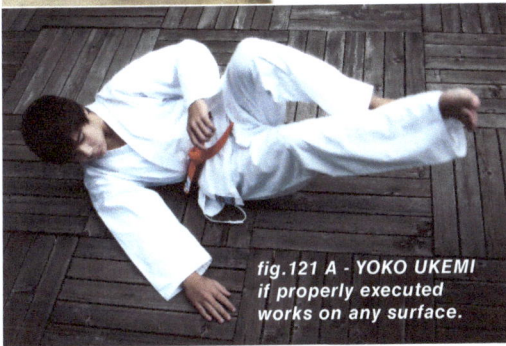

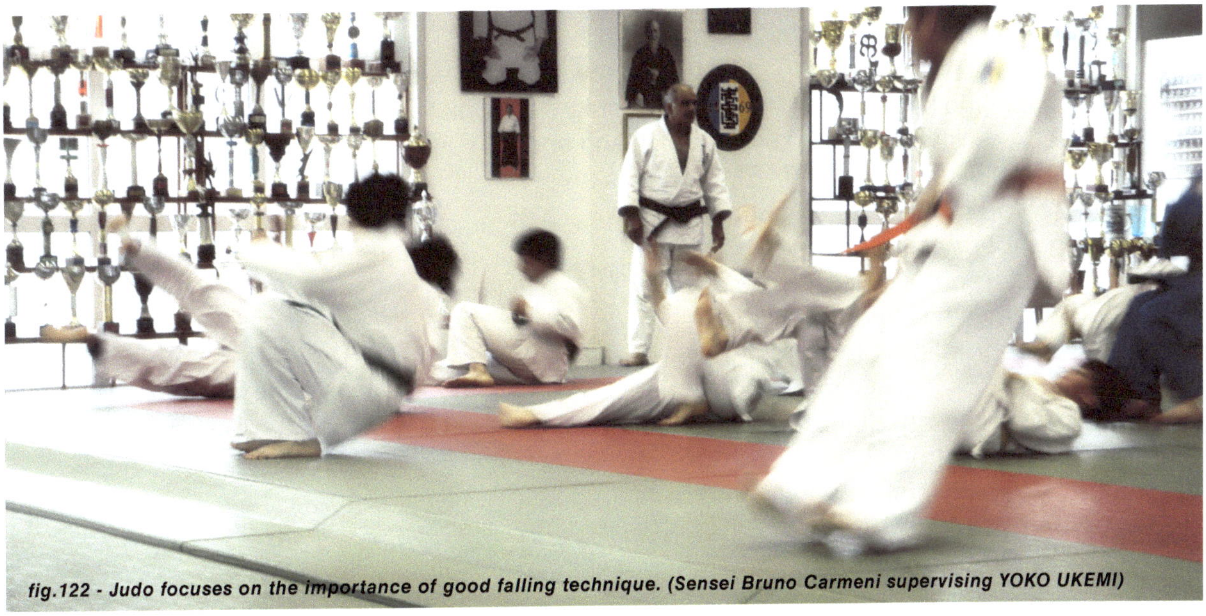

fig.122 - Judo focuses on the importance of good falling technique. (Sensei Bruno Carmeni supervising YOKO UKEMI)

Many different type of sports will cause falls when practicing, such as gymnastics, rollerblading, skiing, football, rugby and so on, therefore even from a young age you must have experienced some kind of falling at some point or other, however it's mostly martial arts that deal with falling and makes an art of

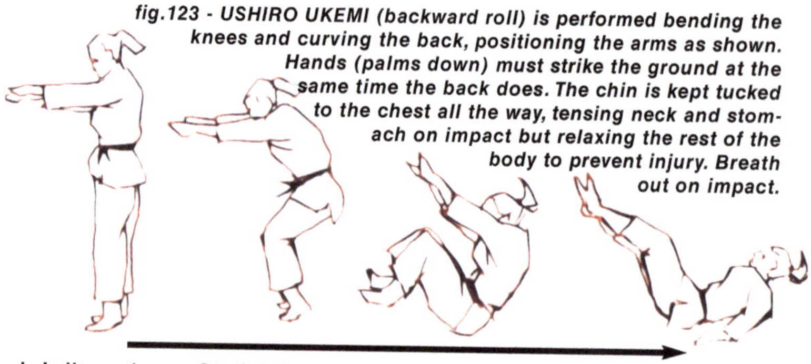

fig.123 - USHIRO UKEMI (backward roll) is performed bending the knees and curving the back, positioning the arms as shown. Hands (palms down) must strike the ground at the same time the back does. The chin is kept tucked to the chest all the way, tensing neck and stomach on impact but relaxing the rest of the body to prevent injury. Breath out on impact.

YOU LEARN TO FALL PROPERLY ONLY IF THROWN TO THE GROUND.

falling, especially Judo and Jujitsu (see GLOSSARY page 198), which have so many takedowns and throwing techniques together with sweeping actions.

It is possible to overcome this fear of falling that his often just a distorted perception of what the outcome will be.

We will discover that controlled falling is not so unachievable after all if we understand the physics behind it.

Of course nobody likes to be thrown to the ground, even the founder of Judo, Jigoro Kano, said so, but to train and learn how to fall can only be learned by being thrown.

This increases your chances of surviving an attack since you are not going to be overcome by the shock of the fall if thrown to the ground or from losing your balance.

The two easy steps that you should take to learn how to fall: initially start from a lower position for instance on your knees and slowly roll onto the floor more slowly and increase speed and height as you progress. Ideally you want to practice with somebody who can guide and ease your fall as you practice. Eventually you can increase in height and increase the speed of your practice and learn how to be pushed to the ground without suffering any damage but especially overcoming the very fear of falling that is quite overpowering for the majority of people.

The other type of fall, the one on your back, called USHIRO UKEMI in Judo (page 236), should always be achieved using your buttocks as an initial point of impact and then rolling on your back, that should be in an arch shape. The best way to break a fall going backwards is to use your body creating the broadest possible surface impacting the ground, distributing the force of the impact towards the gluteus and back muscles.

As for the forward fall it is best to start from a low position such as a squatting position and to slowly let yourself go backwards ideally on a slightly soft surface such as a carpet, and as you fall arch your back, tuck your chin into your chest and spread your arms outwards like in figure 123. This in Judo is called USHIRO UKEMI and it is a very useful all-round fall to apply in all those cases where you fall backward, such as on ice or on slippery surfaces, and once you have mastered it, you can increase the height from which you are falling and eventually practice it from a standing position.

Falling sideways is equally important, especially in a fighting situation when very often you will end up falling laterally, sometimes to avoid a side swing or a sudden push.

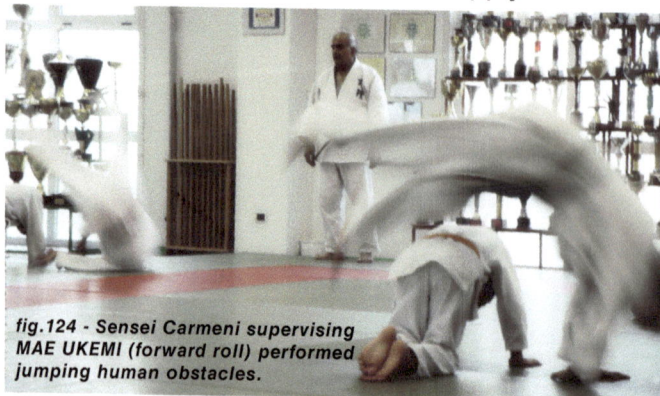

fig.124 - Sensei Carmeni supervising MAE UKEMI (forward roll) performed jumping human obstacles.

fig.125 - YOKO UKEMI (side roll). Similar to USHIRO UKEMI except theroll is onto one side rather than on the back. Curving the body, head off the ground, slapping the arm on the same side one is falling to, slapping the ground on impact. As for the other type of falling techniques is important to breath out as hitting the ground tensing neck and stomach, relaxing the rest of the body to avoid injury.

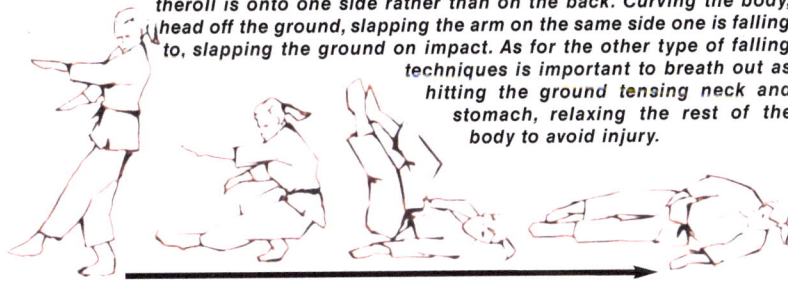

As you fall favour the same side leg to avoid hitting your knee on the ground and as you hit the deck exhale and use the same side arm in a slapping motion to absorb part of the impact. As for the backwards fall start practicing from a squatting position and eventually increase your height. This in judo is called YOKO UKEMI, see figure 125.

All these principles apply because falling is regulated by one very important law of physics: gravity.

You should also remember that it's not necessarily true that a largely built person risks more injuries falling than someone with a small frame and light built.

In fact a person structurally large will have a lot of parts of the body "padded" naturally which will absorb a fall quite well. In any case, big or small, heavy or light we can all fall and it does help if we know how to control our motion towards the ground.

To recap, here is what you SHOULDN'T do as you fall:

DO NOT try to save yourself using a stretched out arm, the wrist will almost certainly suffer damage, often breaking, and the shoulder will possibly dislocate.

DO NOT try to absorb the fall with your elbow or your arm while bent, elbow, wrist and shoulder will suffer damage.

If for some reason you have to break a fall from a greater height, it's worth knowing that if you fall from a height of 30 feet or more (10 meters) you stand basically almost no chance of survival, meaning that the cut-off for fatality is 30 feet. If chased and you have to jump from a height try and choose your spot, land on bushes or trees (conifers are better since they "slope", a big pile of rubbish or cartons, a tent or the top of a truck, sometimes the top of a car can break some of the impact. The best options to land on if possible are snow and soft grass or soft land, ideally on a slope. As you land spread your impact as much as you can on the widest area of your body, and if you can grab something to slow down your fall, increasing the resistance do so.

It is important to learn basic falling techniques not only to avoid injury but to improve the transition from standing techniques to those on the ground.

fig.126 - MAE UKEMI (forward roll) is performed taking one step forward with the right foot. The right hand is positioned on the mat like a knife edge between the feet, pointing towards the back foot. With the head turned to the left shoulder a simple push with the left foot initiates the roll, performed over the right arm with the back curled to form an arch , The body should remain curled up throughout. Once completed the roll the left hand with part of the forearm)???? slaps the ground. Breathing out on impact is essential as well as tensing neck and stomach, keeping the rest of the body relaxed.
It can be performed on the other side as well, just starting with left foot and doing the opposite.
To make the most of the momentum it is essential to end the roll in a standing and ready position.

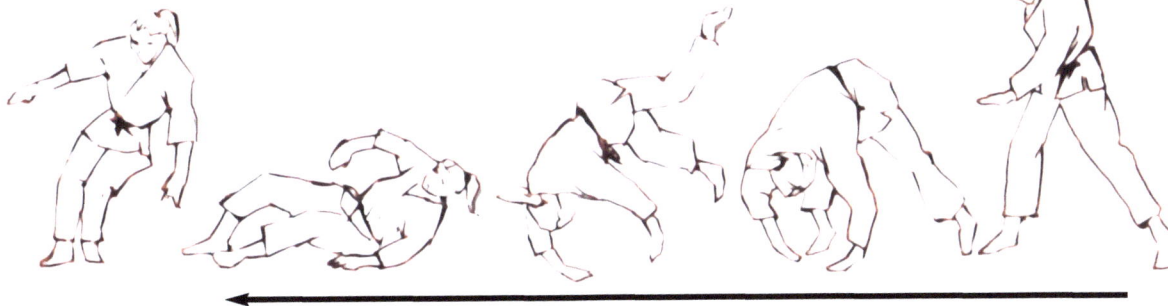

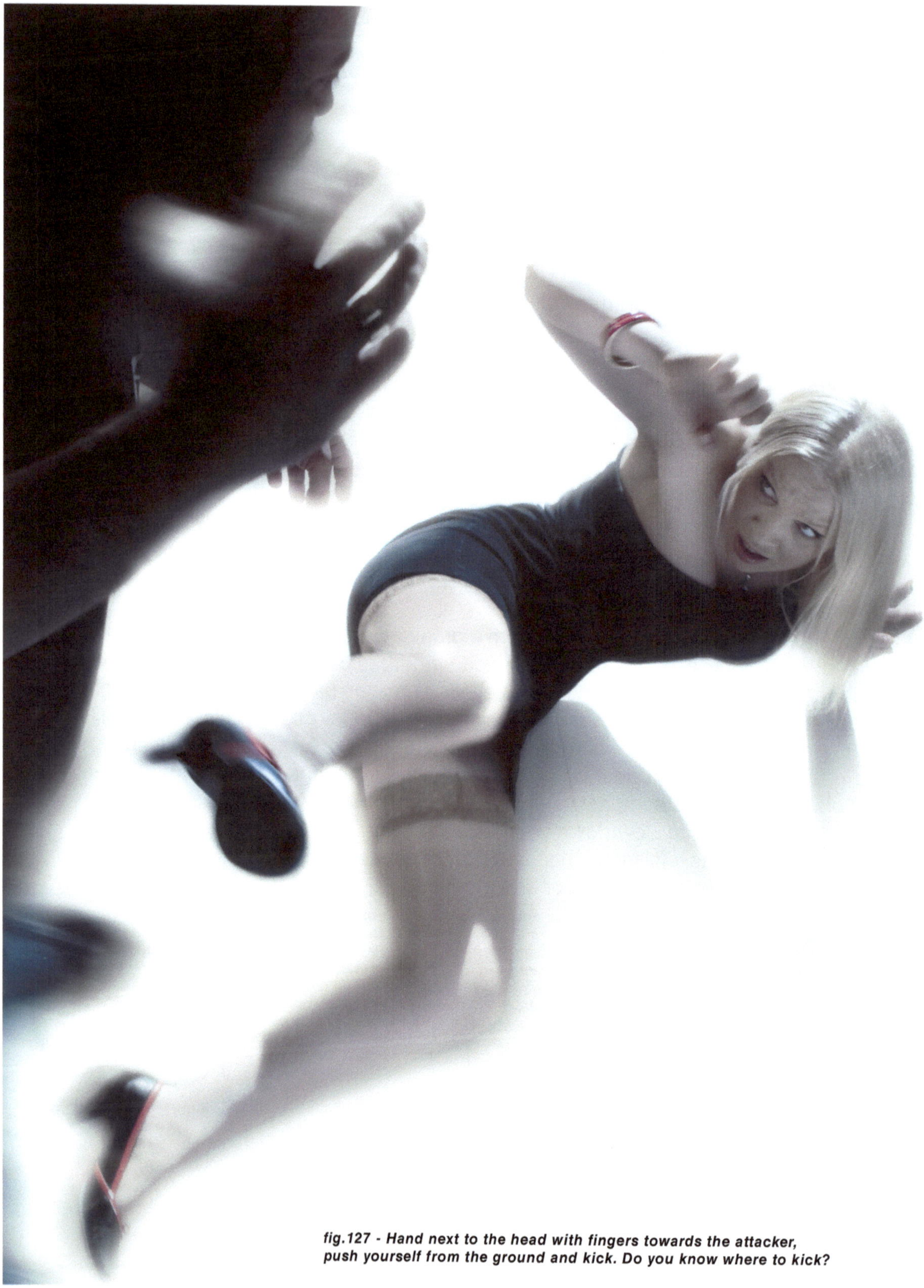

fig.127 - Hand next to the head with fingers towards the attacker,
push yourself from the ground and kick. Do you know where to kick?

groundwork

If you have fallen to the ground for whatever reason, and this is something that you should try and avoid as much as you can, no matter what, you will find yourself in an inferior position, especially if your attacker hasn't ended up on the ground.

We can distinguish two types of groundwork; the first one is where both attacker and defendant have fallen to the ground, and the second when your attacker hasn't.

Let's start with the second situation: your first reaction should be to also get your attacker to the ground, if he's still standing he can control you, and if failing to do so kicks are your first weapon of choice to defend yourself from the ground. As you can see in fig.109, a well placed kick to the groin area or to his knee or shin (fig.110) will neutralise your attacker as he approaches you as you lay down.

Almost certainly once you have fallen to the ground, your attacker will try to kick you on the head, to knock you unconscious and then finish his business.

If you can't reach him and he is moving to control the upper part of your body (your head), you should expect such a kick. Keep your hands in a fist, put your forearms in front of your face, bearing in mind to keep your fists with the fingers facing towards your attacker (see fig.127 and fig.130).

This position allows you to grab his foot, if you are quick enough, and to twist his leg getting him to the ground.

You are also better off if tensing up your abdominal muscles, in case he decides to kick you in the stomach.

If he's going for a kick to the abdomen, you are in the perfect position, to kick him from the ground onto the side of his knee, and you can even hook him at his foot ankle with your other leg (fig.131).

IF YOU FALL TO THE GROUND, PROTECT YOUR HEAD!

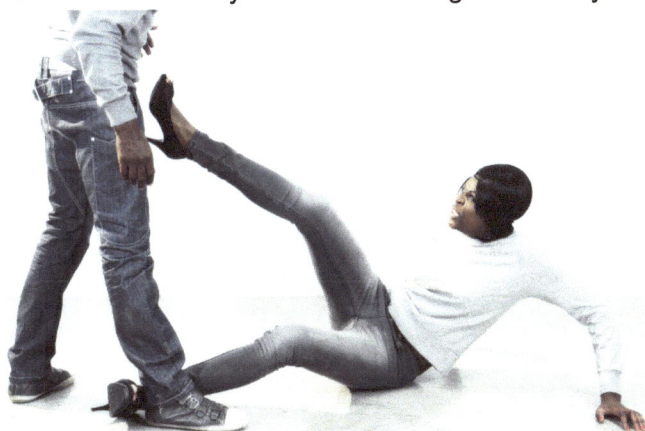

fig.128 - Kick to the groin. Note the position of her left leg.

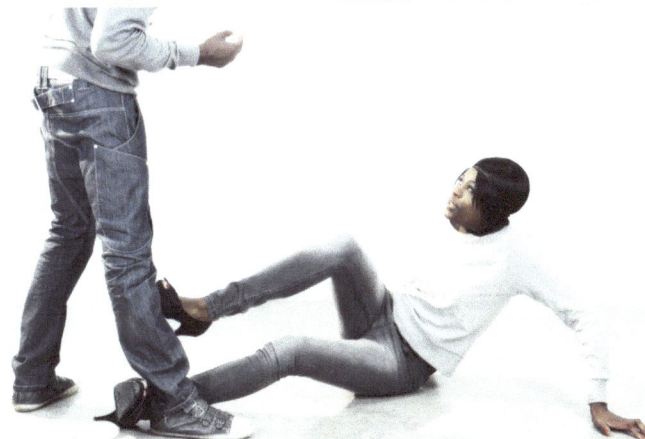

fig.129 - Kick to the shin, your left leg is trapping his leg in place.

DID YOU END UP ON THE GROUND? GET UP NOW!

As soon as you possibly can, you should try to get up and flee. Let's see how to get up from the ground effectively.

If you have managed to get up on your knees quickly, spread your legs a bit wider to make yourself a bit more stable and keep your guard up, and don't forget to rest on the balls of your feet not on your insteps (fig.132).

Being on the balls of your feet, allows you to push yourself up quicker, and gives you more stability, now crouch slightly to lower your centre of gravity and get up at the first opportunity.

If you haven't managed to get on your knees quickly enough, always try to get up keeping an eye on your attacker and having at least three points to balance yourself, as well as being ready to kick his shin or knee if he comes closer (fig.133). Getting up, like in fig.134, the natural, normal way, will expose you to a kick or grab from your attacker with little possibilities to react efficiently. If your attacker starts circling around you to find a way to get to you, pivot on your hip, always keeping a leg ready to kick him. If done convincingly, he will think you are not worth the risk. If you find yourself in the first scenario, where you have both fallen to the ground, things are a bit trickier; the main problem is to have reasonable reach and reasonable balance to be effective with your techniques.

DON'T BE STATIC, MOVE ALL THE TIME.

However there are some simple and effective ways to turn the odds in your favour.

Your very first attempt should be, as soon as he approaches, to grab both his legs at knee height, squeezing them together to narrow the foundation and pushing him with your shoulder just above the knee to the ground. It is important that you keep your centre of gravity low, and don't end up sitting, a very disadvantaged position, because you cannot gain leverage and momentum to counterattack. As soon as possible you should try to get into a position as shown in fig.137, to go for a lower level takedown or if you manage to grab his wrist, applying an arm lock.

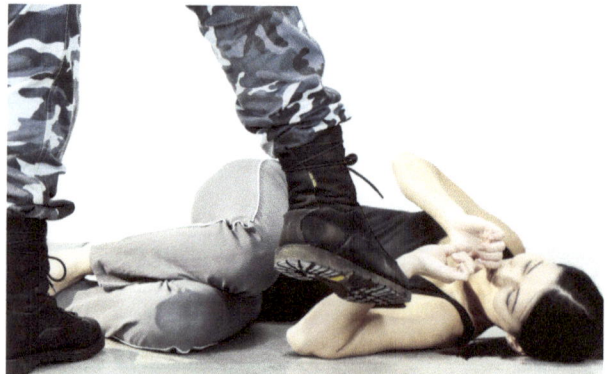

fig.130 - Defending your body once on the ground.

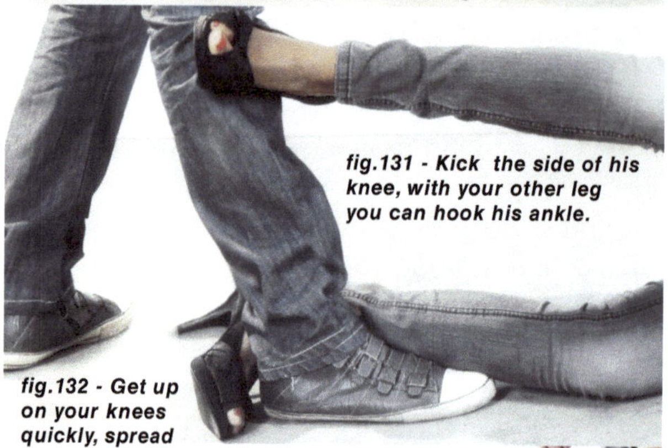

fig.131 - Kick the side of his knee, with your other leg you can hook his ankle.

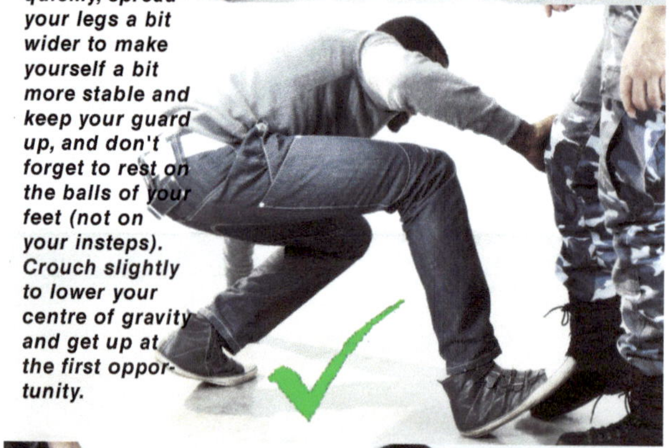

fig.132 - Get up on your knees quickly, spread your legs a bit wider to make yourself a bit more stable and keep your guard up, and don't forget to rest on the balls of your feet (not on your insteps). Crouch slightly to lower your centre of gravity and get up at the first opportunity.

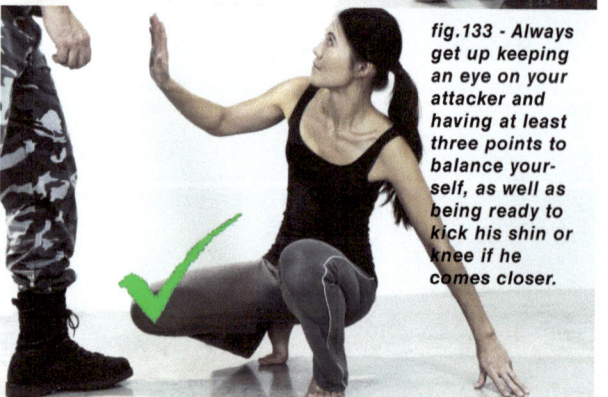

fig.133 - Always get up keeping an eye on your attacker and having at least three points to balance yourself, as well as being ready to kick his shin or knee if he comes closer.

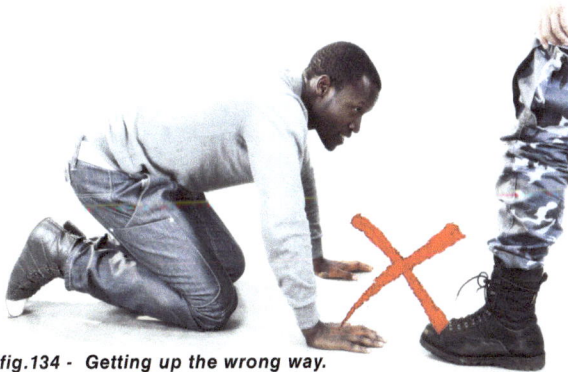
fig.134 - Getting up the wrong way.

Her left foot is firm to the ground, knee bent.

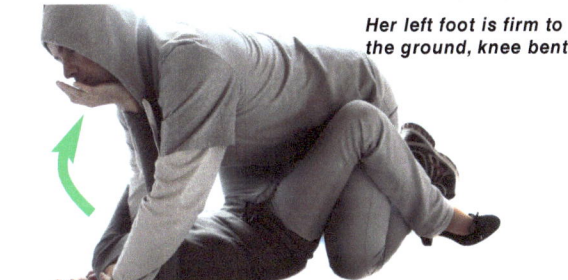
fig.135 - Push-and -pull technique to the chin and back of the head, pointing one foot (left in this case) firmly to the ground. (knee bent)

fig.136 - Keeping one leg (the right in the photo) straight along the ground, push with the other leg, as you push and pull his head and neck, rolling him to the side, pivoting on your hip.

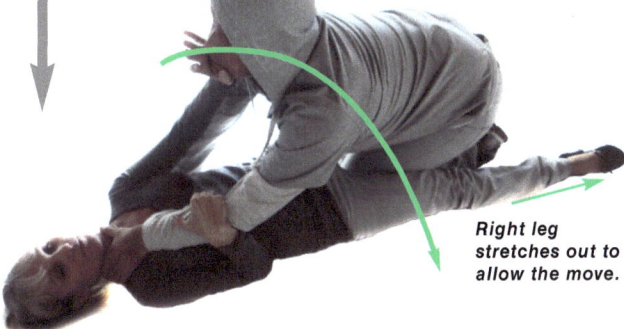
Right leg stretches out to allow the move.

All the techniques that we've seen for TAKE-DOWNS (page 52), apply here. For instance, you can still use the "figure four" lock or crank his elbow, or using the unbalancing or head manipulation techniques shown previously.

You will also find that because his centre of gravity is obviously lower, you will struggle to unbalance him. It is also important that you don't become static, keep moving and grab whatever you can to apply what's described above, and be careful that he doesn't grab your arm, head or leg. You can even use him as a tool to get up from the ground, pushing him down at the same time.

If for whatever reason, your attacker has managed to trap you with your shoulders to the ground and maybe he is on top of you, e.g. knees on the sides of your waist (fig.135), you can still apply the push-and-pull technique to the chin and back of the head, pointing firmly one foot to the ground (knee bent), and keeping the other leg straight along the ground, push with the bent leg and, as you push-pull his head and neck, roll him to the side, pivoting on your hip (fig.136).

If you can manage to grab his arm, especially if he tries to choke you with one or both hands, you can apply a very simple and effective technique, that seems complicated at first but truly is not: grab both his wrists, pushing his arms downwards towards your chest, tucking in your chin in at the same time, now push down both his arms with your left arm, lift your right leg next to his shoulder, and at the same time with your right arm, grab the inside of his knee.

Now bring your other leg under his throat, clamping his neck between your legs, and then pivoting 90 degrees, push him so you end up perpendicular to his body, still holding his arms.

Keep pulling his arm towards your chest, and if he keeps trying to gain control, keep pushing lifting your hips until you break his arm (this lock is called UDEISHIGI-JUJI GATAME in Judo, page 236). Obviously, his hand should be positioned palm away from you to make the lever work against the natural articulation of the arm (see fig.137 for the technique).

This technique relies on torque and two points of balance and don't forget to pull the arm towards you and to push your hips up at the same time. You can see more in LOCKS (page 90).

It looks complicated on paper but in actual fact it is very simple and quite intuitive once you can grasp the principle while practicing it.

Another effective technique that we have been teaching especially in attempted rape case scenarios is the following: as your attacker positions himself between your legs, and grabs you either by the shoulder or by your neck to pin you down, grab both his arms, ⚠ wrapping around your arms and pulling them on your chest, and at the same time, point your feet onto his knees.

ALWAYS TRY TO UNBALANCE YOUR ATTACKER, WHATEVER YOUR POSITION IS. As you straighten your legs, his knees will slip backwards; taking away the only point of balance he has (fig.137).

Leaving one leg straight, push with your other leg still firmly to the ground, pivoting on the side, spinning him to the ground. Now you can get up and run or go into a choking technique (see CHOKES (page 96) or armlock.

While fighting at ground level you can also use other techniques, you can still punch, poke him in the eye, or even better use whatever you find on the ground to use against him, a stone, a shoe, any object, or throw dust into his eyes. You can even use a full Nelson from the front as previously demonstrated, capping your hands onto his face, bending his head to the rear, unbalancing him easily to the back.

Obviously, you should be rolling on one side at the same time, to get your attacker on his side and to reverse positions, in that way, you can become the one in control. Another option is to wrap your legs around your attacker's floating ribs, just above his waist, in a scissors lock and put pressure on his rib cage extending your legs (See also ANIMALS - page 160).

At the same time, you can cup your hands on his chin and the back of his head and twist his head violently to one side (fig.138).

IF PINNED DOWN BY YOUR ARMS, USE YOUR LEGS. The most common mistake one tends to do when pinned in such a position is to push the attacker back by his shoulders and not using the legs, that are much stronger, or using the hands to hit the eyes, or pushing away in the techniques demonstrated.

fig.137 - Grab his wrists, push his arms to your chest, push his knees backwards with your feet .

Raise your right eg to his neck as you pivot pushing him.

See fig.139 for leg hook action in details.

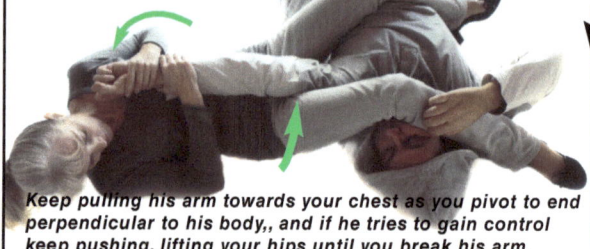

Keep pulling his arm towards your chest as you pivot to end perpendicular to his body,, and if he tries to gain control keep pushing, lifting your hips until you break his arm.

fig.137 A - Attacker on top grabbing you either by the shoulder or by your neck to pin you down.

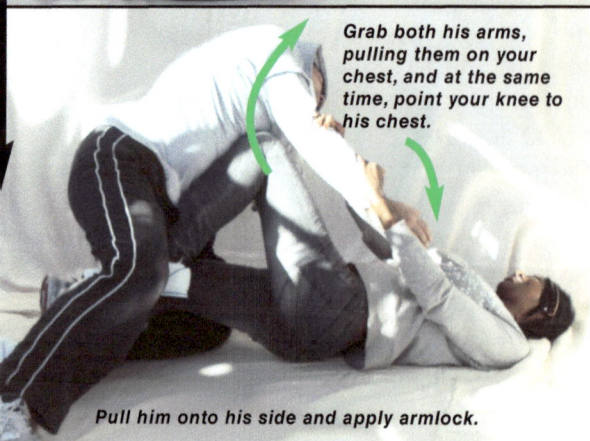

Grab both his arms, pulling them on your chest, and at the same time, point your knee to his chest.

Pull him onto his side and apply armlock.

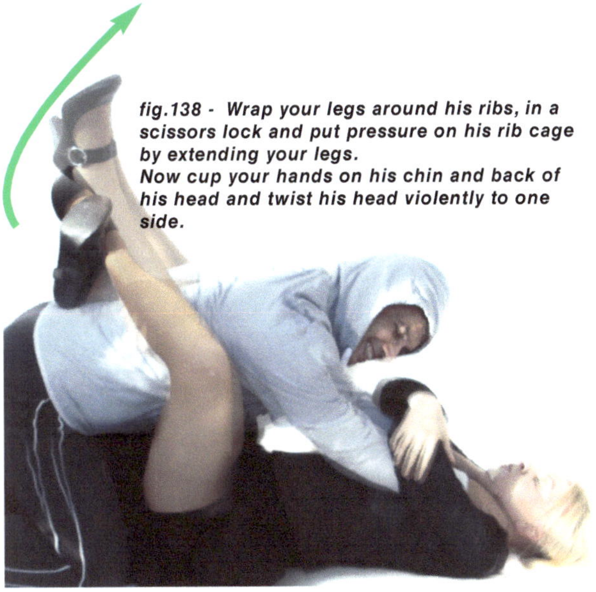

fig.138 - Wrap your legs around his ribs, in a scissors lock and put pressure on his rib cage by extending your legs.
Now cup your hands on his chin and back of his head and twist his head violently to one side.

Don't forget that your legs offer a fantastic leverage to shift positions. In fig.139 you can see how easy it is to overturn or unbalance even a heavier, stronger attacker with such a simple maneuver. It is important to remember that speed is of the essence and hooking your leg around his neck requires a push-and-pull technique. You push, for instance with your right leg (fig.139) and you hook him with your left leg.

USE YOUR LEGS IF YOU END UP ON THE GROUND.

The push allows you to bring his body into a more favourable position for your hooking action as well as, if you add a rocking motion to it, you can revert positions completely.

If for whatever reason, you find yourself completely pinned down, it is worth remembering that you can use a bit of psychology and beg, saying that you are going to do exactly as you are told, so that he relaxes and allows you to do these actions.

You can see more of these techniques in SWITCHING OFF (page 116).

All the techniques that we have seen, obviously, apply in situations where you have been thrown to the ground or as you were lying on the ground, e.g. sleeping, sunbathing, and you are being attacked. These are all techniques that are particularly useful in the case of attempted rape, where most of the time, to keep control of you, he will pin you to the ground.

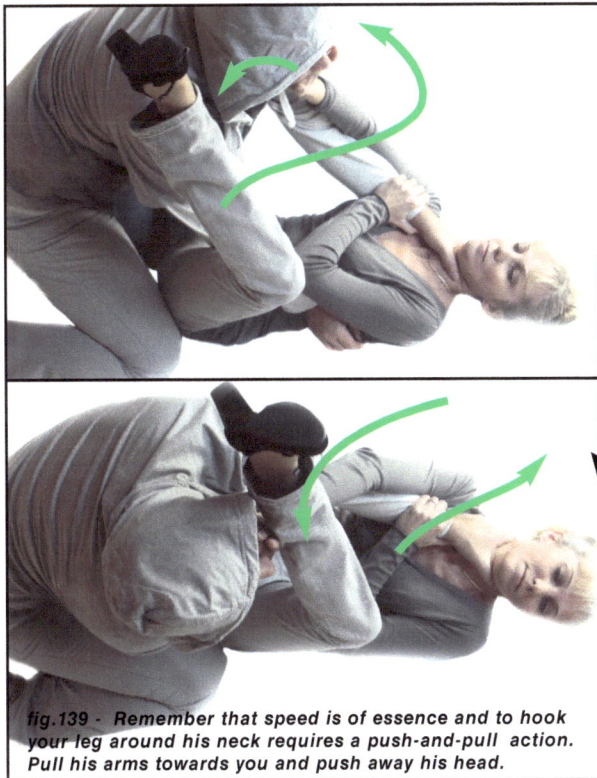

We want to reinforce the notion that if you find your hands free at any given moment, you can slap on your attacker's ears, cupping both hands, and cause ear damage or, if you decide to push or strike him, make sure that you strike him under the chin or in the eyes or just under his nose.

The natural reaction is to push him with your hands off his chest or shoulders: think how useless that is, and that you are going to strain and exhaust yourself, when in actual fact, applying little strength to the right weak spots you can achieve much greater results.

If, as shown in fig.140 he is holding you by your wrists, pinning you down, your immediate reaction should be to hit him hard with one of your knees on his bottom to make him fall forwards.

As you do that add a twisting motion with your shoulders, pushing with your wrists as you hit him, to make him roll on one side.

ADD A TWISTING MOTION TO ALL YOUR ACTIONS.

fig.139 - Remember that speed is of essence and to hook your leg around his neck requires a push-and-pull action. Pull his arms towards you and push away his head.

As he loses his grip, hit him hard on the groin or any other vulnerable point.

Another common attempted rape position is when the attacker holds your throat with one hand, normally his right, using his left to get down to business.

This is a very dangerous hold because as you can see in fig.142, he is using his entire weight on your throat to make you lose consciousness to better take advantage of you or to increase your level of fear to control you better and this requires very prompt decisive reaction.

Bring both hands on his hand, pushing away and at the same time, bring your left leg across his throat (fig.139).

Push-and-pull (pull with your arms, push with your legs) adding a twisting motion to unbalance him on his side, and do not lose contact with his body so you can maximise the leverage (do you remember the principle of takedowns and throws we discussed?).

You will end up in the same position as you have seen in fig.137 (UDE ISHIJI JUJI GATAME), and you now control his arm and lifting your hips, you could actually break it.

You might find it difficult to grab his arm because maybe too thick or too sweaty, but it is important throughout all Perfect Defence system techniques to remember the principles.

Remember that in any case if you can't get a firm hold, if you cannot pull him towards you instead of pushing him away (remember: close your distance).

You can always strike him with your hands, even a simple thumb press to his eyes, holding the side of his head, anything causing severe pain and creating a window of opportunity.

We have seen over the years people giving advice in self-defence to get your attacker into a scarf-hold or other restraining or subduing technique, but to be honest, the average person with no training in martial arts or with average strength will not be able to apply these techniques effectively at all.

There is also a very simple but fundamental question: even supposing that you can achieve a very successful hold, what are you going to do next?

Hold him down on the ground for an hour? Will it be enough to just whisper in his ear to behave?

Realistically speaking everything we teach is based on the principle of breaking your attacker's momentum and switching off either his adrenaline boost or his animal instincts, to give you that precious moment to run for safety.

YOU SUCCEEDED IN YOUR DEFENCE, NOW RUN!

fig.140- If he is holding you by your wrists, pinning you down, hit him hard with one of your knees on his butt to make him fall forwards.

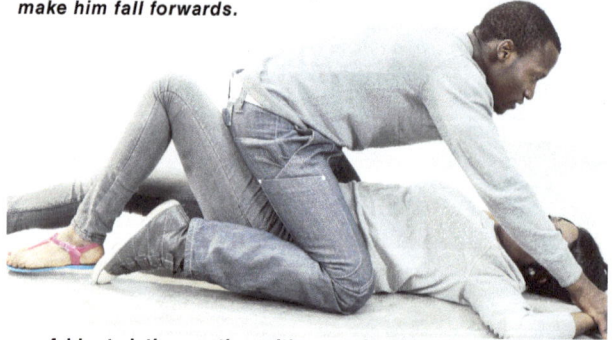

Add a twisting motion with your shoulders, pushing with your wrists as you hit him, make him roll on one side. As he loses his grip, hit his groin.

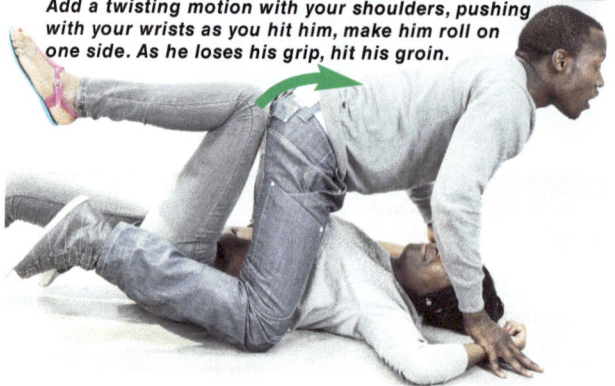

fig.141 - You managed to get on top of him. Now what?

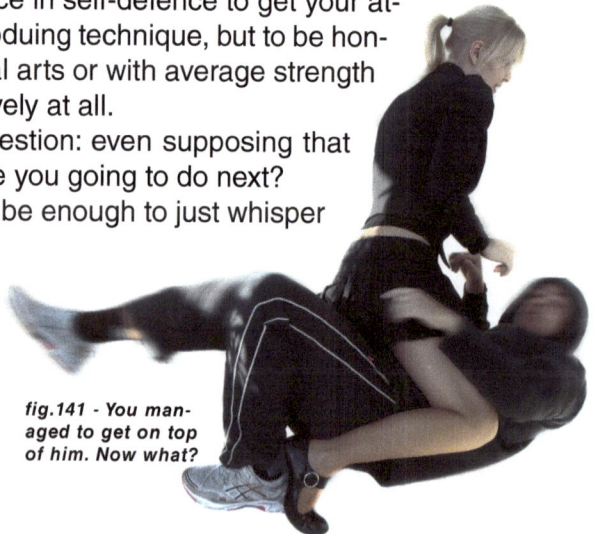

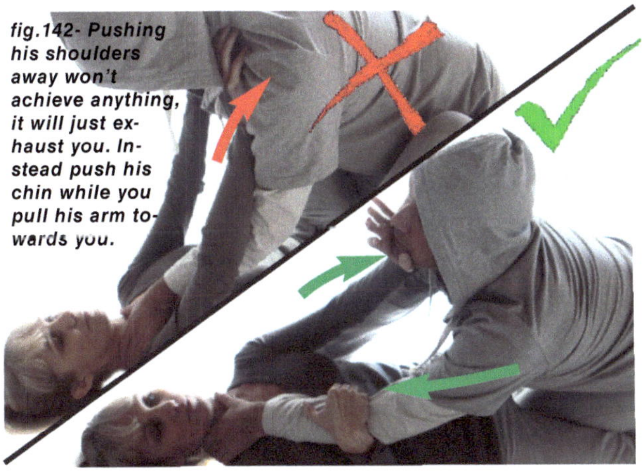

fig.142- Pushing his shoulders away won't achieve anything, it will just exhaust you. Instead push his chin while you pull his arm towards you.

Most of the time, if you are following our techniques you will not be an easy prey he'll let you go.

There have been people attacked by sharks who managed to get away with little or no harm, just hitting them hard once where it hurts (see ANIMALS - page 160).

Do the same, just remember where to.

If you really want to learn how to control somebody in a hold and get them onto the ground, here are a couple of useful techniques, both from Judo.

Osaekomi Waza (holding techniques) are the bread and butter of Jujitsu and Judo's groundwork and they work on a simple principle that is the points of contact.

For self defence purpose you should try to add pain compliance techniques to these holds, since the closeness with your attacker does not work to your advantage.

In actual fact it would be best to break his arm (fig.143), since any promise he will make not to hurt you once you let him go cannot be trusted.

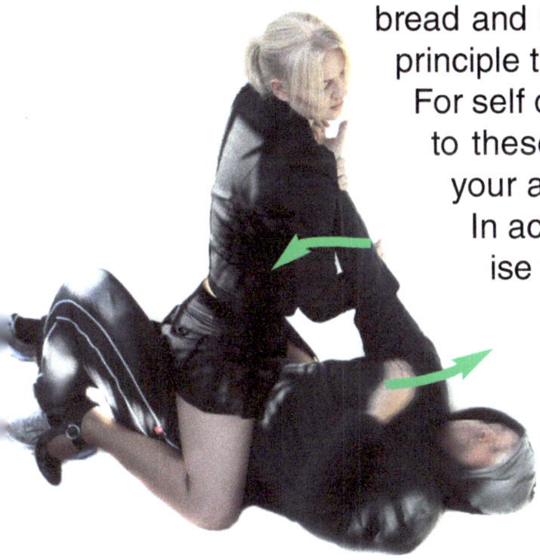

fig.143 - If you manage to get on top of your attacker or to gain control on the ground you should apply a choke or an arm lever as quickly as possible.
Osaekomi waza (ground control techniques). Here we have illustrated the ones that can be most useful in self defence, especially when at the same time applying a joint lock, spine lock or choke.
See page 238 for a more detailed explanation.

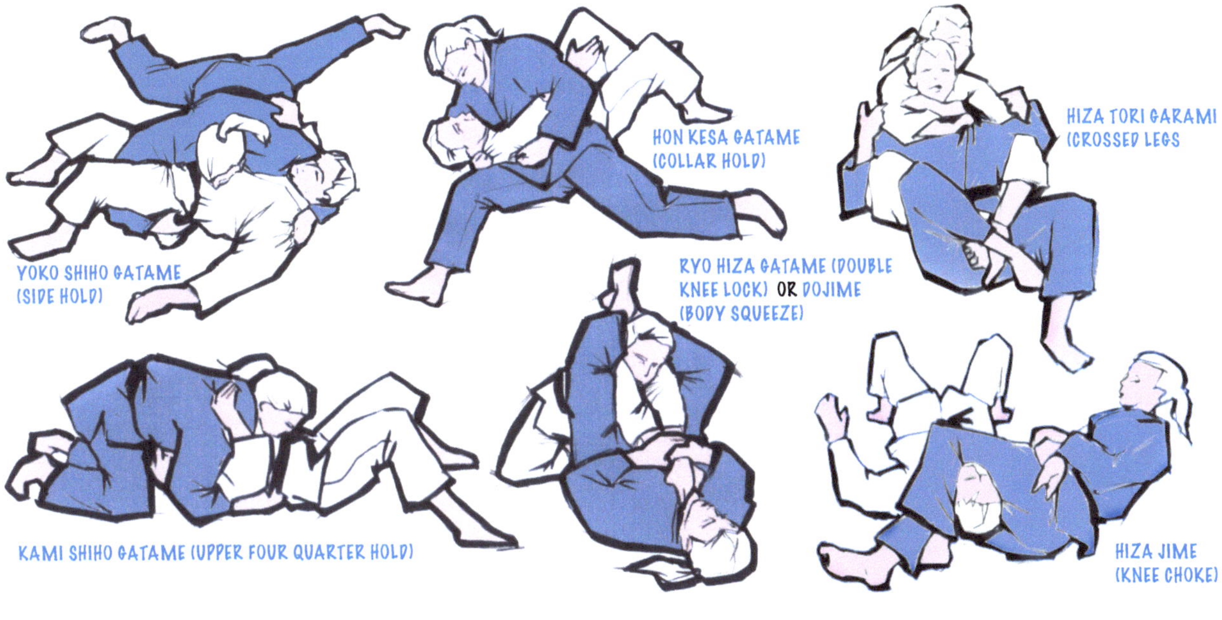

YOKO SHIHO GATAME (SIDE HOLD)

HON KESA GATAME (COLLAR HOLD)

HIZA TORI GARAMI (CROSSED LEGS

RYO HIZA GATAME (DOUBLE KNEE LOCK) OR DOJIME (BODY SQUEEZE)

KAMI SHIHO GATAME (UPPER FOUR QUARTER HOLD)

HIZA JIME (KNEE CHOKE)

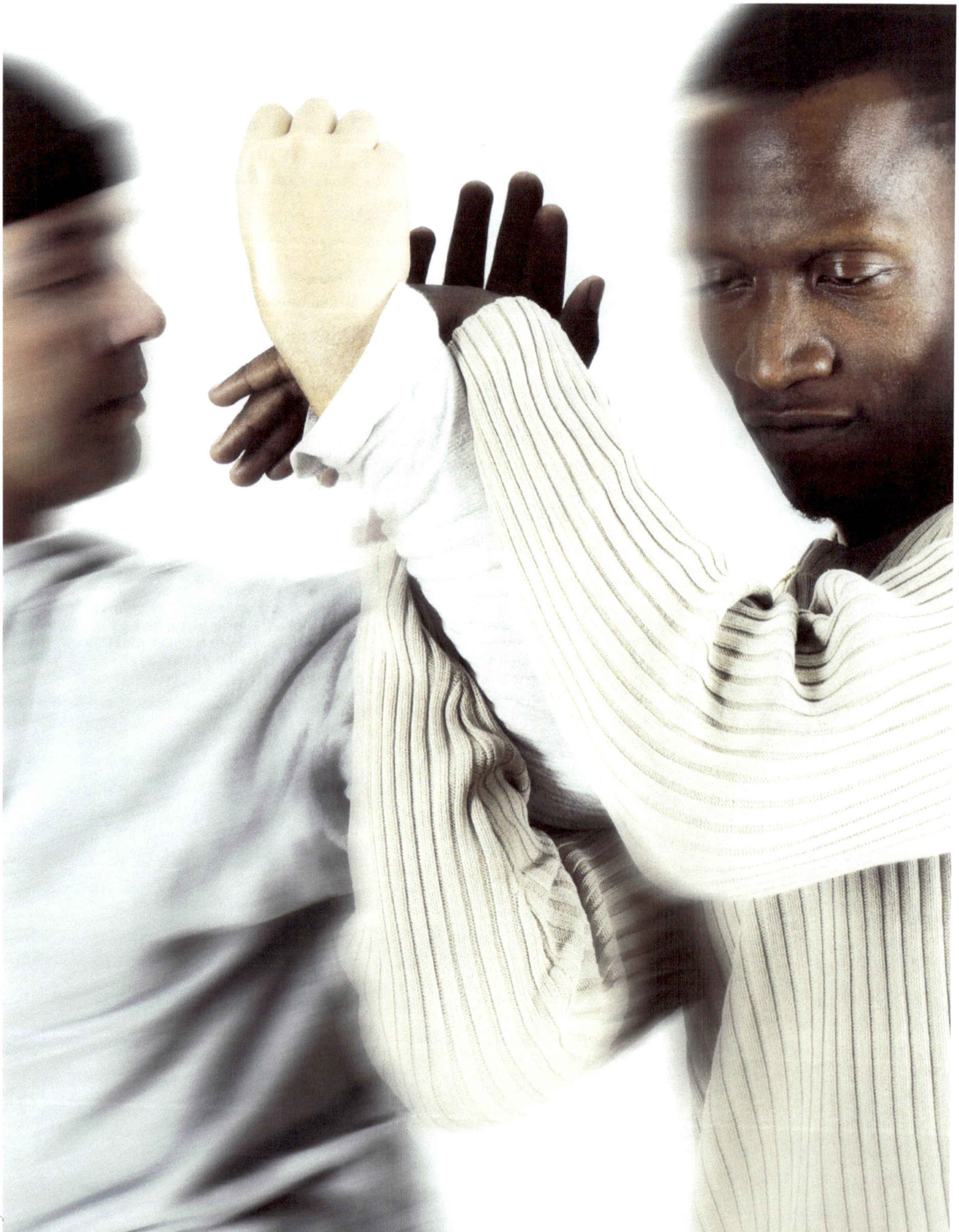

fig.144 - A Figure-of-Four lock is very versatile and easily applied. It looks complicated but it's as easy as one, two, three...

photo by David Tett

locks

A joint lock is the manipulation of a joint by either twisting or bending against the normal direction of movement of the joint itself. Extending or stretching the joint against the natural movement or beyond its maximum bending capability will result in incredible pain or rupture of the ligament and in more serious cases the bone.

Now, I can already feel your excitement, if this was really the case you probably think that all you need to know to defend yourself against an attacker is few effective joint locks and you are perfectly safe: well, not so fast and needless to say not so easy. It is true that locks can be extremely effective and can produce great results even against a stronger opponent, but not in a self defence scenario in the street or outside a training environment because joint manipulations or joint locks require a high degree of training and technique and rarely can be applied against the speed and viciousness of a sudden attack.

JOINT LOCKS ARE NOT THE FIRST CHOICE IN SELF DEFENCE.

Locks are very productive to a trained law enforcement officer who needs to submit someone who has been abusive or violent, in fact to handcuff someone effectively many times a standing arm or wrist lock is applied to "turn" and submit someone in a favourable position to apply handcuffs. Arm locks have been extremely popular in many martial arts, it was the Russians that gave Judokas worldwide a lot to rethink in International competitions when they start using arm locks in Judo tournaments to great effect, but in a street fight or sudden violent attack striking back as we have seen before remain the number one choice.

So why bother writing at all about it then?

Because joint manipulation can nevertheless be very effective, and as we have already seen, knowing certain principles can be applied to other techniques, and knowing certain techniques can give you an edge in some unforeseen circumstances, unpredictability is violence mantra.

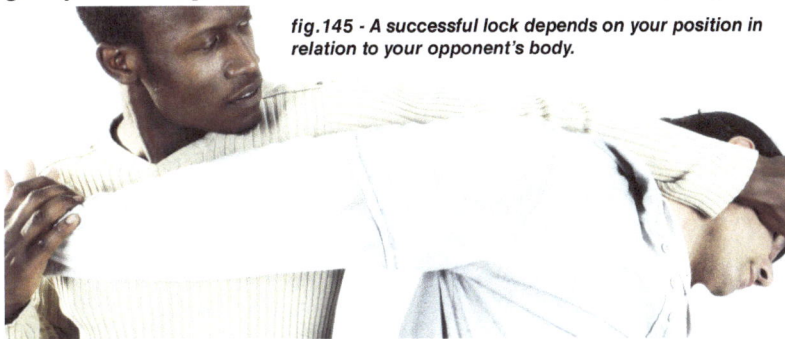

fig.145 - A successful lock depends on your position in relation to your opponent's body.

We do believe in the principle that having too many techniques at your disposal works against an effective defence, always remember that to react promptly is the best defence, not "how" to react, but to "react" pure and simple.

It is also true that arm locks especially, and by arm locks we consider manipulating shoulder, elbow or wrist, can be a lifesaver in some situations, but as most techniques rely on a feel for the action which needs to be applied we emphasise the need for supervised practice, as we have always recommended so far.

fig.146 - Little finger lock.

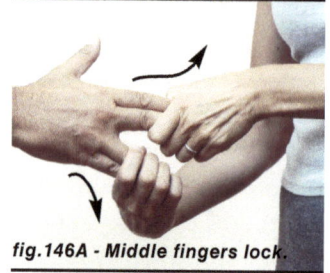

Leverage on the joints causes an unnatural position for the articulation, the point of application must be precise otherwise the technique will not work, this because the lock works on two points, one is as close to the joint as possible where the fulcrum is applied, the other as far away from the joint where force is applied. Force does not mean brutal force, but an adequate pressure applied correctly and continuously, as we'll also see in CHOKES (page 96).

As you can see joint locks take you to very close contact with your attacker. Given the choice it shouldn't be your first choice of action, if you can put enough distance to be safe do so, if already too close or if he is already grappling with you or he has got hold of you, this is the moment that a lock can be useful.

A lock can be useful in preparation for a takedown or to position your attacker where you want him for a follow up strike, to the head for instance: he bends forwards because of the applied lock to his shoulder and you can strike him with your knee to his face.

fig.146A - Middle fingers lock.

Fingers are delicate articulations, they are a favourite target with many self-defence locks but always remember the practicality of it, your hands will be sweating with fear, his hands are probably bigger and grabbing his fingers is not truly practical. However a finger lock as shown in fig. 146 can give you a temporary advantage, or allow you to break his grip, especially if he is trying to strangle you.

The small finger is quite exposed and lends itself to be grabbed easily and very rarely is it a "strong" finger even if someone has a big hand (the thumb is strong). If you manage to grab his little finger make sure you hold his hand as shown with your other hand and apply the lever going out and up, against the natural movement of the joint. This can be quite successful in case you need to free an object from his hand or to make him let go of your clothes. A proper understanding of how the wrist and fingers relate to the arm can help you in escaping a wrist grab (fig.146B).

fig.146B - Fingers manipulation to escape wrist hold.

The same can be applied to his middle fingers, spreading them out as shown in fig. 146A. Remember to use both hands to secure the proper lever of the articulation, two points should always be the target of your manipulation, understanding this principle will always help to readjust a lock the moment you feel it's not working as it should and knowing on what principle the technique is based upon will help in applying a principle and not trying to remember a technique and all its variations. Another very important principle to remember is that you have to make sure that the limb or joint that you are manipulating is away from your opponent's body, increasing the effectiveness of the leverage. Positioning of your own body is fundamental to achieving a good leverage that cannot be stressed enough.

Physics and self-defence go hand in hand, martial arts are based on the laws of physics and their understanding can achieve a powerful kick, a successful throw or a devastating lock.

The fulcrum is what characterises leverage and what makes it effective, the position of the fulcrum can increase or decrease resistance and make the lever more or less effective. (See fig.147A). As you can see the closer the fulcrum is to the point of resistance the better and the longer the lever the less force needs to be applied, resulting in a more effective lock.

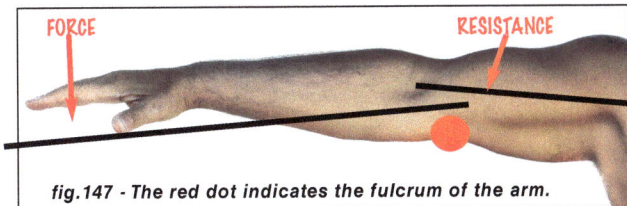

fig.147 - The red dot indicates the fulcrum of the arm.

FORCE

RESISTANCE

Anyone who has ever tried to restrain someone's arm will object that a strong and muscled up arm will resist easily to a lever being applied: in

JOINT LOCKS FOLLOW SIMPLE LAWS OF PHYSICS: LEARN THE PRINCIPLE.

fact it is not so, what is happening is that the lever has been applied incorrectly.

The size of the arm is irrelevant, however what comes into play to frustrate our efforts is clothing. I once had to restrain someone in a restaurant, helping a friend who owned the place: a group of bikers had had too many drinks and they started to misbehave.

I took care of one of the lads, long hair, tattooed, you know the type. I wanted to put his arm in a joint lock but I quickly realized that the thick leather jacket with elbow protection built in was not going to allow me to do that easily. I quickly kept the same principle though and I grabbed his hair and using his neck as a fulcrum. I put him into a headlock and because he kept misbehaving I decided that enough was enough and sent him to sleep for a while.

When he woke up he asked how I did it: the laws of physics were the answer.

We have seen the simplest of joint locks, the one that can be applied to the fingers.

Lets see then aiming a bit further down the arm, that delicate part of the arm anatomy called wrist, rarely strong because it is designed for flexibility? If you haven't noticed it is the one of the very few parts of our body that can move in many directions without any problem. In fact it can rotate easier and with less danger than the neck or the ankle but as most people who roller blade or skate know the wrist is quite delicate, it is a complex articulation and like anything with lots of parts it must be dealt with delicately. This is why a wristlock can be very effective; there are two rows of a total of eight bones called Carpal bones that join the lower arm bones, the radius and

fig.148- Types of wrist locks.

the ulna, to form the wrist. Wrist locks can indeed be quite spectacular, if you have seen AIKIDO practitioners there are some spectacular throws just making the most of the wrist, however in a self defence situation the wrist is not an easy part of the body to grab, hands move very fast and to think they are easy to intercept is simply naive.

SIMPLICITY OF EXECUTION IS ALWAYS THE KEY FOR SUCCESSFUL TECHNIQUES.

Nevertheless there could be situations where this is possible and we examine the most effective.

There are many wristlocks available but most of them do require a high degree of accuracy and skill and some others leave the attacker with the other arm in a favourable position for a strike.

The most useful situation for a wristlock is when your attacker is holding you to drag you somewhere.

As you can see in fig.150 the moment his arms are positioned around your body grab his left hand with your right in a solid grasp and at the same time turn your shoulder and move your elbow as demonstrated in fig.150. The advantage of this particular wrist lock are several: you manipulate his left wrist, probably weaker assuming he is right handed, also you have your elbow in a good position for a strike to his face if necessary and thirdly you can take him to the ground using your body weight easily. Manipulating the right wrist will work equally, just change arm and elbow. As we have said there are other wrist locks (see fig.148) but this is probably the most useful.

WRISTS ARE COMPLEX ARTICULATIONS AND QUITE FRAGILE.

The position of your own body in relation to your attacker's plays a fundamental part to achieve a successful lock: as you can see in fig.145 it is important that your body has keeps a good distance from the opponent's body, you can control him through a lock if his limb is away from his own body and at the same time you keep his limb close to yours.

Don't forget that his applies to wristlocks too.

This is quite visible in applying an elbow lock correctly, especially in a straight-arm lock (or arm bar). To successfully apply leverage to the elbow you must first block the shoulder, this allows you to utilise the fulcrum of the arm, generally located in the hollow past the point of the elbow, towards the shoulder (see fig.147A).

Blocking the shoulder does not allow an escape turning his arm on its axis; also remember that pressure should be applied to the wrist (the lever in this case) in the direction of the little finger, opposite way to the thumb.

APPLY A FAKE TO PREPARE FOR THE LOCK.

An arm lock can be applied standing or on the ground, just remember that applying locks while standing requires a higher degree of training to avoid injury, because your opponent can move more freely increasing the chances of the lock getting out of control causing a dislocation, a serious injury and quite possible while applying leverage to the elbow or shoulder, therefore proper supervised training must be taken.

In any case as soon as the pressure is felt on the joint a signal must me given to make your partner stop. Normally a tap on the mat or on the body is a sign that pressure must be released immediately. Let's now see the most effective arm locks to the elbow.

To initiate an arm lock it is always a good idea to apply a distracting technique to focus your attacker attention somewhere away from what you are doing. A strike with your knee to his thigh, an elbow hit to his ribs can well achieve what you need: good positioning for your lock.

It is also important that while applying the arm lock that you secure his body in a way that he cannot move, escaping the lock, for instance positioning him against a fixed object (wall, lamppost) or using your own body (see fig.149). If on the ground you could use your knee to pin him down or wrap your legs around his body. This lock using your legs (see JUJI GATAME in JUDO - page 236) has many variations and it is one of the most widely used in groundwork.

It can be effective if someone is pinning you down holding you by the shoulders or by the wrists. We have already seen this technique in fig.137 page 85, is very effective if pinned down with an aggressor on top.

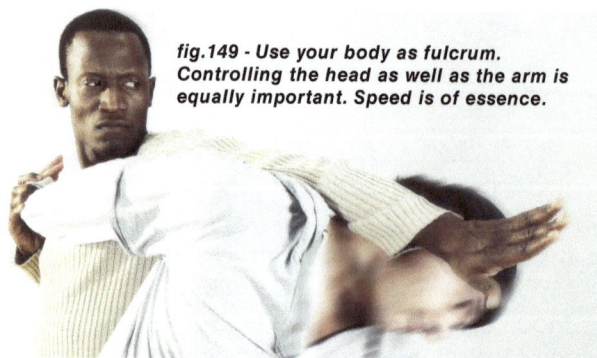

fig.149 - Use your body as fulcrum. Controlling the head as well as the arm is equally important. Speed is of essence.

fig.150 - This wrist lock allows you great control of your attacker on many levels, as well as positioning you for further techniques.

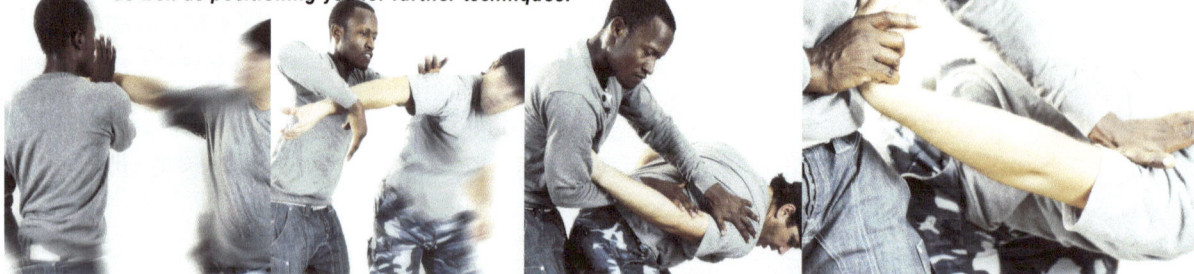

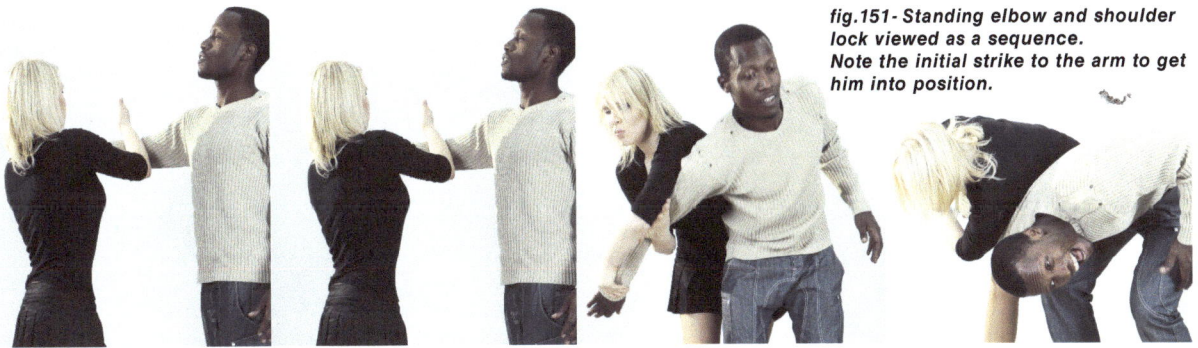

fig.151- Standing elbow and shoulder lock viewed as a sequence.
Note the initial strike to the arm to get him into position.

It is quite difficult to clearly separate a wristlock from an elbow lock; often the two joints are involved closely in the lock. However we can differentiate elbow locks in two types: straight and bent arm. The elbow is quite limited in movement compared to the other body's joint; it's more similar to the knee in that.

USE A DISTRACTION TO INITIATE YOUR TECHNIQUE.

The most efficient elbow lock is UDE HISHIGI ASHI GATAME or HARA GATAME if using your abdomen (see fig 151 and JUDO - page 236).

Both are very effective straight-arm stand locks, but rely in a good distraction maneuver to get into good positioning. A strike to his triceps can effectively give you the opportunity to initiate the lock, turning his arm so his palm is facing towards you (if you are positioned as in fig.151) and then using your other arm to push onto the elbow's fulcrum blocking his shoulder at the same time.

Remember that you must adapt your position so you achieve control, keeping his hand away from his body, close to yours. Push and pull to achieve the hyperextension of the joint.

In the case of bent arm locks the principle remain the same but they are more difficult to achieve because the attacker's body is closer to yours, however these types of locks manipulate also the shoulder and that is useful when you cannot move away from your attacker's body.

The shoulder can rotate in all directions thank to the ball joint of the humerus, the only joint that has really almost complete movement in all direction.

However the shoulder is limited in back extension, and that is the direction for an effective lock.

As you can see in fig.152 there are many types of joint lock, far too many to remember in a stressful situation away from a training environment, however the principle is the same for all of them, independently by the specific technique, remember that.

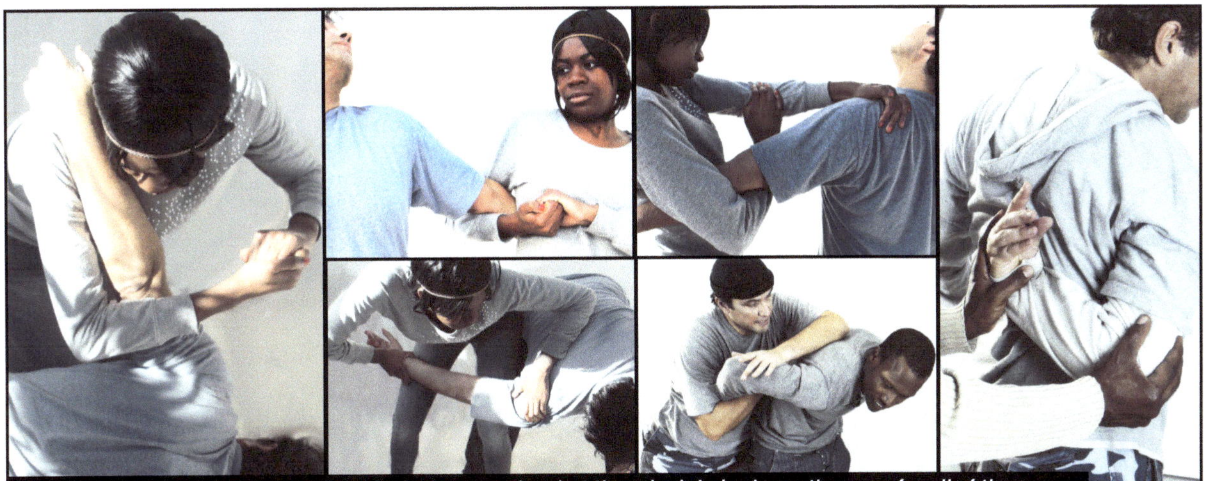

fig.152- There are way too many joint locks to remember, but the principle is always the same for all of them.

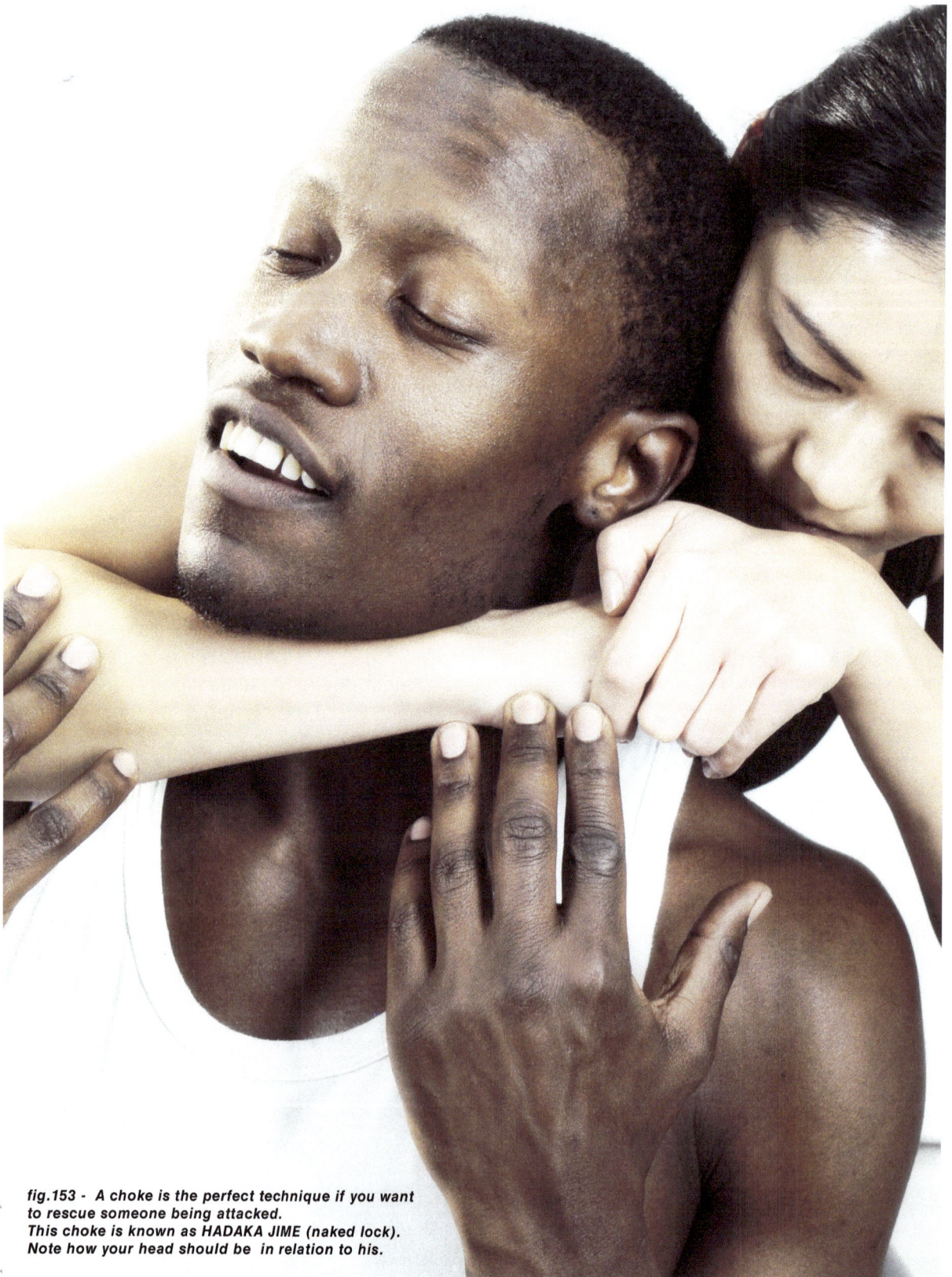

fig.153 - A choke is the perfect technique if you want
to rescue someone being attacked.
This choke is known as HADAKA JIME (naked lock).
Note how your head should be in relation to his.

Let me be absolutely crystal clear here: a choke or strangulation, if correctly executed, will, let me repeat it louder; WILL kill someone in fifteen seconds after he loses consciousness Now fifteen seconds is a very short period of time, especially when there is a lot of adrenaline flowing. It takes just past three seconds for someone to pass out if strangled, and about fifteen to die. I stress this fact because of all the techniques that we explore in this book, some lethal, the choke is the one that can be easily overlooked or misunderstood and the results, either in practice or training or in a real life scenario are irreversible.

I hope I made this absolutely clear, and don't be surprised if I will mention this again further on. Many martial arts have encompassed strangulation techniques in their practice and many if not all of the Special Forces manuals and training worldwide teach this important skill, this alone should make chokes an important chapter learning self defence.

A choke can be carried out from several different angles, standing or lying on the ground, from the front or from behind, using just arms and hands or with the aid of batons or other objects, including belts. You can even choke someone using the lapel of his own jacket.

It is important to remember though that strangulations are by definition carried out at close range, and therefore are very effective when you are either grabbed or onto the ground with your attacker on top of you. We'll see how that works shortly; lets see first

CHOKES MUST BE CARRIED OUT AT CLOSE RANGE TO BE EFFECTIVE.

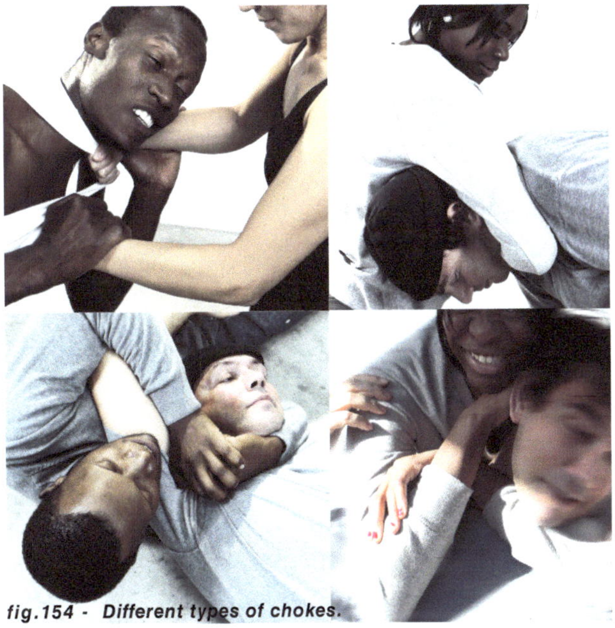

what makes a choke effective.

Of all martial arts it is in Jujitsu and obviously Judo that strangulation techniques achieve greatest effect, concentrating in accuracy and not strength.

This has made the majority of choking techniques (shime=constriction-waza=technique - in Judo) highly accessible in their simplicity and effectiveness. Fundamentally we can distinguish two basic ways of strangling someone: stopping the flow of blood to the brain putting pressure on the carotid or impeding the flow of air to the lungs blocking the trachea, (larynx or windpipe).

Small variations are irrelevant, such as blocking the mouth and nose, and we will concentrate on the simplest and easiest to perform.

YOU CAN STOP BLOOD FLOW TO THE BRAIN OR AIR FLOW TO THE LUNGS.

fig.154 - Different types of chokes.

Unconsciousness can also be achieved applying compression to the nerves near the carotid, a known pressure point amongst martial artists.

The majority of effective strangulations concentrate in compressing the carotid artery, that requires little pressure to stop the flow of blood and the fact that is quite exposed on the neck and also adds simplicity to the application of the technique, as well as the fact that stopping the flood of blood to the brain provokes loss of consciousness much faster than trying to restrict breathing applying pressure to the windpipe (trachea), as well as allowing more control.

All this sounds very exciting but there is one huge problem affecting the teaching of strangulations or neck holding techniques: safety.

In practice within the gym or dojo environment there are trained professionals that will supervise your techniques and there are measures agreed and put in place to guarantee everyone's safety. When a choke is starting to take effect the person on the receiving end will signal with a tap (to the mat or onto the opponent) when it's time to stop, and as soon as the tap is heard or felt the choke is stopped.

Feeling the choke or strangulation being applied to you is an important part of the training especially to learn when to submit during a competition.

BEFORE YOU STRANGLE YOU SHOULD FEEL BEING STRANGLED.

An added danger is that if a choke is improperly applied or too much force is used, the windpipe can collapse, with almost irreversible consequences.

Therefore the first and foremost rule when commencing the strangulation and choke techniques is to keep control of what you are doing and be aware at all time of the status of the other person. How? Well if you are standing and the person goes limp and stops trying to get out of the choke you know that he has probably passed out (probably though, he might be faking it).

If on the floor you'll know either because you can see his face going red (the onset of face flushing is caused by the change in pressure in the carotid arteries and jugular veins), or because he stops struggling, obviously because he has lost consciousness.

This has made chokes very popular with Police forces worldwide as an effective way of tackling violent subjects who refuse to submit, without the use of weapons.

Unfortunately on the contrary to Judo where there have been no deaths during practice or tournaments since Jigoro Kano founded judo in 1882, there have been an increasing number of deaths caused by Law Enforcement Personnel in some countries subduing violent persons using choking holds or other controlling and restraining techniques including a choke. Examining the majority of these cases there is one factor that seems immediately evident, all these fatalities allegedly caused by "bar-arm" and carotid artery control hold techniques seem caused by poor control of the technique or the fact that the person being choked was often under the influence of drugs.

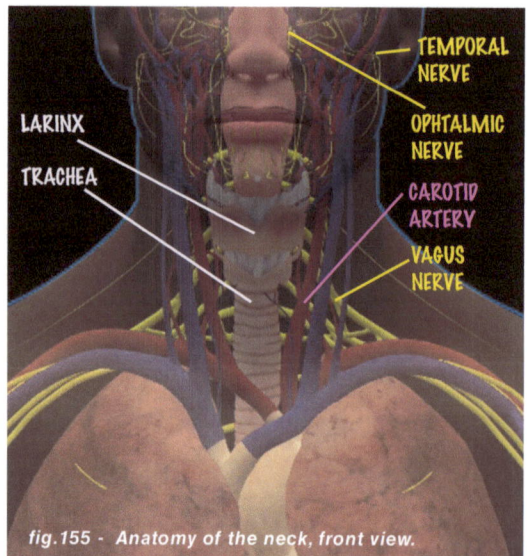

fig.155 - Anatomy of the neck, front view.

TEMPORAL NERVE
OPHTALMIC NERVE
CAROTID ARTERY
VAGUS NERVE
LARINX
TRACHEA

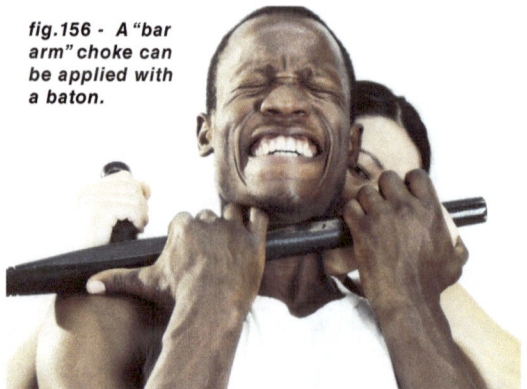

fig.156 - A "bar arm" choke can be applied with a baton.

97

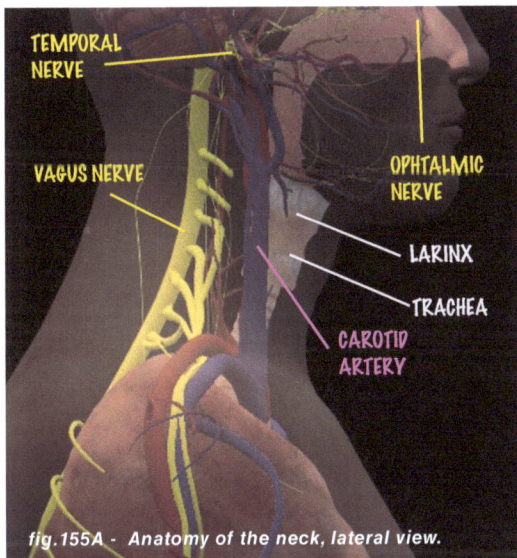

fig.155A - Anatomy of the neck, lateral view.

TEMPORAL NERVE

VAGUS NERVE

OPHTALMIC NERVE

LARINX

TRACHEA

CAROTID ARTERY

This should make us think twice before applying a choke to someone, as it is evident that things can get out of hand pretty quickly if the person cannot comply.

THINGS CAN GO BAD VERY QUICKLY WITHOUT SELF-CONTROL.

The advantage of a chokehold is also psychological, very few people have experienced been choked and it can be an extremely frightening experience for anyone at the receiving end.

A woman of averagely strong build can quite easily subdue a man twice her size if she can apply a choke with good technique. What makes a good technique then? There are a few general things to remember and then we'll see individual techniques.

First of all make sure that you can put your entire body's power behind the choke, meaning having a good position in relation to your opponent, in a way that you use more than just the strength of your hands. If on the ground you should arch backwards, away from your opponent, and straighten your body to maximise the choking action.

Once you have committed yourself to perform a choke or strangulation make sure you go all the way, without releasing your hold or slackening, quite the opposite, apply increasing constant pressure on the neck until your opponent looses consciousness.

Using excessive strength is a bad technique; very little pressure is required to achieve a perfect result in all chokes, especially if directed at the carotid.

TECHNIQUE IS EVERYTHING, STRENGTH WORKS AGAINST THE EXECUTION.

Let's examine some of the most popular chokes and strangulations that can be used in a self-defence situation. As we have discussed we can apply a choke from a variety of different positions, using one hand, two hands, your legs or part of our attacker's clothes or using objects such as batons or other similar tools.

The most basic choking technique is called HADAKA JIME (naked lock) in Judo (page 236), and takes its name from the fact that it does not require using anything but your arms.

As we can see in fig.153 your arm should be positioned across his throat from behind, applying direct pressure with your forearm onto his trachea, and because of the pressure applied to a

fig.157 - Going to someone's rescue you can use a belt to apply a choke and control the attacker. Note the rescuer's knee position.

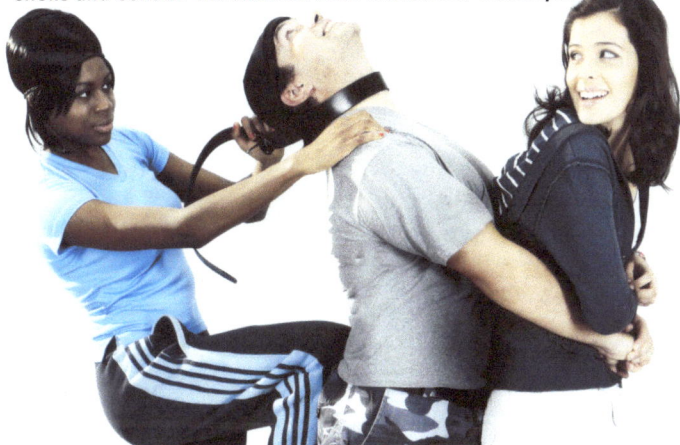

frontal wide area, it is very painful, adding the shock of sharp pain to the choking action.

Clasp your hand at the same time (if it is the right arm across his neck use your left to do that) and now pull backwards using both hands.

Now keep pulling backwards, and even if you fall on your back keep pulling until your attacker loses consciousness It is important that the area of the forearm used to apply pressure on the neck is the hard "bony" part, not the soft one.

IT IS IMPORTANT TO APPLY PRESSURE USING YOUR BONY PART, NOT THE SOFT ONE.

To make sure that the right part of the forearm is used make sure your palm is facing down, also be careful that his neck does not slide towards your elbow, allowing a gap to be formed where the elbow bends.

To avoid this from happening make sure that you position your shoulder behind your attacker's head and move your head to the side of his head to keep his head in position (fig.157). There are few variations of this choke (see fig. 158 and 159) changing hand position or using part of your opponent's clothing to secure a better hold and all these variations can be applied if clasping your other hand is not practical or not feasible, for instance your opponent has grabbed part of your arm or your other hand is slippery with sweat.

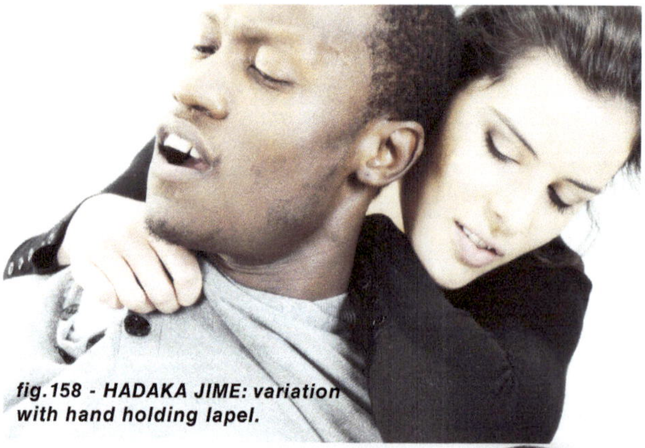

fig.158 - HADAKA JIME: variation with hand holding lapel.

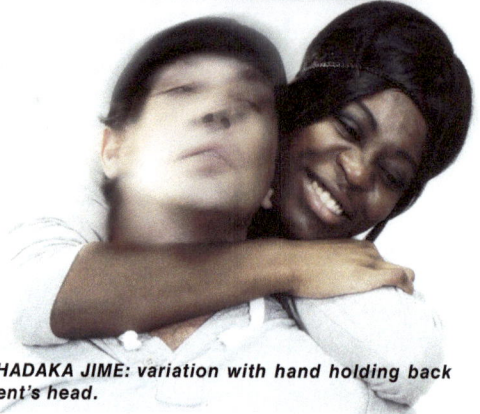

This choke is effective also coming to someone's rescue, because it is most effective from behind: it can be performed standing, kneeling or while on the ground. To escape from this particular hold, in case you find yourself being subjected to it, turn your head towards the elbow of your opponent to free the airway and at the same time insert your hand between his arm and your neck, pushing hard up and if he moves to adjust his position, head butt him.

fig.159 - HADAKA JIME: variation with hand holding back of opponent's head.

TO ESCAPE STRANGULATION YOU MUST BE EXPLOSIVE WITH YOUR REACTION.

The majority of defence techniques against chokes must be conducted quickly and swiftly, you only have a couple of seconds before loosing consciousness and your response must be explosive. If strangled from behind sometimes is best to spin around towards his elbow and hit him on the ribs with your elbow (see fig.160).

Strangulations are very effective even when standing and when your attacker tries to grab you by the waist, the guillotine choke hold (called Mae Hadaka Jime in Judo (page 236) is quite effective in this case and you can even drag your attacker to the floor, or in any case if he pushes you to the ground, with the impetus of his attack, you know that you can choke him with this technique (fig.162).

As we have mentioned you can also use his clothing to perform a choke, for instance the lapel of his jacket, using the lapel like a cord wrapped around his neck or to get a more effective grip. There are several chokes using lapels, the most useful is known in Judo as Kataha Jime (page 236) if from behind, while if you need to apply it frontally, even with your attacker on top of you, you should perform any of the so called cross locks (Juji Jime).

fig.160 - Spin around towards his elbow and hit your attacker hard with your elbow any- where.

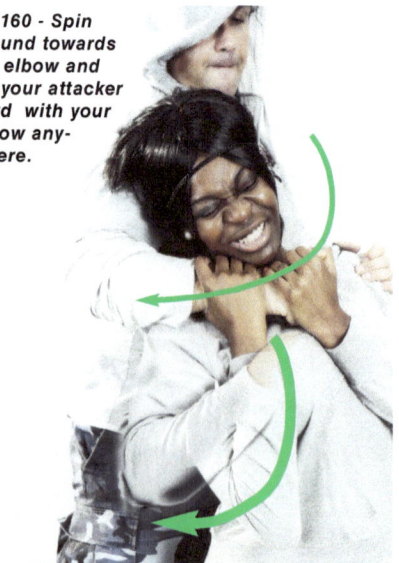

fig.161 - Nami Juji Jime. Notice the way the elbows are positioned.

There is Nami Juji JIme (palms down), Gyaku Juji Jime (two palms facing up) or Kata Juji Jime (one thumb in and one thumb out), all very similar except that the exact position of the hands varies.

The easiest and most natural to execute is Nami-Juji-Jime (fig.161) where both hands are in the normal position, palm downwards, that you would have going for his neck, thumbs in the jacket, fingers out.

Your left hand grabs his right collar pulling slightly to your left, to get a deep grip with your right hand, using full thumb inside, on his right collar as close to his neck as possible.

Then the left hand goes underneath your right hand and gets a deep grip on the opposite collar, again with your thumb inside.

Positioning your head beside his head so he won't be able to escape as you spread your elbows sideways and choke him.

Pulling him towards you (to the ground) will bring his centre of weight to your chest, preventing him from creating distance.

REMEMBER TO PULL YOUR OPPONENT TOWARDS YOU TO ACHIEVE A GOOD CHOKE.

His reaction would be to pull himself up, away from you so your entire weight is now applying a choke. Continue until he passes out, this is important to achieve an effective strangulation.

Gyaku-Juji-Jime has the hands in the reverse position, palms upwards and both hands have fingers in the jacket and the thumbs outside.

All three strangulations use the elbows spread outwards to apply pressure to the carotid, and all cross chokes are very effective even when you are pinned to the ground with your opponent on top of you.

The reason why I prefer carotid chokes to windpipe chokes is because it takes less strength to put pressure on the carotid and lost of consciousness is achieved much earlier.

Also, pressure to the carotid can be applied from different angles, while a choke to the larynx is more effectively controlled when applied from behind.

Knowing that both type of choke can work effectively even against a far superior opponent should give you an advantage in case your life is threatened and you want to survive.

Fig.162 - Guillotine choke ending on the ground. In Judo this choke is known as MAE HADAKA JIME. You can drag your attacker to the ground and wrapping your legs around his torso get him in a scissor lock at the same time.

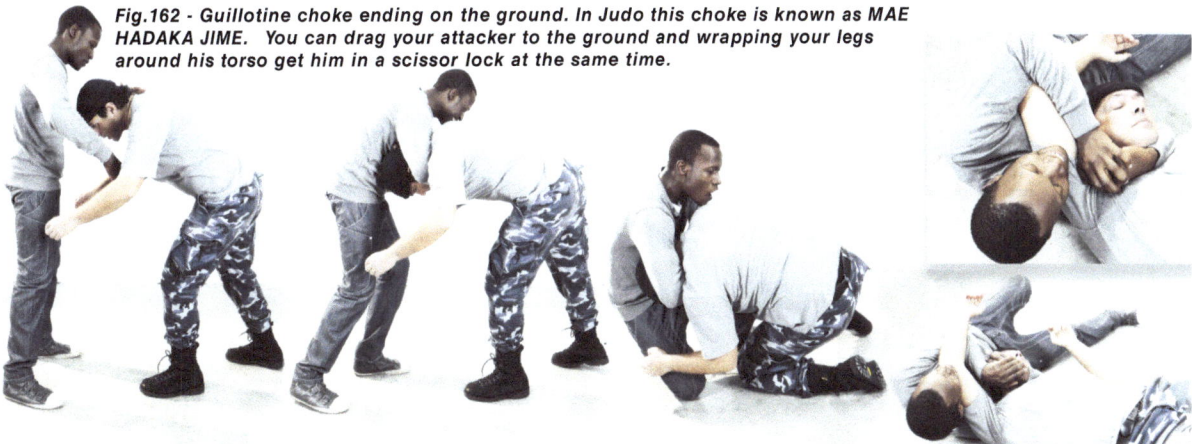

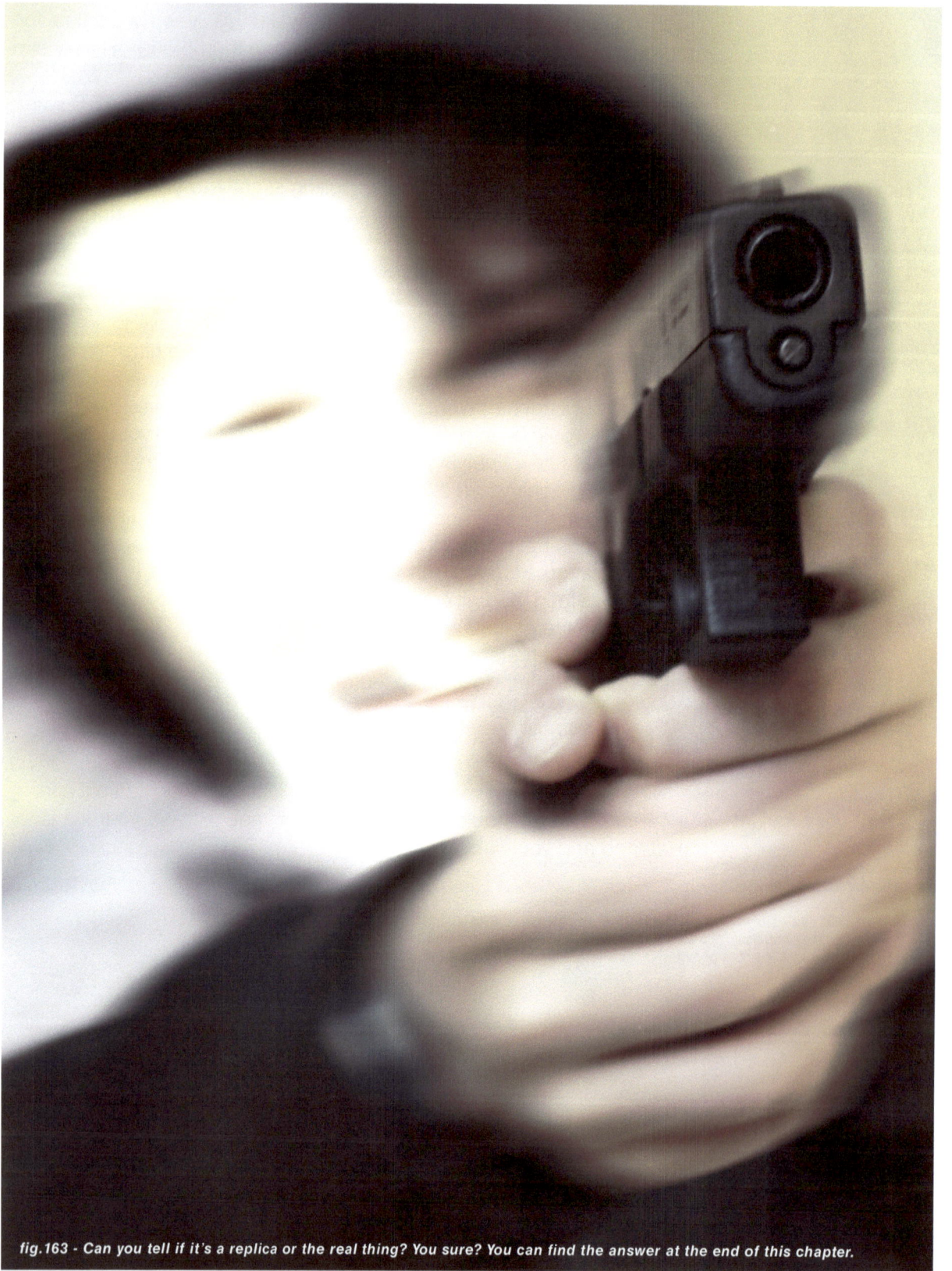

fig.163 - Can you tell if it's a replica or the real thing? You sure? You can find the answer at the end of this chapter.

weapons

When facing someone threatening you with a weapon, either a knife or a gun, I would always strongly suggest that you do as you are told unless you know that you are about to be killed. At the end of the day, if it's only a wallet or a bag that is the object of the threat you can always replace it but reacting to an armed assailant just to protect material possession is not a smart move. A completely different situation is if you fear for your own life or someone else's.
In that case, you have no choice but to react either to remove the weapon or neutralise the attacker. Let me make it very clear: if someone points either a knife or a gun at you, in the majority of cases he's prepared to use it.
We can identify two types of attacker, the expert well-trained type, for instance ex-military, and the improvised, desperate, quite often under-influence-of-substances-type of person. The first type is normally someone that keeps a safe distance, is calm and determined. Quite often you find this type of attacker in a bank robbery scenario.
I would suggest that you do not tackle him unless you think he is about to harm you.

A TINY WINDOW OF OPPORTUNITY IS ALL YOU GOT IF FACING A WEAPON.

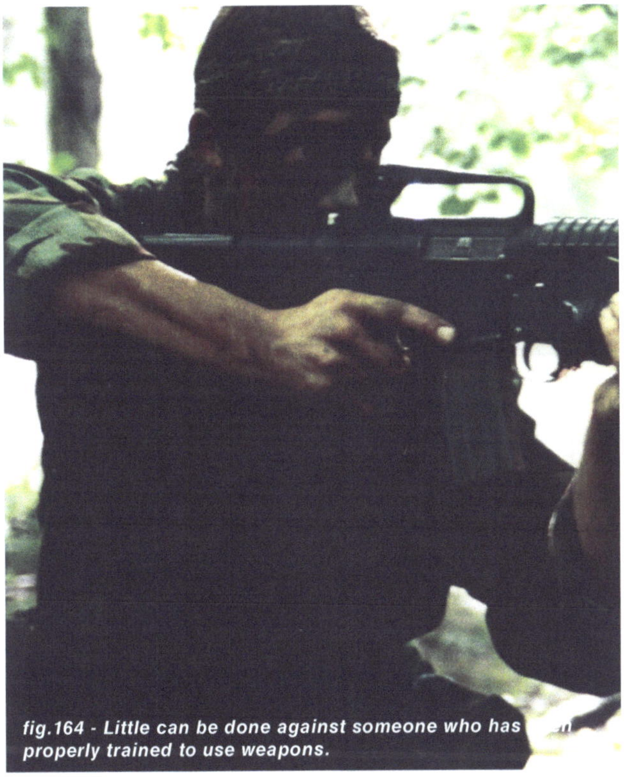

fig.164 - Little can be done against someone who has been properly trained to use weapons.

The second type is quite often very agitated, possibly close to you and very edgy, almost spirited, off his head so to speak.
Due to the unpredictability of the latter, don't underestimate the danger he can pose even if he appears untrained to you.
As a general rule comply doing as you are told if someone is pointing a firearm at you, don't think you can dodge or outrun a bullet, you can't. Keep calm (I know, easier said than done) and do not make any sudden move, don't try any moves you have seen in a movie, reality is different.
All this is the best advice you can get if someone only wants your valuables.
A completely different matter is if the person holding the gun wants you to follow him somewhere or forces you to drive somewhere or wants you to get into a car/van and so on.
This is a different scenario; all you have to do is ask yourself what this person will do once has finished with you.

This is why I am happy to show what can be done if the threat is not just to your valuables but also to you as a person, or to your loved ones. As we have just seen

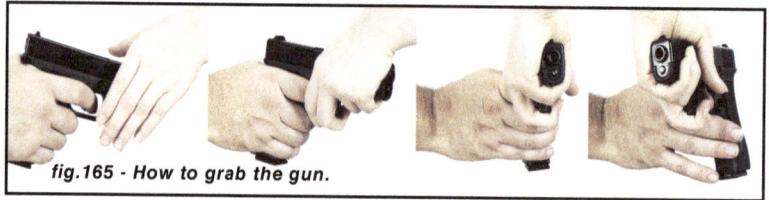

fig.165 - How to grab the gun.

the distance and stance of somebody holding a gun defines who he is.

We distinguish the position of the attacker in relation to you because somebody who is trained in the use of weapons, especially firearms, will keep a safe distance, normally twice an arms length to avoid being disarmed, what law enforcement people call "reactionary gap", a 9 feet (3 meters) distance. This is just a rule of thumb and should be taken as such.

There is no guarantee that it is always like that, however the advantage that you have is that someone holding a gun feels very powerful, almost invincible, and that makes him quite careless and this will give you quite often a few windows of opportunity that as we see throughout this book constitute a prerequisite before you initiate any reaction to a threat.

ONCE YOU HAVE INITIATED AN ACTION YOU CANNOT STOP.

It is very important and we cannot stress it enough that when reacting to defend yourself you do it with sheer determination and lightning speed. However there are several things that are absolutely fundamental when defending yourself against an armed assailant if you want to increase the chances to succeed.

Once you have initiated an action in reaction to a armed threat, you have to follow through, and if you miss or mess up, you cannot stop.

You have to carry on, changing to a different action but always with the same purpose of neutralising your assailant. Let's stick with firearms to start with, since strangely enough it's simpler to discuss those than knives that I prefer to treat later on. If somebody is pointing a gun at you, always assume it's real. Let me tell you straight that very rarely replicas or toy guns are used, even though, it is this kind that makes the news more than the real stuff, however even to a trained eye, it's almost impossible to distinguish a real from a fake, and in these kinds of situations, your judgement is probably impaired by adrenaline.

Also do not necessarily assume that somebody pointing a gun at you necessarily intends to kill you, so try to stay calm, remember that your window of opportunity normally comes the moment the person speaks either to tell you what to do, answer a question that you asked or reacts verbally to a verbal prompt you offered.

This tells you that you can create a window of opportunity by asking him a question or saying something that will prompt him to reply, such as "Please don't hurt me". The moment he starts speaking, is the moment to initiate your action. It is a good idea not to stare at the weapon.

CREATE YOUR OWN WINDOW OF OPPORTUNITY.

As we have said before it is not good idea to "telegraph" your intention to your attacker, warning him that you are about to act or react. The burning question now is: do you grab his arm or the gun?

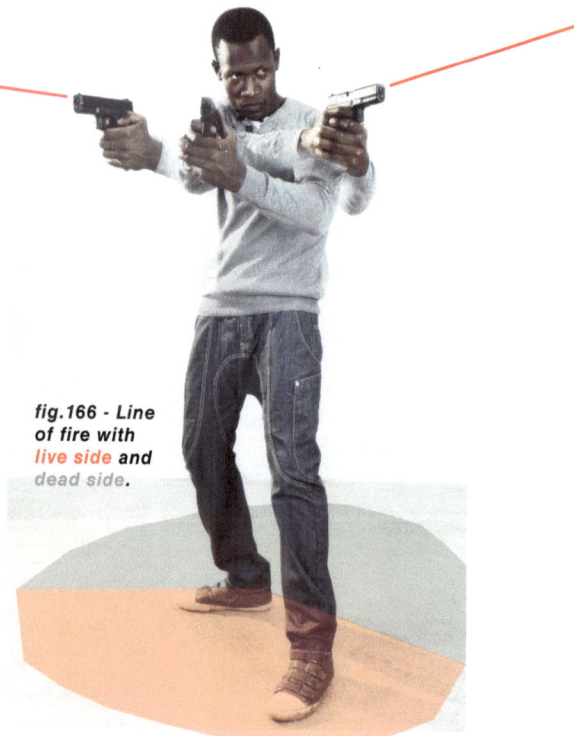

fig.166 - Line of fire with *live side* and *dead side*.

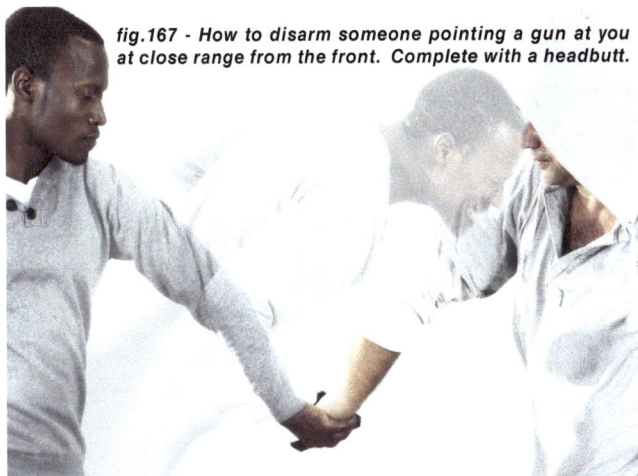

fig.167 - How to disarm someone pointing a gun at you at close range from the front. Complete with a headbutt.

Even if you are tempted or it seems easier to grab his arm remember that he can always flex his wrist and shoot you, or worse, grab the weapon with his other hand in no time.

Therefore, you should grab the gun and in fig.165 we show you how. As you can see when grabbing it, assuming your attacker is holding it with his right hand, you should grasp it with your left hand deflecting the weapon to the side, not up, not down but to the side, in a decisive and extremely fast action, because what you have to worry the most about is the line of fire, in other

ALWAYS DEFLECT THE BARREL AWAY FROM YOU, TOWARDS THE DEAD SIDE.

words, where the bullet will go if the trigger is pulled (see fig.167 for the whole action). When somebody points a gun at you we can distinguish between a live side and a dead side (see fig.166) and you should always deflect the weapon onto the dead side.

The idea is that when deflecting the gun, whatever or however you do it, the barrel should always point away from you or towards your attacker, so that any reaction from his side to bring the gun to point at you becomes really hard.

For instance, it's much easier to lower an arm if somebody is resisting you than raising an arm if the same action is applied. While deflecting the gun away, add a twisting motion working against the articulations of his wrist to which he cannot resist, (see fig. 165) and the only outcome can be him letting go of the weapon: we have seen that extensively in VULNERABLE (page 30) discussing articulations and in LOCKS (page 90).

IF YOU GRAB THE GUN BE PREPARED TO USE IT.

The same principle applies here; you must work against the natural movement of your attacker's articulations, even when he is holding the gun with two hands, law-enforcement style. You have to consider that once you initiate this maneuver you have to expect that the attacker will fight for his own life, and what you also have to be prepared for is what you are going to do with the gun once you've got it: are you prepared to use it? Are you really?

My honest suggestion is that if you get it, point it at him and step backwards, shouting not to move or you will shoot. You had better be prepared for when he walks towards you, probably not believing that you would carry out your threat. In this case, fire into the air by simply pulling the trigger and

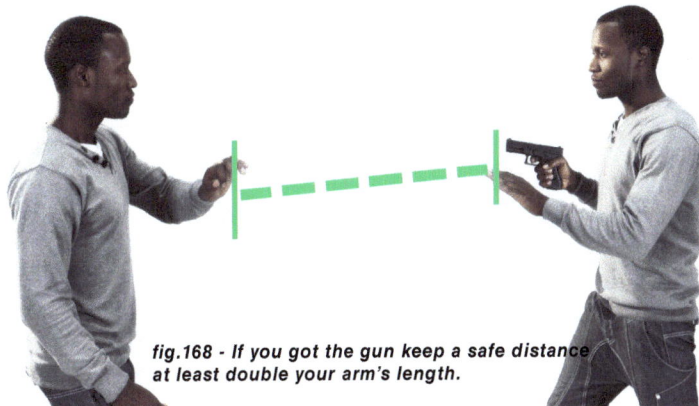

fig.168 - If you got the gun keep a safe distance at least double your arm's length.

prepare yourself for the bang, it is going to be very loud.

You should also be prepared that there is going to be no bang, either because there is no ammunition or it is a fake, or the safety is on (fig.174).

To recap, first move away and keep your distance (fig.168), secondly be prepared to fire or fire if he ignores your commands to stay away.

Keep him in the line of fire and if he doesn't want to leave be firm in your commands, tell him to "GO ON YOUR KNEES"! And "LIE DOWN, FACE TO THE GROUND!"

Once this is achieved keep him in the weapon's line of fire and call the Police stating that you are holding your attacker's gun aimed at him, when the Police arrive do exactly as told.

Do not get complacent because you now have the weapon and if for whatever reason you cannot call for help, move to safety without ever losing sight of your attacker.

Personally I don't think that the majority of people would be keen to hold a gun against somebody or are prepared to pull the trigger, and thank God for that, but that's also why I think if you suc-

IF YOU GRAB THE GUN AND CANNOT USE IT THROW IT AWAY SAFELY.

ceed in grabbing the gun, run away and throw it where he cannot recover it easily (river, pot hole, bin, under a car, on top of a roof, or simply hide it, and obviously it would be better if completely out of reach once disposed of.

Once you have managed to grab the gun's barrel as shown in fig.169, it is important that you slide your fingers and hold the weapon as shown, also because such movement naturally should make you turn and position your entire body on the dead side of your attacker.

fig.169 - Slide your fingers along the barrel.

Body language is very important: always remember that even a slight weight shift or flinching can give away your real intention, and if somebody has his finger on the trigger, he might react with disastrous consequences. The first few seconds of being threatened at gunpoint are the crucial: the attacker assumes you might react and he is ready to pull the trigger.

DOUBLE ON YOUR MOVES.

As you can see in fig.170, it is not a bad idea to add a punch or a hit to his throat as you go for the gun, as we repeated a few times throughout, someone can only resist one action at the time, and doubling up on your moves will always give you an advantage. You can also add a kick to the shin, which is always very disabling.

As stated before, get close since getting closer to your attacker makes manoeuvring the weapon more difficult and more than ever, when it comes to guns, your reaction has to be explosive and fast: resist from just pulling the gun, it never works and quite often you are actually making your attacker pull the trigger just to hold onto it. Your action should be to rotate the gun, always away from you, remember, against the natural movement of this articulation. It's an action impossible to resist.

fig.170 - Add a sweep as you go for the gun.

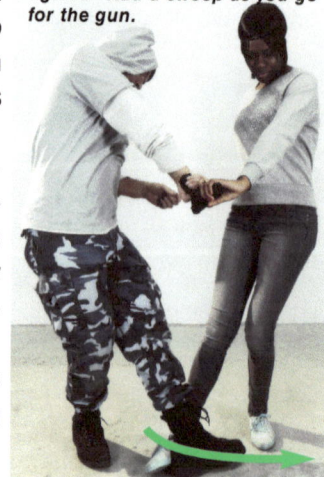

All these techniques need to be rehearsed under proper supervision, you should try and get a feel for a gun, using a replica as realistic (especially in weight) as possible, and the majority of people always find that guns are heavier than they thought and quite slippery

PRACTICE WITH REALISTIC WEAPONS AS MUCH AS POSSIBLE.

too. Practicing with equipment as real as possible is important; there really is no substitute to that.

A technique that always impresses people who sign up to self-defence courses is disarming someone of his gun using a double slap to hand and wrist simultaneously.

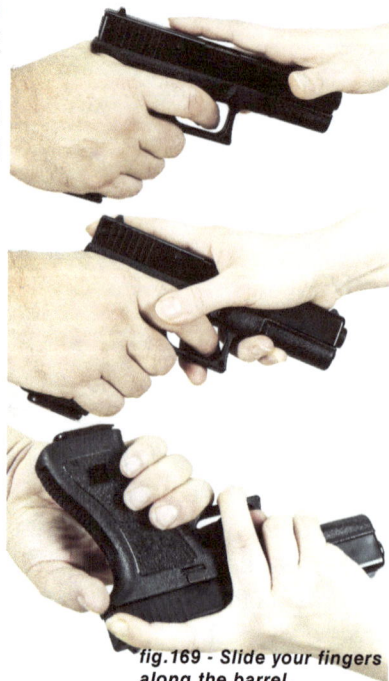

The effect in a demonstration is quite spectacular, the gun literally flies off the holder's hand, this is why it's a popular move in action movies and why it makes self-defence instructors look cool, however it very rarely works in real life. This particular move is done slapping with you left hand the hand holding the weapon and with your right his wrist. The strike has to happen perfectly simultaneously and hitting right through it, meaning without stopping on point of contact.

The result is springing the gun away (fig.171).

In reality this technique, designed to work obviously at short range, presents two problems: the first one is that it requires great accuracy, missing the exact points of impact will result in disaster.

GIVEN THE CHANCE IT IS BETTER TO CONTROL THE WEAPON.

The second problem is that, even if succeeding, the gun falls within a short distance and nothing stops the attacker grabbing it again and this time shoot you: for this reason I prefer to focus on techniques that are simpler to apply and give you control of the weapon, instead of relying on luck. Where weapons are involved you'll have one chance and one only, no point messing around. Since we are discussing firearms I am sure that some readers are expecting that a distinction be drawn between a weapon with a short barrel, such as a handgun or revolver and a long barrel type such as a rifle, shotgun or submachine gun.

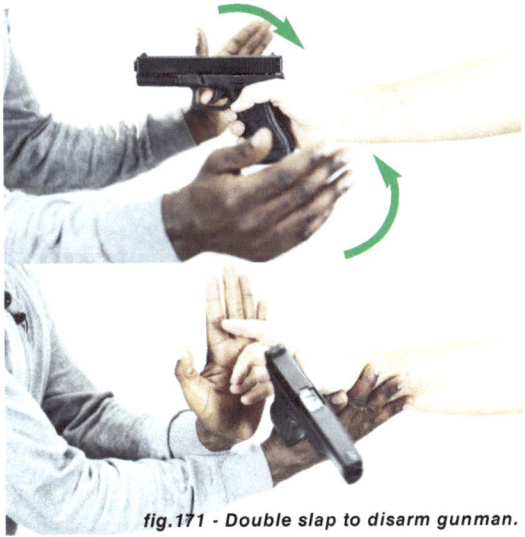

fig.171 - Double slap to disarm gunman.

It is true that the techniques to disarm someone holding a handgun differ from techniques used in case you are facing a rifle, but I would like to point out that the second situation is unlikely unless you are in a war zone. Criminals prefer small guns, easier to conceal and quicker to operate.Criminal activities involving guns are normally over in few seconds, and more often than not (think bank robbery) all they are after is the money. If you assist an armed robbery, inside a building or on the street, just stay out of harms way, ideally sheltering behind something solid, a car, wall etc, and don't play the hero, unless you are sure that they want to harm you. Try to remember what you see and if safe enough either record everything with your mobile phone's video camera or try to remember faces and registration plates, but only and exclusively if you are sure that you will not be spotted or expose yourself to harm doing so. Let's see then what you can do when you have a barrel pointed at you at close range. Remember that reacting might get you hurt or killed, so you should apply the techniques that follow only when you are sure that you have no other choice.

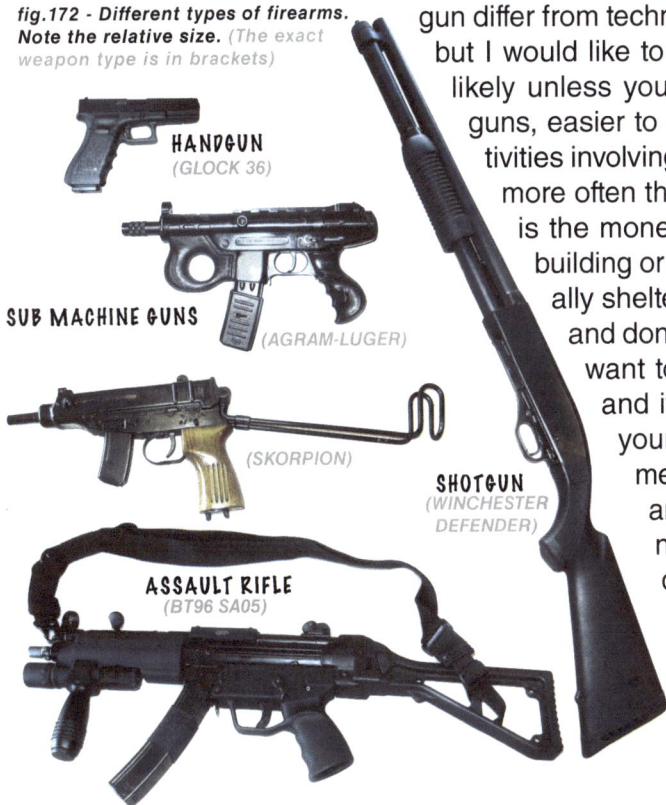

fig.172 - Different types of firearms. Note the relative size. (The exact weapon type is in brackets)

HANDGUN
(GLOCK 36)

SUB MACHINE GUNS
(AGRAM-LUGER)

(SKORPION)

SHOTGUN
(WINCHESTER DEFENDER)

ASSAULT RIFLE
(BT96 SA05)

In the case of a long barrel (fig.172) weapon (shotgun/rifle) close your distance stepping to the dead side, then embrace the rifle firmly under your (right) arm and use your free arm to hit the attacker in the groin or to the face, adding a sweep with your leg too (see fig.173), make sure that you hit hard and furious.

The disadvantage of long barrel weapons is the very fact that they have a long barrel, and it can be wrestled because it gives you a long lever, provided that once you have grabbed it, you do not let go at any cost, no matter what. Always remember, if you decided to grab the gun, there is no way back, you have to go through it determinedly. Many times throughout this book we have stressed the fact that there is no substitute for practice, well, once more, and stronger than ever, you must have practical sessions under the supervision of an experienced instructor: a gun is heavy, slippery and has many sharp edges, extensive, supervised and repeated practice can only help, just reading how to is surely not enough.

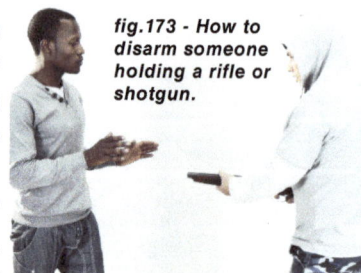

Let's now discuss short barrel firearms such as a pistol or handgun. There are two types, the (semi automatic) pistol (fig.174) and the revolver (fig.175).

KNOWING HOW IT WORKS CAN MAKE IT WORK.

Why do I need to know this you might ask?

What difference does it make? Loads, is the answer.

A pistol is a semi-automatic weapon, meaning a gentle squeeze of the trigger will fire the gun; the gases emitted by the exploding cartridge are used to reload the chamber with the next cartridge after a round is fired. As the slide moves the spent casing is ejected and a new round from the magazine reaches the chamber This allows another shot to take place immediately.

If the spent cartridge is not expelled or the slide cannot move the pistol cannot fire again (see fig.165). A revolver has a rotating cylinder with chambers where the cartridges are loaded.

Every time the trigger is pulled the hammer hits the cartridge firing the bullet and a mechanism linked to the trigger rotates the chamber into position in a new ready firing position (double-action).

Knowing these simple notions can give you an advantage once you manage to grab the gun, just imagine that if you are struggling with someone over a handgun, knowing that pressing certain levers can release the magazine or put the safety on could make a difference. Unfortunately I speak from experience.

GET YOUR BODY OUT OF THE LINE OF FIRE AS YOU REACT.

Obviously this section cannot be a treaty on firearms handling or go into too many details on handguns, however if you are unlucky enough to be threatened with a firearm and you have the feeling that you should react or else, you have sufficient knowledge that gives you a better chance to survive.

This makes even more sense if you consider why once you have grabbed the weapon you should slide your hand up the barrel, giving you better control of the weapon itself.

Most attacks involving weapons are normally over in less than a minute, a store robbery or a street robbery carried out by criminal holding guns are over quickly.

fig.173 - How to disarm someone holding a rifle or shotgun.

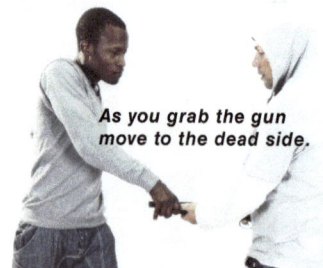

As you grab the gun move to the dead side.

Keep hold of the weapon and strike hard.

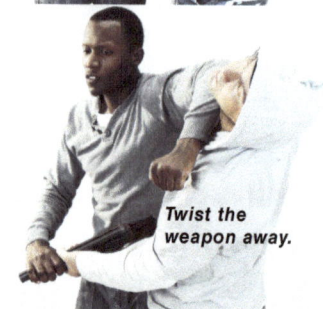

Twist the weapon away.

fig.174 A - The cartridges are in the magazine.

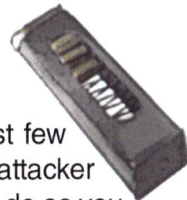

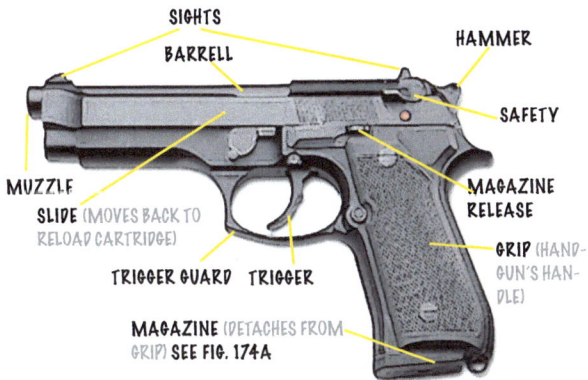

SIGHTS
BARRELL
HAMMER
SAFETY
MUZZLE
SLIDE (MOVES BACK TO RELOAD CARTRIDGE)
MAGAZINE RELEASE
GRIP (HAND-GUN'S HAN-DLE)
TRIGGER GUARD   TRIGGER
MAGAZINE (DETACHES FROM GRIP) SEE FIG. 174A

fig.174 - Semi automatic pistol explained.

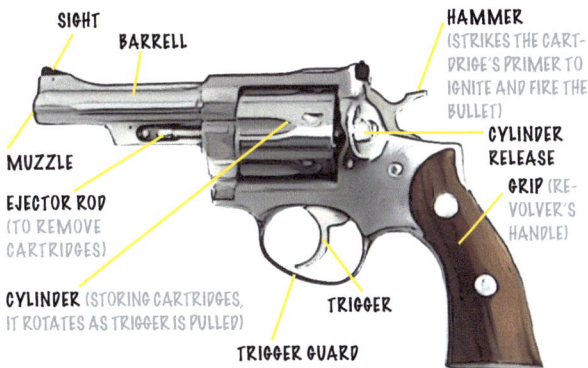

SIGHT
BARRELL
HAMMER (STRIKES THE CART-DRIGE'S PRIMER TO IGNITE AND FIRE THE BULLET)
MUZZLE
CYLINDER RELEASE
EJECTOR ROD (TO REMOVE CARTRIDGES)
GRIP (RE-VOLVER'S HANDLE)
CYLINDER (STORING CARTRIDGES, IT ROTATES AS TRIGGER IS PULLED)
TRIGGER
TRIGGER GUARD

fig.175 - Double action revolver explained.

For this reason, because the first few seconds are the ones in which an attacker expects a reaction, do not react and do as you are told, it is not worth risking your or someone's else life or for money or some jewellery.

Only if you are forced at gunpoint to follow someone somewhere might it be worth reacting at first given chance. When the handgun is pointed from the front, from a distance, let's say just beyond the reach of your arm, (fig.167) dart your left hand to grab the gun (as shown in fig.165) and at the same time push the gun down and onto the dead side (towards his opposite knee). This action will naturally position your body at an angle. It is important that the arm that reaches the gun does not telegraph the move in advance and keeps the elbow locked straight: now is the time to lunge forward landing an almighty punch to his face or throat or an open palm strike to his chin.

Keep twisting his hand until you get the gun out of his grasp, use both hands if necessary, do not let go and keep twisting against his wrist's natural direction (fig.165).

When you grab the gun lock your elbow and put all your weight into this move, to avoid him disengaging himself from your grasp. The same technique applies if the gun is pointed at your stomach or your head just make sure you grab the gun as shown. Moving your body sideways as you move decreases the chances of getting hit. Practice is what makes this technique work, and in practice the instructor will try and catch you out if you telegraph the move. It takes only a few pounds of pressure (between 5 and 7 depending on gun models) to pull the trigger, and that is not much at all: all moves must be carried out together as a continuum and with fast-determined execution. If the attacker is left handed perform the technique shown in fig.167 in the same way, grabbing the gun with your right hand, moving your right leg forward and striking with your left hand.

If you are performing the move in fig.176 and you find yourself at the wrong angle (attacker is also at an angle) then use your leg to kick your opponent instead of hitting him with your hand.

PULLING THE TRIGGER REQUIRES VERY LITTLE PRESSURE.

fig.176 - If disarming someone threatening you from the side don't hesitate, if you find yourself at the wrong angle, to add a kick and go for a takedon. In any case do not stop , just change action using a different technique, keeping to the same principle.

fig.177- Action to take if threatened at gunpoint from behind. You can finish with a strike to his throat or an elbow lock like in fig.149

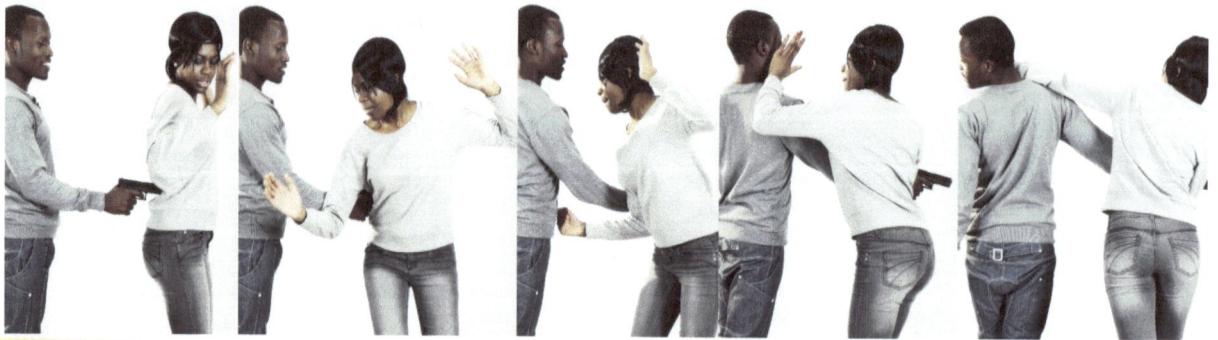

ALWAYS ASSUME A GUN IS LOADED.

The important thing is that you rotate the handgun in his hand as previously shown, the technique applies in the same way.

What about if the gun is pointing at you from behind, at close range? In actual fact, contrary to common belief this is one of the easiest defences.

If you look at fig.177 your natural reaction if feeling a gun would be a slight turn, and in doing so you can use your left arm to deflect the attacker's arm holding the pistol, at the same time trap his forearm under your forearm, striking his jaw or throat with your elbow or right forearm.

By now you should have control of the gun.

For this technique to be effective you must be sure of your attacker's position in relation to yours, since if you deflect the wrong arm or cannot secure his gun holding arm he can easily shoot you.

Any correction should be aimed at his face, grabbing the gun at the same time.

The same applies if the gun is aimed at your head (fig.178). If you ever find yourself handling a firearm, even if just a starter pistol firing blanks, remember the following:

> 1- Always assume a gun is loaded, even if told it is not.
> 2- Keep the gun pointed in a safe direction, possibly to the ground.
> 3 - Never point the gun at anyone or anything you do not intend to destroy or kill.
> 3- Keep your finger off the trigger until ready to shoot, do not walk or run with the finger on the trigger.
> 4- Do not rely on the gun's safety mechanism.
> 5- Keep the gun unloaded until ready to use.
> 7- Even a gun loaded with blanks can kill, treat blanks as real bullets.

It might be reassuring to remember that Police figures in the United Kingdom for the year 2008-09 indicate 39 firearms-related deaths of which seven involved a shotgun.

This total figure is the lowest recorded by the police in 20 years. Guns are present in just 0.3% of all recorded crimes, one in every 330 incidents. It is a different story though in the USA or South Africa, where guns are more available.

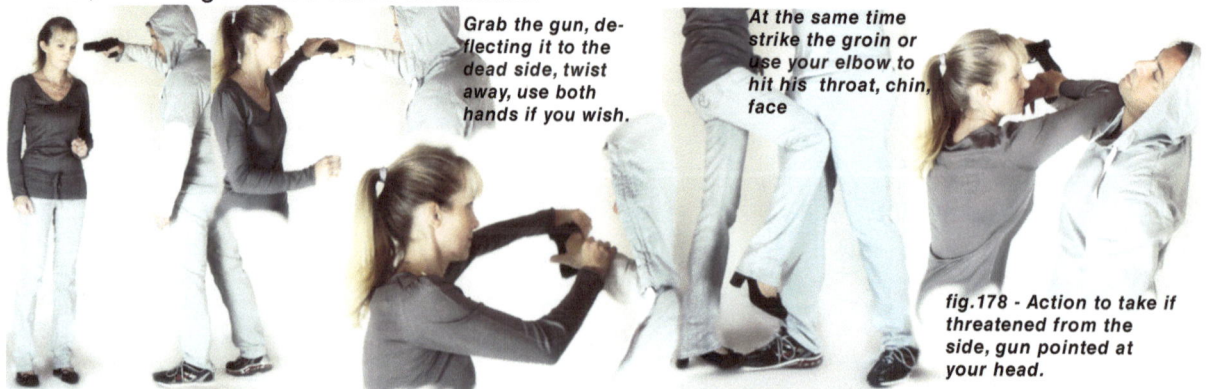

Grab the gun, deflecting it to the dead side, twist away, use both hands if you wish.

At the same time strike the groin or use your elbow to hit his throat, chin, face

fig.178 - Action to take if threatened from the side, gun pointed at your head.

fig.179 - The dynamics of a knife fight mostly see a side stabber joining in after someone else starts the action. Did you spot the knife?

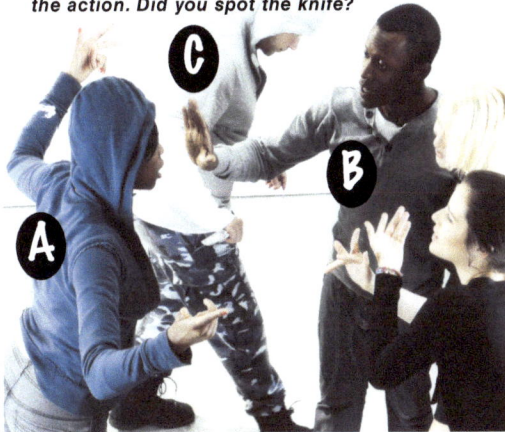

Personally and from past experience I find a threat carried out with a knife much more difficult to handle. First of all a knife is rarely used as you see in films, with the attacker coming at you, knife drawn and assuming a challenging posture, quite the opposite, a knife is normally used from a concealed stance, and you realise you have been stabbed long after the event, the majority of people that have been stabbed, myself included, thought they were punched.

So how can anyone defend themselves against a concealed knife? The honest answer is that you can't, the only defence is avoiding a possible scenario or trouble spot at the first sign of trouble.

The main difference between a knife and a gun is actually how fast a knife, yes you read correctly, a knife, can be employed to harm someone. The US Police have conducted numerous tests to calculate what it takes to respond to someone using a knife in a violent attack, and the results are not very encouraging.

What has emerged is that by the time an assailant has extracted a knife and lunged at an officer the average Policeman is still extracting his weapon and he's not ready to fire, unless the distance is more than 21 feet (6.4 meters). If the distance is about that or less the chances of getting stabbed before being able to use a firearm are almost 100%. This why there is the saying "rush a gun, run from a knife", meaning that you do have more chances to disarm someone holding a gun if you move closer, lighting fast, but the only serious option against a knife is to run. Don't worry about someone throwing the knife at you as you run away, it only happens in films.

fig.180 - Different types of knives: can you guess which one is a mugger's favorite? The answer can be found at the end of the chapter.

Let's be absolutely honest about knives, the majority of people carrying a knife do so because it's part of a certain street culture, a credo. Forget about people carrying a utility knife or the odd teenager that carries it because he thinks it will make him safe. I am talking about people, thugs if you prefer, who consider the knife to be an instrument of daily intimidation and are happy to use it without thinking twice. They use it, not just to threaten someone but actually to stab him: their language is the knife.

A common myth believed by people who have no experience of "knife" culture is the notion that when people fight with knives they do it "duel" style, like they have seen in "the wild one" or "rumble fish". That is total fiction. When people fight with knives, mostly rival gangs, it's all over in seconds, a few seconds, not minutes and all these fights are dirty and ugly, there is no honour or square fight, it's vicious and a cowardly act. Often confrontation of this kind will have subject A distracting subject B, while a mate (C) of A stabs B from the side (fig. 179). All this considered, how can anyone expect to fight someone with a knife just empty handed? Every time I come across anyone teaching blocks and moves to par a knife I get really frustrated, because it is totally unrealistic.

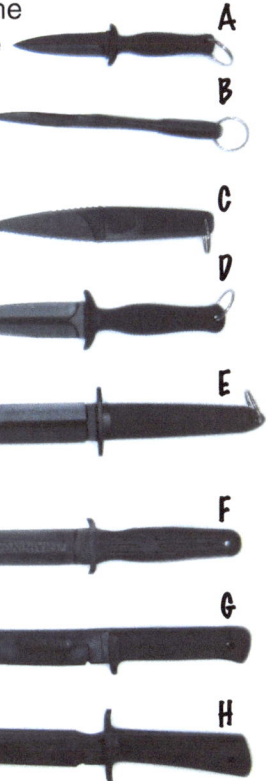

KNIFE FIGHTS ARE OVER IN JUST A FEW SECONDS.

fig.181 - A simple exercise: how many markings are there in red? How many in green? Would you get none?

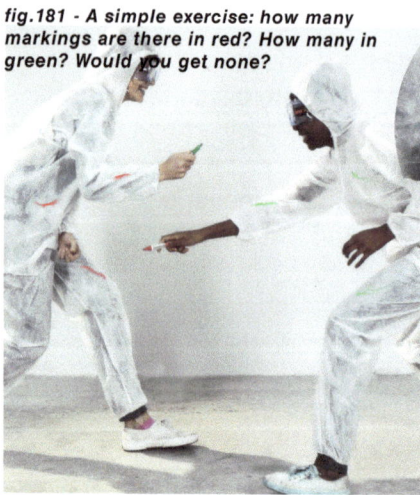

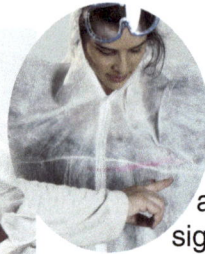

One of the exercises I normally use to demonstrate this is having two people wearing white overalls, the paper thin ones, and safety goggles. Then I arm them in turn with large and long red and green felt markers, the type used to write big signs, and then I tell them to attack in turns pretending the marker is a knife.

fig.181 A - Knife concealing technique.

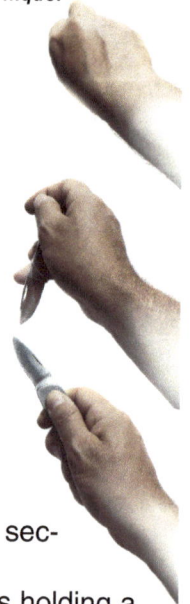

After few seconds is very clear by the number of red or green strikes on the overalls what are the chances of not getting cut, zero (fig.181). I am also aware though that in case you are fighting for your own life and you cannot run from the knife you should at least know what the options are in terms of ultimate survival, because as we have seen you do not defend yourself from a knife attack, yo u survive one. Just consider what protocol and guidelines law enforcement personnel, especially in the USA, have in place when dealing with a knife-wielding individual. After the usual voice commands to drop the weapon and so on they shoot the knife carrier, before the attacker gets closer than 21 feet. This because they cannot take any chances, especially because Police officers are taught according the so called Tueller Drill, by the name of the Police sergeant who demonstrated that drawing your weapon and firing at an assailant holding a knife does not result in a stopping maneuver, because an adrenaline fuelled aggressor would cover seven meters (21 feet) in an average 1.5 seconds, way too short to react with a weapon effectively.

KEEPING A DISTANCE OF AT LEAST 7 METERS IS THE SAFEST OPTION.

(!) The conclusion of the Tueller study was that anyone with aggressive intentions holding a knife at 21 feet or less is a lethal threat. Lets not forget that any blunt sharp edged tool should be equip rated to a knife, be a screwdriver, razor or Stanley knife.

As we have examined before throughout this book, one of the most difficult if not impossible factors to replicate in training is the rush of emotions, fear, confusion etc that a real life situation will bring into the scenario in a very debilitating way.

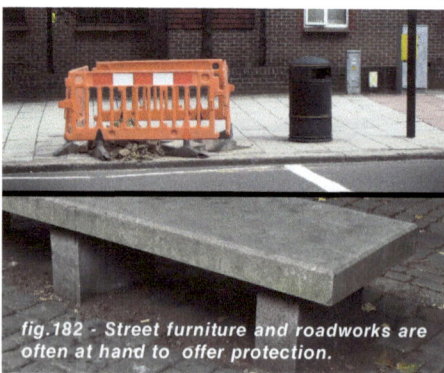

During training I have seen accomplished martial artistes fighting empty handed multiple assailants wielding knives and batons, and hear later on of even more accomplished fighters or experts dying of stab wounds. In a training scenario, even if real knives are used it is always a controllable and predictable environment, while real life is by definition unpredictable, unorthodox, chaotic and unfair, at super speed pace. In any case lets see what can be done, failing

fig.182 - Street furniture and roadworks are often at hand to offer protection.

(!) the chance to run away to safety, and there are some techniques used in knife attacks effectively for a number of reasons, and knowledge of what can be done has contributed sometimes to a successful escape.

As we have seen previously there is no point discussing a defence against a concealed knife, prevention is the only defence.

But if the knife is out rule number one is to keep as much distance as you can from it, treating any move towards you as an attempt to stab you, keep your distance with kicks to the shins, do not grapple, or try to disarm the knife, this is just plain suicide.

Also it's important that in the event you do get stabbed you must keep fighting, do not assume that because he has stabbed you he will leave you alone, the opposite is more likely to happen, that he will carry on stabbing: fight with all your might to stop him. The fact that there is no defence that can theoretically succeed against a knife-wielding attacker does not rule out that you might land a lucky kick to his face or hand, disarming him or knocking him out.

Kicks are more effective than any attempt to try to grab the arm or parrying with your forearm. Keep kicking him away, your shoes offer better protection than anything else that you might have on you.

Do not waste time wrapping up a coat around your arm and nonsense like that. It will just make you slow and more vulnerable.

By all means if you have something to put between you and the aggressor do so, a chair, a table, a briefcase will do, anything to keep him away from you. You can throw sand, plants, use a fire extinguisher or try to place a big object between you and your attacker, a car or a pillar, a railing, street furniture (fig.182). In any case, do not lose sight of your attacker and keep yelling to him to go away and leave you alone.

At all times keep your throat protected (chin down to chest) and upper torso protected or out of the way.   As we have seen before keep your vital organs protected (see VULNERABLE - page 30).

I have seen people falling on purpose on the ground to fend off an assault with a knife, lying on their back and kicking like mad. It might work, but I am not sure I feel ready to advise people on using that as a tactic until I spend more time looking into it. The advantage could be that it makes it more difficult for the attacker to stab you in the stomach or throat, he has to overcome your feet and legs kicking wildly, also most people seem quite reluctant to bend and lean to the ground while fighting, but as I said I haven't tested it properly yet (see GROUNDWORK at page 82 for appropriate techniques).

There is one situation though when empty hand technique can produce results while under threat from a knife, and it's not as uncommon as we might think, especially in rape scenarios, specifically when the threat comes from behind, knife held at the throat, being dragged somewhere.

fig.183 - Different types of knife holds.

ice pick hold

straight hold

oriental hold

concealed hold

fig.184 - Attack from behind, knife at the throat.

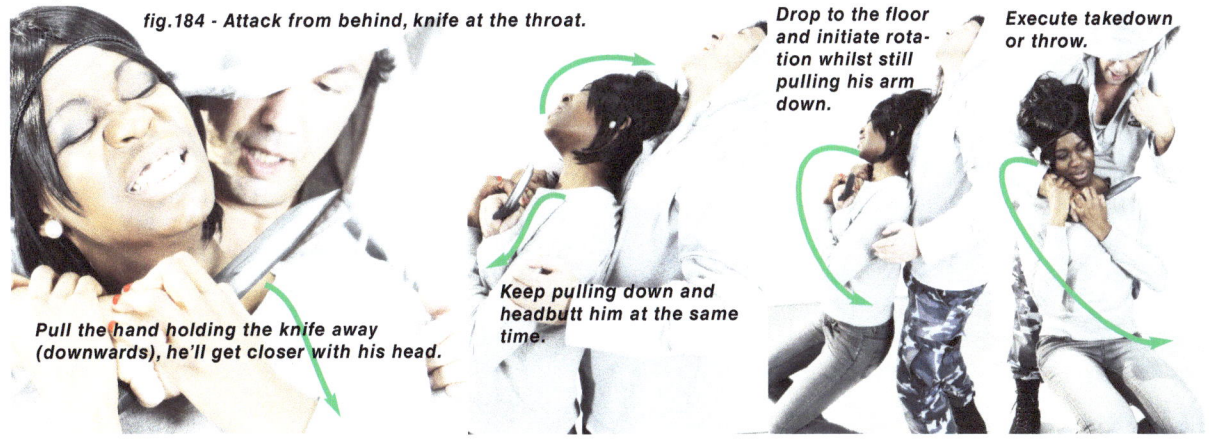

Pull the hand holding the knife away (downwards), he'll get closer with his head.

Keep pulling down and headbutt him at the same time.

Drop to the floor and initiate rotation whilst still pulling his arm down.

Execute takedown or throw.

FULL FORCE

This is a situation where the victim is suddenly taken from behind, and a knife held to the throat. Clearly if the attacker wanted to kill it would have happened already, therefore it is obvious that he wants to drag the victim somewhere (van, car, a secluded spot) to abuse or kidnap his victim.

Since there isn't an immediate intention of killing there's a chance that reacting properly can save your life: remember, acquiescence is no guarantee you'll be spared afterwards, quite the opposite.

fig.185 - Force is transferred towards the opposite end of the hand holding the stick.

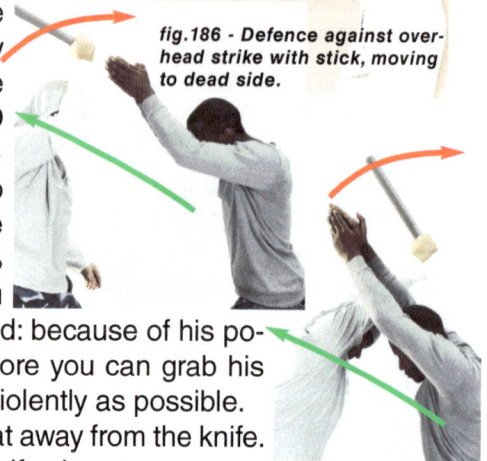

So let's see what can be done: once the initial surprise is gone (yes I know, a bit of an understatement) keep calm but mostly ignore what you are told, almost certainly something on the lines of "SCREAM AND I'LL CUT YOU" or "BE GOOD AND YOU'LL BE OK". Do not believe that is the case, almost certainly it won't be. The main difference in this case compared to what we advised earlier is the fact that the knife is very close and the chances of the situation worsening are almost 100% once you comply. The technique is the same as that you would use to defend yourself against a head lock from behind: because of his position, the attacker cannot control or see your hands, therefore you can grab his wrist and at the same time pull down and head butt him as violently as possible. As an added bonus head butting him will also move your throat away from the knife.

fig.186 - Defence against overhead strike with stick, moving to dead side.

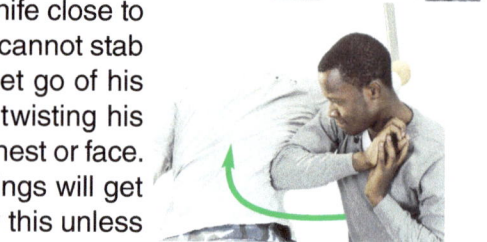

Lift your right shoulder (to make it more difficult to keep the knife close to your throat) and keeping his hand firmly to your chest (so he cannot stab you) turn inward as you bend to release his hold, but don't let go of his hand as you turn. Once you have completed the turn keep twisting his wrist until he releases the knife, and add a knee strike to his chest or face. (fig.188). This is a high risk technique, but if you feel that things will get worse you should go for it, however it is not possible to apply this unless properly supervised by an instructor, the variables are too great and the technique must be repeated many times to perfection.

fig.187 - Defence against stick swung horizontally.

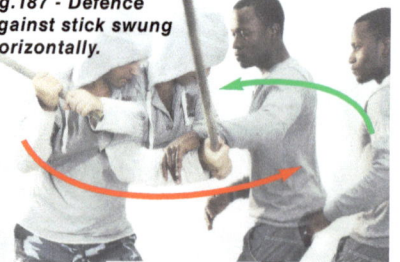

The same thing applies if you are attacked with a stick or a baton: your defence in case someone attacks you with an overhead swing is to move closer, lifting both your arms as shown in fig.186. This position has a double purpose, deflecting the blow to the side (fig.187) and getting you ready to strike the attacker. Your head should be leaning forward, towards the attacker, keeping it between your arms to protect you from a sudden change of direction.

fig.188 - Finish with a knee strike.

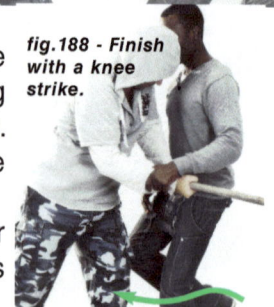

You can advance with either foot, the important thing is that you close the distance fast the moment your attacker raises the stick, avoiding being at a distance where the stick will impact with full force (see fig 185). Your hands (even one hand in position is effective) must aim towards the hand of the person holding the stick.

It should come naturally because our immediate instinct is to raise our hands, but instead of parrying (highly dangerous) you should lean forwards as shown (fig.186).

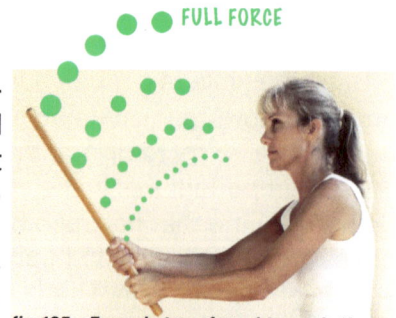

fig.189 - Twist the wrist against the natural movement.

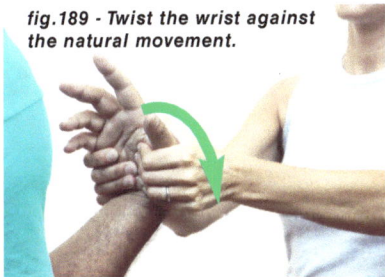

Your position in relation to the direction can be the attacker's left or right, the important factor is how you then finish the move.

If you have moved onto the "dead" side (fig.186) that is the attacker's right side, then you should grab the stick as close as you can to his hand and forcefully bend his wrist to make him lose his grip (fig.189). If you are attacked from the side just spin around to face the attacker and thrust your hand as per fig.186.

The fundamental principle remains the same if the stick is swung "baseball style" horizontally, as seen before, close the distance and with your left arm (if attacked by right handed) go under his armpit to grab your right hand as you swing your elbow onto his face (fig.187). Finish with a knee strike to the groin (fig.188) All these techniques can be applied even to a swing carried out with two hands, the principle and dynamics are the same. If attacked by someone wielding a syringe, threatening to infect you, treat it as a knife attack, keep your distance or use anything to put between you and the syringe. A syringe's needle is very fragile and hitting it with a bag or a kick will easily break it. In any case bear in mind it is a type of attack carried out by people under the influence and they are highly unpredictable and dangerous, often near or in withdrawal, and to bear in mind that if you manage to break the needle they'll try to attack you with something else (for example a broken bottle). Be aware of this possibility. Any attack that is carried out with a blunt instrument is potentially lethal, a knife, machete, screwdriver, Japanese sword (katana) broken bottle, razor, syringe, are all weapons that cause lethal damage easily.

Prison officers know that too well, and most of the training they receive deals with improvised sharp objects, called "shank" in prison jargon. What they learn quickly is that you are either able to put some distance or an obstacle between your vital parts and the knife or you close the distance in a way that you can stop the "stabbing" action, preventing the attacker taking swings at you.

Discussing weapons I am often asked about Pepper sprays: these devices, often sold as little canisters, are made using an extract from chilli pepper suspended in an oily solution that doesn't wash off easily. They are illegal in many countries and can be effective only if the person carrying it has been trained to use it. Just carrying it doesn't help, in actual fact it can be counter productive, you might end up spraying yourself. If sprayed directly into the eyes at a distance of 3-7 feet, the person will be incapacitated for up to 45 minutes, eyes watering copiously, temporarily blind, feeling nauseous and suffocating, accompanied by incontrollable coughing.

A burning sensation to the skin is also common, rubbing the eyes will make it worse, and the only relief is through washing it with baby shampoo and running cold water. Pepper spray is not effective unless ready to hand anytime, the majority of people will lose it inside their bags, and when needed it they won't find it on time.

Often they will spray themselves by accident or their children will hurt themselves playing with it. If someone suffering from asthma is sprayed they can suffer serious damage or even death.

The same applies to stun guns (also known as tazers) or other self-defence tools, most of the time illegal to possess and difficult to deploy. Before carrying or buying one, ask yourself if you REALLY need it.

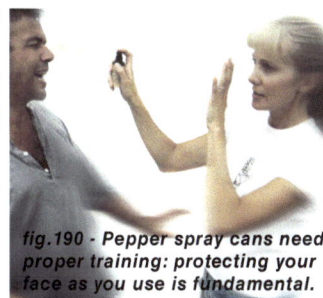

fig.190 - Pepper spray cans need proper training: protecting your face as you use is fundamental.

ANSWERS: The handgun in fig.163 is a real gun modified and made safe for film work. The knives in fig.180 are the following types: A) military vest knife. B) throwing knife C) concealable knife, a mugger's favorite. D) combat knife E) bayonet F) diving knife G) utility knife H) Bowie or hunter's knife.

fig.191 - Understanding body language and a sense of humor can help you getting out of a threatening situation. If you can't beat them, humor them.

switching off

There are fundamentally two types of aggressive behaviour, one so-called "instrumental", meaning any behaviour motivated by obtaining a result, for example defending yourself. The other type, called "hostile" is when the only purpose is to cause damage to a person physically or verbally.

We can also distinguish between an active aggressiveness, where the damage comes from an action like a kick or swearwords and the passive type where the damage is caused for lack of action, for example not helping someone.

Several schools of thought, from Freud to Lorenz, have described man as a naturally aggressive creature because he often obeys strong genetic impulses either sexual or dictated by hunger or predatory instincts.

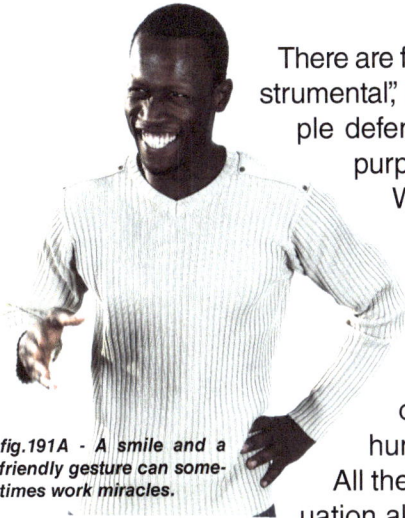

fig.191A - A smile and a friendly gesture can sometimes work miracles.

All these instincts accumulate and discharge themselves when the situation allows. However, there are also other factors affecting man as a human, not just an animal: the environment, personal experience as well as education.

Environmentally we should consider any influence, physical or psychological, surrounding the individual, affecting in different ways and intensity certain aspects of our personality, thus common to everyone, more than others.

If someone has had to fight physically since childhood to survive, he doesn't really consider verbal confrontation as an option, physical force is his language.

Often parents who abuse their children come from a background of abuse themselves, and they apply what they consider their "normal" system of education according to the education received and the values learned.

AGGRESSIVE BEHAVIOR IS OFTEN A PRODUCT OF FRUSTRATION.

Aggressive behaviour is often the product of frustration, coming from many factors like deprivations, punishments, physical impediments, anything that makes the individual feel inadequate or in any case surfacing when he cannot satisfy his needs or desires.

This often translates into channelling anger towards the perceived cause of the frustration.

Typical is the case when the boss is assaulted by a member of staff who perceives him or her as a source of personal frustration at work. The wife is often the unfortunate target of rage induced by frustration and this is the reason why fathers often punish their children with excessive force because they add their frustration to the punishment.

We are discussing this to understand that very often-aggressive behaviour is unplanned, or poorly planned, often unconsciously produced.

Of course, there are exceptions (for example serial killers) that plan every detail very carefully but this is not the right forum to look at that in detail, even though self-defence techniques still apply.

In any case, knowing the basic psychological mechanisms producing aggressive behaviour will allow you to know what to hit psychologically to neutralise an aggressive threat effectively.

Any attacker knows how to have a superior position, because of the surprise factor.

Very often he feels very strong and he feels strongly motivated, almost on a mission. If you are just defending yourself you can only be effective if you don't let the situation (scenario) overwhelm you but you adapt to regain control.

We are perfectly aware that this is easier said than done, we have stressed already that prevention is better, and the first reaction to a threat should be a verbal disengagement. There are some well proven techniques to achieve that, let's see what really works.

A firm tone often works, especially when a date goes in a direction that makes you uncomfortable. If

fig.192 -Turning your back and running away from an attacking dog is the worst thing you can do.

you have gone out with someone and quite fancy him but you are not quite ready to have sex with that person then avoid sending signals that most men will tend to misinterpret. If he takes you back home and you ask him if he wants to come up for a cup of coffee you can expect that what he understand is "come in for wild sex".

If you really want him to come in for a while it is better to state very clearly that coffee is all he is going to get. This is when self-defence, if taught properly, can help, as a general state of mind to understand and prevent. Don't think of learning how to defend yourself just as a series of striking techniques, joint locks, or throws. Think of it as an attitude that allows you to think and react properly in response to a threat of any kind, including a dog attack.

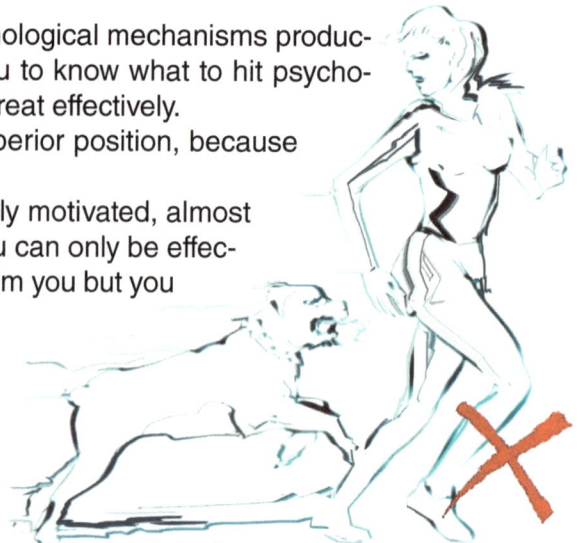

Turning your back on the dog and running, or freezing and falling to the ground are common reactions for the untrained person but if you are trained, in other words if you know how to, you can handle the situation.

In this case, you know that running is bad, it will provoke the dog into attacking you, while standing your ground and wrap anything around your arm quickly offering as a target, can save your life.

These reactions are the product of experience-derived techniques, knowing what works best in that given scenario (see also ANIMALS - page 160).

To stand your ground when somebody physically grabs you will surprise him, putting you in a superior position. This doesn't necessarily mean reacting physically every time. Reacting also means using a firm tone to stop the aggressor in his tracks, again surprising him. Don't forget that an aggressor perceives his victim as incapable to react, verbally and physically. This is why when somebody is subjected to abuse repeatedly, over a long period of time there is a vicious circle where the more he or she is abused the more insecure and withdrawn the victim becomes. Also you shouldn't rely, and I say this with great sadness, on other people coming to your rescue.

There is a phenomenon called "COLLECTIVE INERTIA" studied by psychologists and sociologists alike all over the world. Basically, before somebody would help somebody under attack or when threatened, he wants to make sure that the threat or attack is real, meaning not a game between lovers for instance.

This happened to me a few years ago, tackling someone who was chasing a woman in the street. As I tackled him and pinned him to the ground the woman came back, yelling at me in tears to leave him alone. It turned out they were just messing around and being foolish. Apart from being hugely embarrassed I nearly got into trouble for assault. Would I do it again? Yes, maybe though I would probably wait a bit longer, just to make sure my judgement is correct. Generally speaking quite unfortunately the common perception is that if several people are present everyone will think it's up to the others to intervene, therefore nobody does.   So the general belief is that because nobody is intervening there is no need to do so.

All this helps you to understand what goes on psychologically in a threatening or aggressive situation. I have witnessed someone succeeding in throwing a big man onto the floor and being shocked at how easy it was.

YOU CAN IF YOU WANT, IT'S AS SIMPLE AS THAT.

This tells you that we often tend to overestimate the aggressor and we just become passive because we think there is no point resisting, we are sure that we cannot succeed and then it's not even worth trying.

Think about two athletes competing against each other, having the same build, the same diet, the same training. Only the one with the will to win is going to win.

We have seen in VICTIMS (page 14), that we shouldn't feel sorry for ourselves and we shouldn't think that resisting is futile. Instead we should learn to conquer fear and not let other people intimidate us only because we think that they are stronger: you become a victim the moment you think of yourself as a victim. Based upon these notions let's see how SWITCHING OFF works in practice. One of my favourite techniques when confronted by someone who is trying to pick a fight, has always been answering to his threatening behaviour with a big smile, raising my hands in surrender, saying something like "Sorry, I don't really want to cause any trouble...Really sorry" and as I

IF YOU THINK YOU ARE A VICTIM, YOU ARE MAKING YOURSELF A VICTIM.

am turning away, carry on my turn transforming into a spinning side-kick to his stomach (see fig.58 - page 45).
So why is such a fancy kick suddenly effective?

fig.193 - As I am turning away I transform my turning into a spinning side-kick to his stomach.

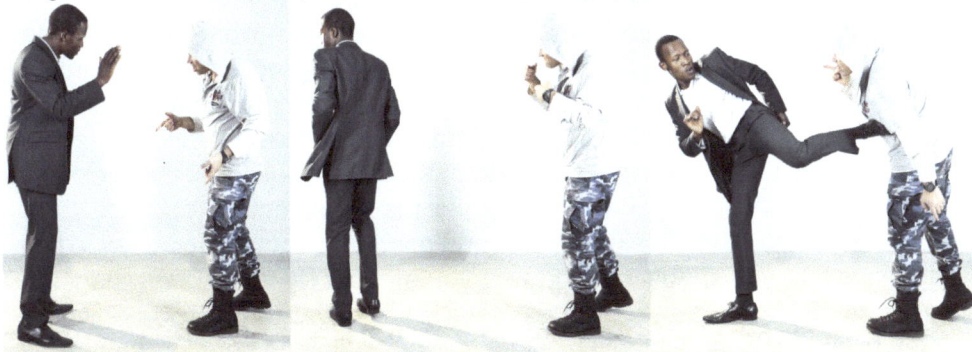

The reasons rest on several factors. He's moving towards me to control me and probably throw a punch; he is angry, full of adrenaline and prepared for a fight.

If I react in the same manner we are both going to get hurt.

So first of all I have to switch him off, meaning stop the flow of adrenaline and anger that increases his strength, raise the pain threshold and gives him fast reactions.

As I smile and apologise, he immediately perceives me as a coward or in any case not as a threat, so his defence and aggressive mechanisms go down, relaxing.

He's less alert and probably will keep moving towards me to mock me as I walk away.

As I turn I carry on my action tensing up as I kick him, doubling the effect of the kick since he is walking right into it. This is an extreme example but it summarises from start to finish what the switching off technique is about.

Personally, I take great pride if I succeed in diffusing a volatile situation with words and body language only, believe me I'm not an aggressive person and I believe violence should only be used to defend your-self when everything else fails.

But that is often not possible and I have a verbal sequence that will "make" me hit the aggressor no matter what. In other words because deciding to hit someone is quite difficult, especially if you are a decent human being, decide that in case you will be facing a potentially violent confrontation you will have a phrase that you will use that will make you hit that someone.

Ideally use something that engages his brain for a period of time just long enough to "switch off" his adrenaline or alertness.

A good example is something that has nothing to do with the situation at hand, for instance "tell me why you are so handsome?" This kind of question does two things, confuses him because it has nothing to do with the situation and at the same time cannot be answered with a simple "yes" or "no", meaning you make him talk.

That is when you strike. Delaying or trying to talk your way out of it is plain suicide.

However if you think it can be resolved with an apology then do so.

BODY LANGUAGE DETERMINES YOUR APPEARANCE.

I just apologise even at the classic "what are you looking at?" This ends aggressive behaviour towards me and I am happy to say sorry without feeling hurt.

Sometimes though, like when you turn your back on an attacking animal, this behaviour is perceived as an identifying mark for easy prey and turns into an attack, often with a sucker punch (fig.196).

As we have seen before in other sections, a softening technique, like a trick or creating a distraction, could help you to build your window of opportunity.

To understand this, we should examine the importance of body language.

We normally think that words define us. Instead what really describes best what we are the way we move and carry ourselves. Somebody who has bad intentions will select his target carefully, he wants no fuss, and prefers somebody who is submissive and doesn't cause any trouble.

Next time you are in a busy place have a look around and think who would you challenge to an arm wrestling contest? I really don't think you would stop the passing bodybuilder or the occasional burly man, and now you can get the idea of how potential victims are selected.

IF YOU KNOW WHAT TO DO, YOU CAN DO IT.

Ask yourself if, as you walk, you look assertive and confident or timid and easy to bully. I'm not suggesting that you should change who you are, but try to avoid constant fidgeting with your hands, looking away all the time and walking with your chin down. Force yourself to feel that with a bit of knowledge you can defend yourself, if you know what to do, you can certainly do it. So the first rule to apply effective switch-off techniques is becoming more self-assertive, relaxed and confident. Imagine a teacher going through the lesson to her pupils and being very insecure, nervous and fidgety.

What kind of atmosphere would you have in such class? There would probably be total chaos with the odd paper plane landing on the teacher's desk.

So if you have to confront somebody for whatever reason, if they are threatening or molesting you, think of them as children that need to be told off. Use a polite but firm tone, and speak to them as a police officer or a teacher would, leaving no chance to answer inappropriately.

If you don't know what to say, maybe because you have been outsmarted, smile politely and don't say anything, in order not to provoke further reactions.

What has worked in the past for a few people is pretending that you know a relative well, for instance you look at the group or at more than one person at the same time and say "I know your mother/sister and she won't be pleased when she finds out".

If the answer that comes back is "My mother died three years ago" or "I don't have a sister" point to someone to the group you were looking and say "not you him!"

To do this you need to be bold though and it only works if there is a group.

If you are one to one or have been abducted it will make things worse and he might decide to kill you so you won't tell. An effective and well-known technique is to repeat in a very firm voice the same set of words over and over again, like a "broken record".

For instance, if somebody is insistent upon following you, your best line of action will be to turn around, standing your ground and repeating at first a couple of times "Stop following me, go away." Without adding anything, repeating exactly the same words a few times with the same tone, truly like a broken record. This normally has the effect of disarming the other person; it is not a reaction he or she would expect. It is equally important to show no anger and only confidence and assertiveness; your message should be that you are not accepting the other person's behaviour.

STOP FEELING SORRY FOR YOURSELF, BE CONFIDENT, BE BOLD.

Confidence doesn't come from one source; it is a feeling that grows with you, increasing with training, experience and keeping an attitude of not feeling sorry for yourself. Basically what you want to show is that you are not an easy prey, and to let someone who has bad intentions that he is not welcome. As we've said before people that would attack another person, especially the sexually motivated types, are more often than not cowards with serious sexual problems, incapable of having normal relationships (we are keeping this simple, in fact it's obviously much more complicated). We have seen in VICTIMS (page 14), how the shock of actually being attacked makes you freeze and unable to react. People who have been subjected to attacks and were unable to react, usually suffer huge guilt, thinking they should have reacted and fought back. In fact, they were only reacting that way because they have no previous experience of violence or similar situation. They had no time to react and their main state of mind was of denial, thinking, "This is not happening to me." To sum it up, you can switch off someone with bad intentions showing a calm, confident approach, watching your body language; avoiding doing anything that gives away signs

DO NOT FEEL GUILTY IF YOU FAILED TO REACT.

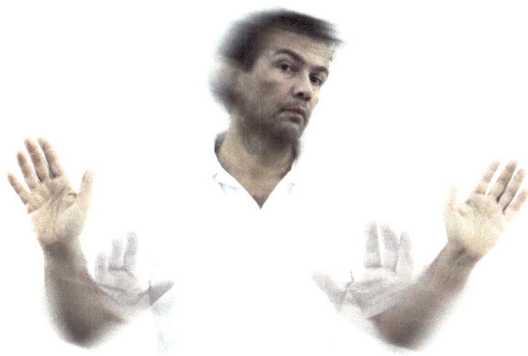
fig.194 - *Raise your hands and apologize.*

of fear, such as looking down, quivering or high pitched voice, sweating profusely. Repeat mentally many times "I can do this... I can do this. I can do this".

If somebody cuts you up while driving, your reaction immediately is to blow the horn and mouth some unpleasant epithets. As most of you know it can cause the other person to get out of the car with seriously bad intentions. Raise your arms, smile and mouth with your lips "I am sorry" and then gesture at the same time to go ahead and not block traffic. Also pointing your right index at your temple and gesturing a trigger being pulled, as if saying you are at fault, works effectively.

The same applies if somebody in a bar or pub spills a drink over you, of course your first reaction would be to swear, but even if that person was trying to provoke you, try to diffuse the situation and especially when alcohol is involved remember that everything feels amplified and louder, and most people under the effect of alcohol become very aggressive.

AVOIDING CONFRONTATION IS ALWAYS THE BEST ATTITUDE. Avoiding confrontations is always better than resorting to physical action, even if you are just trying to defend yourself.

You should always try to make someone who is threatening you think and in a calm tone appeal to his heart or feelings.

You could try for instance if someone is trying to rape you, or if you think you are in danger of it, to say things like "please stop, what if someone would do this to your sister, mother, girlfriend." The aim is to create either a window of opportunity to strike or to flee, but maybe you might be able to make him stop altogether and he might even apologise. It has happened.

Always report a rape or attempted rape to the authorities; you might save someone else from going through the same ordeal or worse.

A calm approach to most heated moments is always the first line of defence, and it does help adding a bit of humour, if you are naturally good at it.

A few years ago, I was crossing the road with a friend and a car came out of nowhere at a crazy speed and nearly ran us over. As we jumped to safety, my friend yelled something I cannot write here. The car came to an abrupt halt, and reversed manically to where we were. The man that came out of the car was huge and very intimidating. I stood up, smiled, and said

WHAT IS THE POINT OF ARGUING WITH SOMEONE ANGRILY? "You don't earn many points running over average guys, you should try with old ladies, crossing with a Zimmer frame."

The man stopped in his tracks, laughed nervously and then suddenly grabbed me and started crying, holding me tight to his chest, my feet inches off the ground. His wife had just left him, he hated his job, and he was tired and lonely.

Gasping for air I managed to breathe out "Let's go for a drink".

We are still friends after all these years. Remember, violence calls for more violence: your first line of defence, prevention aside, should be de-escalating a situation.

You shouldn't try to outsmart somebody who is trying to intimidate you, do not patronise him. At the same time do not argue, but still make your point.

Be polite but firm and keep you're hands down without gesticulating, that certainly irritates most people. Don't raise your voice and listen to what he has to say, keeping your distance. Do not turn away or show him that you are not really interested in what he has to say, that could really inflame things. Just repeat, "Please calm down, I can't hear if you shout ", and maybe ask him to sit down for a second.

APOLOGIZE EVEN IF YOU FEEL IT'S NOT YOUR FAULT. If all this doesn't work just say, "Listen if you keep shouting and swearing at me I won't be able to answer". For instance, you are minding your own business, lost in your thoughts, and suddenly someone says, "Are you looking at me?" or similar.

Quietly, firmly, without showing distress, politely reply, "I really don't see why I should, can you?" This will make him realise the stupidity of his behaviour and often that will be the end of it. You didn't say "No I'm not", you didn't apologise, and basically you didn't submit.

You simply stood your ground and gave him no chance of using your answer against you.

Another good answer would be "Yes, I was: you look like a good friend of mine, but obviously I was mistaken." His only reply can be "Yes, you are." and it ends there.

This last particular answer has worked well in cases when someone is trying to use skin colour or other race related issues to provoke a fight. If you find yourself threatened by someone of a different race, letting him know that you have friends like him will make him realise you are not staring at him because of the colour of his skin (were you?).

Using switching off you also have the ability to distract your opponent in all sorts of ways.

The classic trick in Western films pretending somebody is coming to your rescue from behind your opponent always works and always gives you a good window of opportunity.

Similarly, you can call to a passer-by, pretending you know him, ask him to come here or quickly run to him, pretending you are joining him.

That person might think you are a bit weird but in any case it will help you getting out of a potentially harmful situation.

MAKING A FOOL OF YOURSELF IS A GOOD DEFENCE.

If you are being threatened, even at gunpoint, you could even pretend you are having an asthma attack or a heart attack and fall to the ground, shouting to call an ambulance, it has been used and it always works, for some reason people can't cope with that and flee. When it comes to survival anything counts.

Are you worried about your dignity or about making a fool of yourself?

Years ago I survived an assault by armed bandits in Africa, stripping myself naked and jumping around pretending to be a monkey. They were laughing so hysterically that they didn't notice that I grabbed one of the machine guns and they fled as soon as I started firing into the air. It worked.

Embarrassing? Not at all, a good sense of humour is a very good defensive weapon.

There are countless cases when behaving in a funny way managed to resolve the threat.

The latter approach is a good way to defend yourself against a madman, or somebody who is drunk, since in both cases there is a huge flow of emotive status in their mind.

Given the chance and the proper environment you can act drunk (you can wobble and assume the classic lost look with your eyes). For instance if you end up upsetting somebody in a bar situation and he's threatening you, you can just say "I'm sorry, I had too much to drink, I didn't mean it." and stagger your way out.

Switching off relies heavily on distracting techniques, so think on your feet about what you can do to distract and divert the attention of whoever is threatening you.

Normally, standing your ground if outnumbered won't work. If there is a mob, like a small crowd, angered for whatever reason or simply fuelled by alcohol, you might try and dispatch the first one who is laying hands on you, and the others might have second thoughts but most of the time this might just have the effect of pouring petrol over flames, you are just going to make things worse. So in this particular case, try to escape early enough, if you can't then back yourself up to a wall and make yourself small, pretend you are sick and throw up, and if you can make yourself cry, do so. The angry mob will think you

MAKE YOURSELF SMALL IF IT'S A BIG MOB.

are not worth it, most probably you will feel ashamed and embarrassed at your behaviour afterwards but at least you are alive and unhurt.

If you spot a gang of teenagers or school children fighting it is better if you don't intervene, you might end up hurting them and end up in court for assault.

Call the police if you think it's not just play fight, and shout that you have just called the police and that they should stop NOW. In the case of two men fighting, (including when one is a friend or a relative) it is a potentially very dangerous situation, and if they don't stop at your requests call the police and just keep an eye on them from a safe distance.

HIT YOUR ATTACKER'S PERSONALITY.

Switching off in an attempted rape scenario relies on making yourself seen as a person, not just an object.

An attacker who is using violence towards you does not want to know your name, cannot see you as a person and does not want to see you as a person. So remember in this and similar cases, try to appeal to the attackers' heart, tell him you are a mother, sister, anything that you can see that can appeal to his "good side" if we can call it as such.

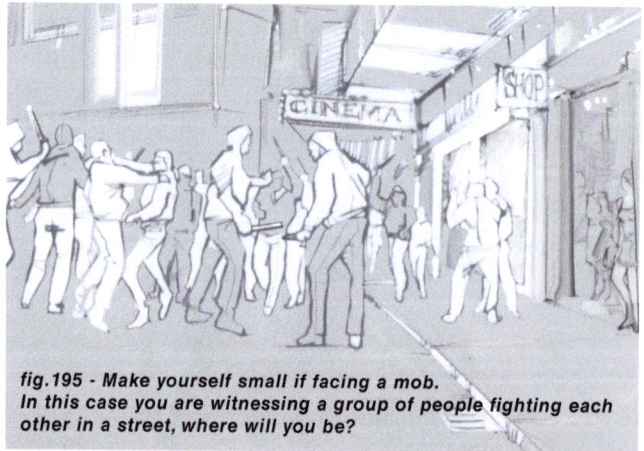

fig.195 - Make yourself small if facing a mob. In this case you are witnessing a group of people fighting each other in a street, where will you be?

There have been cases where a woman subjected to rape managed to convince not the actual person on top of her but one of the others in the group to stop the violence, simply by saying "What about if somebody did this to your sister, mother, girlfriend?"

CREATE A DISTRACTION, ALL YOU NEED IS AN OPPORTUNITY TO FLEE.

This tells you that even when you might think the attacker is only driven by his barest instinct, you can still hit some part of his personality that might switch him off.

Another technique, in this case, is to pretend you are sick, or sticking two fingers down your throat, throw up. As we have seen in other sections this might also create a window of opportunity and allow you to strike back. In any case not complying might be the best solution. In many cases of violent rape when the attacker was interviewed later on by Police he said that because the victim "complied" they needed to be punished because he saw her submission as slut's behaviour.

If confronted by a group, especially teenagers, don't try to outsmart them, their reaction wil be to feel patronised and they will attack you.

Instead, calmly tell them to stop behaving like children and act like men.

The most common reason for loutish behaviour is to attract attention and look tough, that in the youngster's mind is synonymous with being grown-up.

There is always a leader in any group, and you can address the leader in a calm, firm manner saying something like: "Stop, there is no need for this!" and giving a half smile, quietly leave,

BE VERY AWARE OF THE SUCKER PUNCH, KEEP YOUR DISTANCE!

always keeping an eye on what's going on around you, because as you leave there is a good chance that you'll be on the receiving end of a "sucker punch".

A sucker punch is when without any warning and often delivered from close range, your aggressor or one of his mates hits you. Very often it is given while smiling or talking, and it is not necessarily a punch, often it can manifest as a head butt or worse. It is a technique to end a fight before it even starts, and it is difficult to avoid.

fig.196 - Beware of the sucker punch as you walk away. Often coming from a mate of the person you argued with.

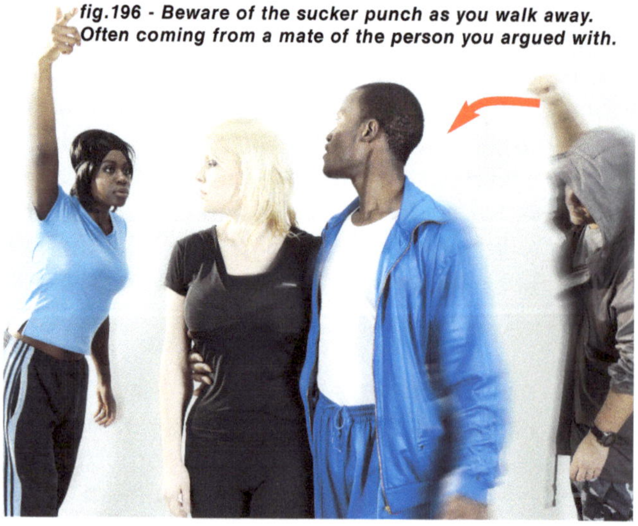

The only form of defence is to keep your distance at all time, at least one and half metres (4-5 feet). It is sometimes thrown feigning fear or submission, very often also when you are walking away certain that all is resolved.

That is the reason why you should never lose sight of someone who has shown aggressive behaviour, especially if and when in the company of a few mates.

As soon as you walk away he will go for a sucker punch, intended to cause maximum damage and using surprise as the main factor. Sadly I need to add that sometimes unfortunately the sucker punch takes the shape of a knife strike.

Switching off means de-escalating a situation, avoiding confrontation, and using distracting techniques, always bearing in mind that it is not just what you say verbally, it's your entire body language that is also communicating with the people threatening you. A fight is decided before punches are exchanged, just by body language.

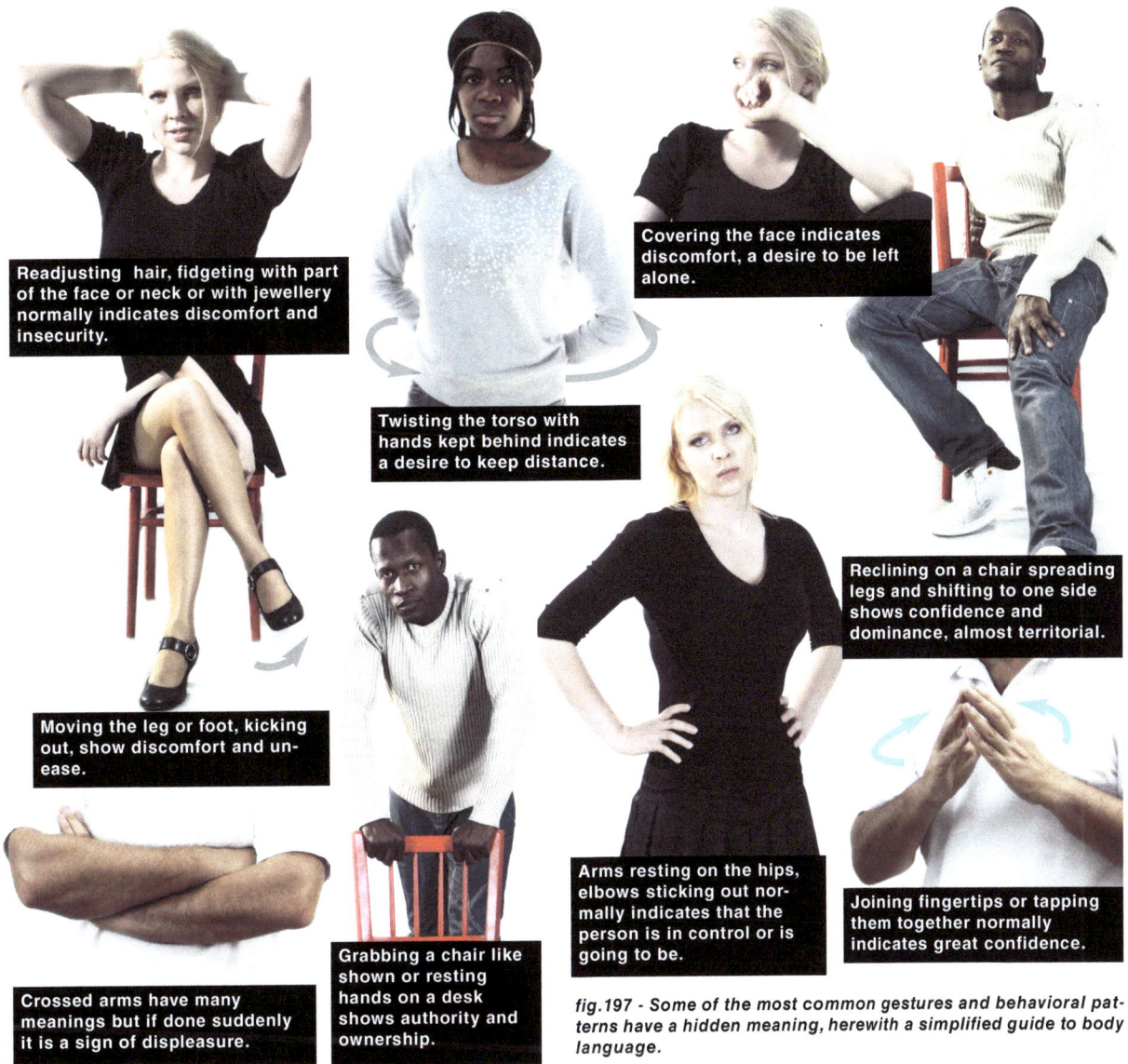

Readjusting hair, fidgeting with part of the face or neck or with jewellery normally indicates discomfort and insecurity.

Covering the face indicates discomfort, a desire to be left alone.

Twisting the torso with hands kept behind indicates a desire to keep distance.

Reclining on a chair spreading legs and shifting to one side shows confidence and dominance, almost territorial.

Moving the leg or foot, kicking out, show discomfort and unease.

Arms resting on the hips, elbows sticking out normally indicates that the person is in control or is going to be.

Joining fingertips or tapping them together normally indicates great confidence.

Crossed arms have many meanings but if done suddenly it is a sign of displeasure.

Grabbing a chair like shown or resting hands on a desk shows authority and ownership.

fig.197 - Some of the most common gestures and behavioral patterns have a hidden meaning, herewith a simplified guide to body language.

fig.198 - White on white? Or a small black number?

blending in

We have briefly mentioned in VICTIMS (page 14), how important it is not to stand out, but instead to blend in with the environment. The attention you are likely to get if you turn up dressed to kill wearing your best jewellery at a posh party, is the one you would expect, compliments and envious looks, but dressed in the same way walking downtown late at night will certainly get the kind of attention that you rather never experience. Obviously?

You'll be surprised at how many people walk or come back from a fancy do dressed up wearing expensive items without considering the safety of the location where they are walking It is better to wear a normal coat and normal shoes and put your smart shoes in a bag, so that you don't attract attention.

DRESS DOWN IF YOU CAN. ESPECIALLY IF EVERYONE AROUND DOES.

You can leave everything at reception or take off the coat and replace your shoes just before you get in. Consider the route you will be taking, and plan how you'll get back, especially if you think you might have a drink or two. It is always wise to organise something with a couple of friends and travel together; you can always return the favour when they need the same.

"Blending in" also means that if you sit in an empty carriage on the underground or a train, not to sit right in the middle with empty seats all around you but to close the door at the end of the seats' row, ideally within reach of the alarm. In that way you avoid standing out as well as having people with bad intentions sitting on both sides of you and jamming you amongst them.

If you are driving to a party or other venue in your own car, on top of locking yourself in it is wise to take off expensive earrings and anything that you might consider tempting that can be seen through the windows of your car.

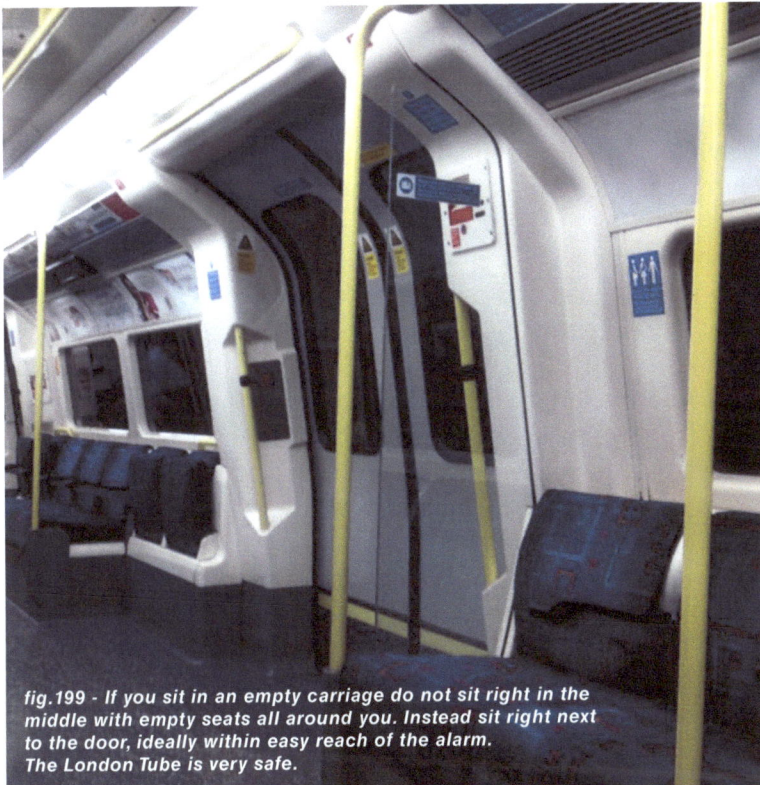

fig.199 - If you sit in an empty carriage do not sit right in the middle with empty seats all around you. Instead sit right next to the door, ideally within easy reach of the alarm. The London Tube is very safe.

If you are taking a taxi remove expensive jewellery including your watch before getting in, it might even save you some money on the fare: generally speaking, "blending in" means to avoid attracting attention and dress appropriately.

For instance, if you are on holiday and you are going to a country where tourists are often a target, see what the locals wear, and buy something similar or the same from a local shop to blend in and it also makes a nicer souvenir than the usual bag almost certainly made in China.

ARE YOU DISCRETE WHEN YOU TALK ON YOUR CELL PHONE IN PUBLIC?

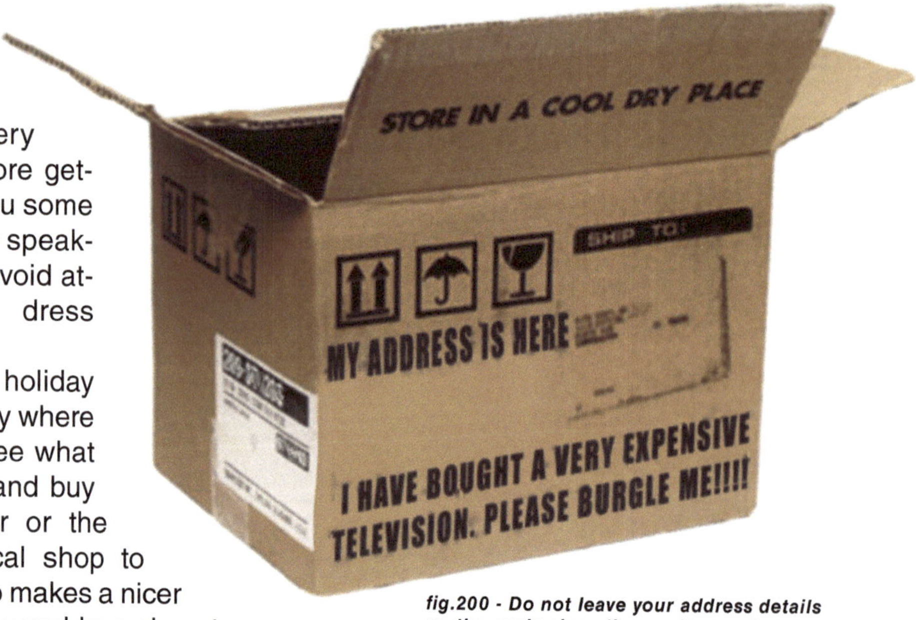

fig.200 - Do not leave your address details on the packaging, dispose it away from home, in this case ideally in a recycling centre!

DO NOT DISPLAY YOUR LIFESTYLE OUTSIDE YOUR HOME.

Avoid in general talking loudly on the mobile phone as you walk, especially if you are discussing wedding arrangements or moving house or that brilliant new laptop you just bought. Avoid anything that might shout "I'm loaded, come on burgle me".

You can blend in at home as well: if you have just bought a new fancy TV set do not put the cardboard box with massive Japanese logo outside your house. Doing so is an open invitation to check out the new TV, probably when you are not in. To be on the safe side remove or deface your address details on the box and dispose of the box away from home, ideally in a recycling centre. Simple, you might think, I already do that, you might add. Really? Think again, because a few of the lines of action that follow might actually surprise you.

The general attitude should be to be aware of your surroundings, and act accordingly, just think that Special Forces when they work in certain countries happily grow a beard and wear what everyone else wears, hiding their hi-tech armament under it.

Blending in is very useful also when panic strikes in a crowd.

We have said many times panic is the killer and you can imagine a crowd in a confined environment turning into a stampede if for example there is a fire or anything else happening perceived as dangerous.

It is good practice if you attend an event where a large number of people are involved, such as a concert, big conference, even at the cinema, to familiarise yourself with escape routes and emergency exits. It is also a good and wise practice to see if there is something close to you that can shelter you if the crowd suddenly tries to run over you, for instance, a large column or a pillar, a niche behind a statue, anything that can shield you from a stampede.

AVOID EYE CONTACT WITH PASSERS BY, BUT STAY VIGILANT.

In other words, blending in with the wallpaper is what you want to do; chameleons have perfected throughout evolution their camouflaging.

If you have to go through a "rough area" or in any case an area where people are dressed in a certain way, we recommend try at least to match the general look if you want a chance of not becoming a target.

Not attracting attention, that is the principle of blending in, also means avoiding eye contact: next time you walk through a busy street in a modern metropolis, such as New York for instance, you will notice that people walk keeping their eyes down, deep in their thoughts, busy within their daily routine. People walk fast and with a purpose, walking around in an enchanted stupor state will attract attention.

All they are thinking of is going from A to B in the shortest of time with the least possible hassle: we will notice that standing out from most people are the tourists with their eyes transfixed to anything that catches their curiosity.

To really blend in, just pretend you live there, so look around and make a mental note of body language, pace of walking and if in a foreign country, buy a local newspaper and put it under your arm even if it is in Cyrillic or Arabic, it is also a lot of fun.

If somebody stops you and talks to you in the local language pretend you lost your voice, make some guttural sounds and point to your throat.

You might think that if you are blonde and fair skin and very tall it will make you look a bit ridiculous walking around with a Chinese newspaper, but in fact it will give the impression that you have been working there for quite a while and you speak the language and have connections and friends, it will say in any case that you are not lost or unfamiliar with the surroundings.

When you travel to countries where the language is very difficult for Westerners, such as in Asia or Russia for instance, a set of cards that have simple phrases written on it with the translation in the appropriate local language can be useful, and ones which show pictures too are even better. If you own a so called smart phone you can download useful applications that can do just that.

Such extreme behaviour might seem funny to you in the comfort of your armchair in your own house reading this, but believe me I'm very serious about it.

Just think of a black rabbit in a snow-covered field with birds of prey flying over his head. What colour would you really like to be if you were the rabbit?

Let's see how blending in works when it comes to more practical aspects of your life, such as a job interview or, if you are an actress or model, just starting out or with some experience, how to go to auditions and be safe at all times.

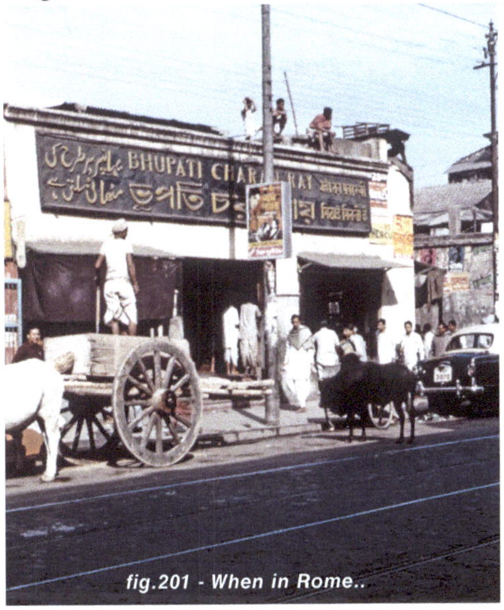

NEVER... NEVER EVER GIVE YOUR HOME ADDRESS TO ANYONE.

fig.201 - When in Rome..

The first rule is that you should never give out your personal details, such as your home address and home telephone number, it is better if you provide your agent's details, this is also what an agent is there for, to act as a filter. If you don't have one, ask a male friend if he doesn't mind pretending to be your agent.

Never meet anyone, director or producer or whoever, at their home, neither in a pub, restaurant or tube station. If they are professionals they will set up a proper casting call in a casting suite or at the very least at the Production office during normal working hours.

Be very wary of casting calls or adverts asking to turn up in a "sexy" outfit. If they are legitimate (check them out in any case) turn up "normally dressed" on the outside and "sexy" underneath.

If you can you should try to talk to a real person on the phone before the meeting, get a feel for it and if it doesn't sound right just don't go. Do not accept a lift back or accept to be picked up to go to the meeting, it will send to the interviewer the wrong signal.

Also, make sure that your details are not on the web already: do a search on Google and type your "name and surname" in quotation marks, see where and what comes up with it and amend accordingly, and make sure your curriculum vitae has no home address on it. It doesn't take much time and you might even find some seriously interesting things.

If you need a portfolio or book to be returned don't give your home address but set up a mailbox. Preferably have it collected.

WE ARE JUDGED BY APPEARANCES

In the same way that body language can reveal a lot of what you really think; your dress code and accessories can reveal your social status or financial situation to a trained eye.

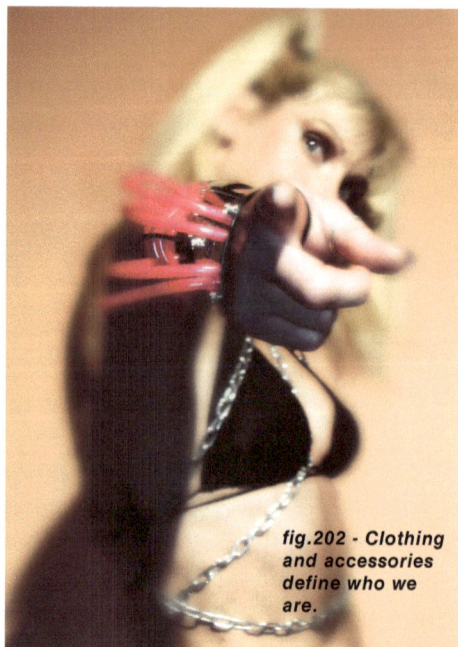

fig.202 - Clothing and accessories define who we are.

As a fun exercise observe people walking past you and try to imagine what they do for a living, how much they earn, and so on. It is not as difficult as you might think, and it can reveal far too much information to people with little or no scruples.

So, how do you blend in? Does this mean that you have to dress down all the time?

By all means surely not, just dress appropriately and make sure that if you are travelling to a location and you have to go through a particular area you don't do so in a way that attracts attention. One of our everyday "accessories" that attracts a lot of attention and can reveal a lot about ourselves is our car.

A friend of mine moved to a neighbourhood in Los Angeles and the first word of advice that she got was to change the doors of her car with the same type but of different colour, that was the best way not to have your car stolen in that area.

This tells you that we are what we drive: if you see an expensive looking sports car parked outside a modest looking house you can well imagine that the owner of the car probably has an expensive watch and expensive stereo inside too.

IMPROPER BEHAVIOR IS SEEN AS PROVOCATION.

If you live in a neighbourhood were the majority of the parked cars are quite plain and you cannot resist having that "flashy little beast" I would suggest that you cover it at least at night time.

There have been cases when opportunist criminals have smashed their way into the house of someone who had an expensive car in their driveway and took the keys and obviously the car too, sometimes beating up whoever was at home at the time.

The same applies if you own a motorbike: if you can only park it in the street, at least make sure that you always secure it with a good chain and lock it to a lamppost or other permanent feature, throwing a motorbike cover over it. For recommended chains and security devices see HELP (page 246).

In modern society we are defined by what we wear, where we live, our accessories and what we drive and we shouldn't change our taste solely on the basis that we may attract unwanted attention.

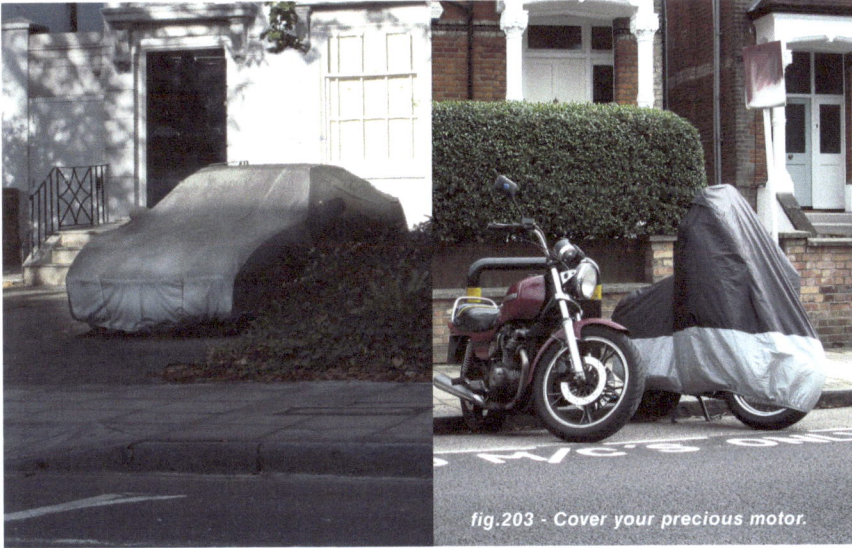

fig.203 - Cover your precious motor.

However, we should always make sure that we do not turn up in certain places dressed or behaving inappropriately because this can be seen by some as a provocation. It is up to us and our common sense to avoid standing out and consequently becoming a target of crime.

Simple precautions that we can easily implement into our routine can make the difference. Look around you and see who stands out as a potential target of crime and try to understand why. Is it the wristwatch that he is wearing? Is it the earring shining in the sunlight or is it the loud irritating conversation he is having on his mobile phone about how much money he is making?

Understanding all this and avoiding inappropriate behaviour will make you not only less of a target to a criminal but also a nicer person.

Several years ago I used to spar in full contact karate with someone who was a very good Karateka but at the same time was someone with a big over inflated ego, always boosting about his black belt and fancy moves. He considered himself a tough guy and he was a bit of a bully too. Once, while out on a tournament with the rest of us, he upset someone in a bar and instead of apologising he told him to f*** off and watch out because he was a Karate champion. The other guy knocked him out cold with a single punch, and he then carried on drinking his coffee saying "Yeah? I am only a truck driver."

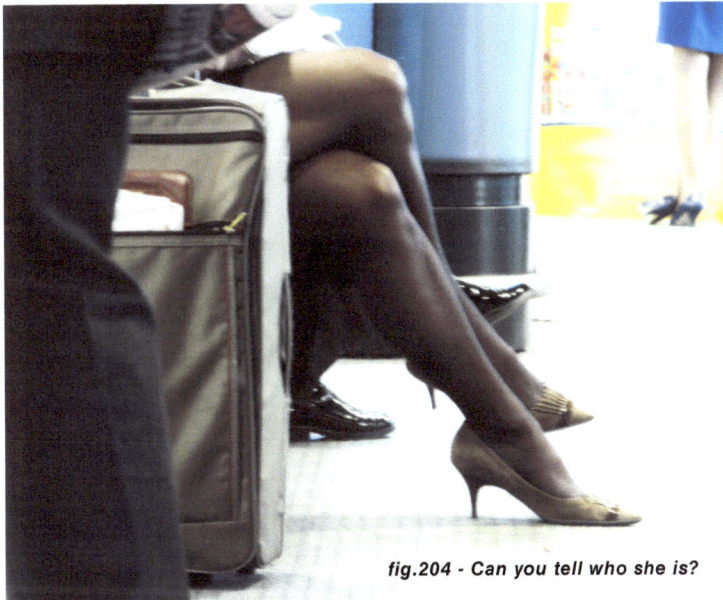

fig.204 - Can you tell who she is?

None of us present intervened, in actual fact we were all quite pleased with the outcome.

If he had blended in as a general rule and not always tried to attract attention to himself he wouldn't have made a fool of himself or worse.

We are defined not just by the way we behave and our relations with others, but also by the accessories that adorn us and the objects that accompany us in our everyday life.

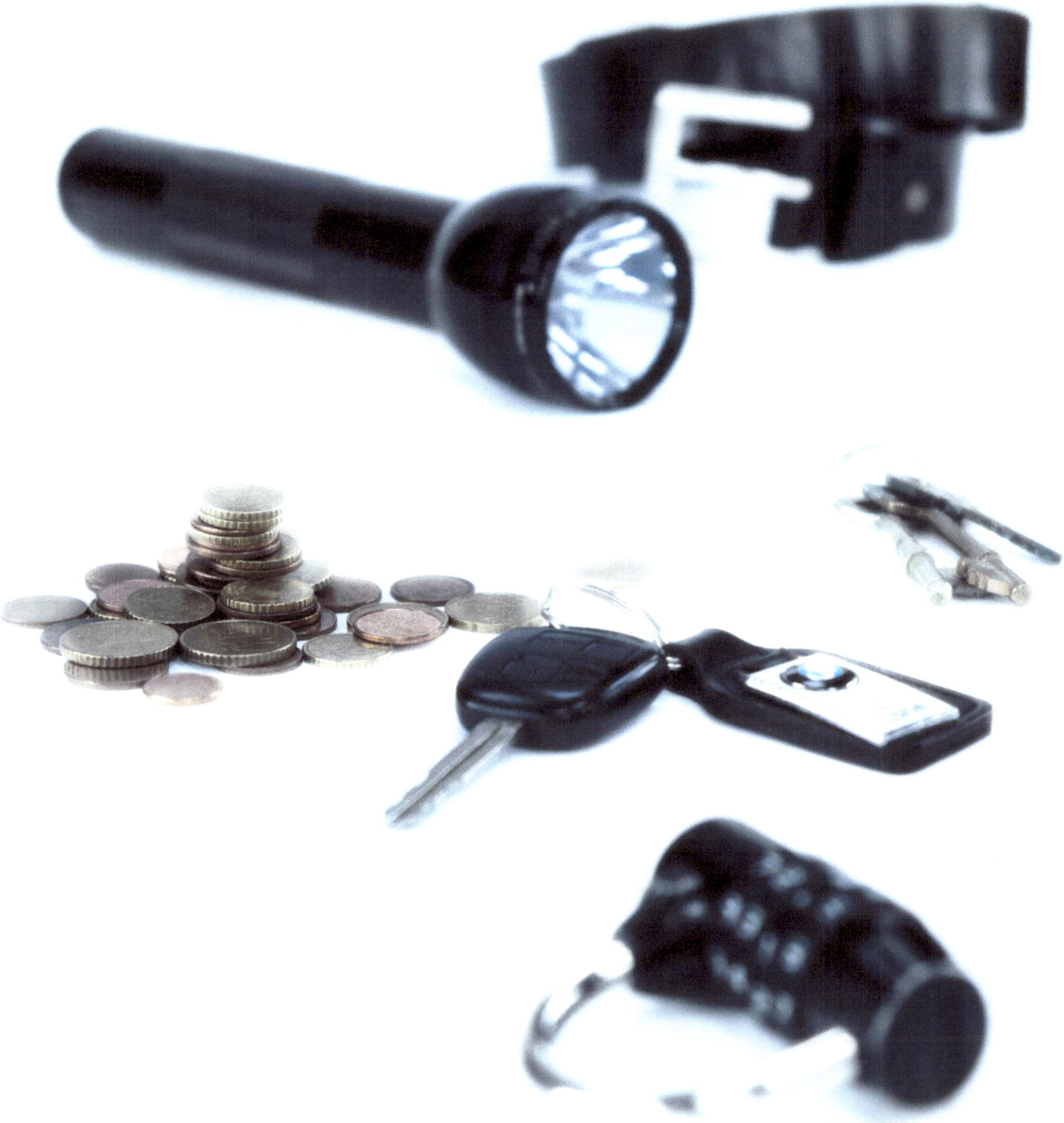

fig.205 - Check in your car, bag or pockets, you have more than enough to defend yourself effectively.

objects

While watching self-defence demonstrations or scenarios where great emphasis is put on kicks, punches and evasive techniques it is easy to forget that we always have something on our person or at close range that we can use as a defensive weapon. For instance, as you are reading this page, just examine what you are wearing right now: a watch on your wrist? Rings on your fingers? Do you have on a belt with a buckle? Are you wearing glasses? Have you got some coins in your pocket?

And if you are a woman please empty the contents of your handbag, and you'll see what I mean. Quite often, the moment you hold something in your hands with the obvious intention to defend yourself, like a bunch of keys or an umbrella, an attacker might think twice before carrying on with his action. I have seen in some self-defence books pictures illustrating techniques to use against rape, where the woman was lying right next to a fireplace, with the fire poker well in view and well within reach and not a word is mentioned on how good that could be as a defensive weapon.

We can distinguish everyday objects in two categories: shield types and striking types.

Objects that can be used as shields are for instance: chairs, bags, cases, coats, lampposts, road barriers, and doors. You can use anything around you or on you to shield yourself from somebody attacking you with a knife, syringe or stick (fig. 53).

Striking type objects are anything that you can use to either hit the attacker (remember: only to defend yourself!) or to throw at him to create a window of opportunity, either to flee or to strike.

It's the classic sand thrown at the baddy's face in Western films, so remember that if you fall to the ground, picking up stones or dust or anything that you find and throwing it back is always a good thing.

Holding small objects in your fist can actually increase the power of your strike, a bunch of coins, a stone; even a mobile phone will actually harden your fist, and make your punch more effective.

Objects always surround us, or we always have something on our person that we can use as a defensive weapon.

fig.205A - Women are often expensively armed.

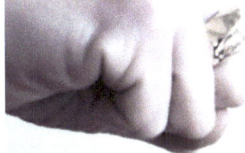

It is important that if you are walking around an environment that makes you feel weary you should actually find something in or around you to hold in your hand as you walk through it, ready to use.

To carry it in your bag or case won't be of much use if attacked by surprise. If you always travel using the same route, from your home to the office for instance, at least once you should consider what there is along the journey which can be used in case somebody tries to attack or harm you. A newsagent stand could be thrown at an attacker, and the ever-present road works always offer plenty of material that can be used.

In a city in particular, there are always plenty of things that can be of help in an emergency.

fig.206 - Using a chair like a shield.

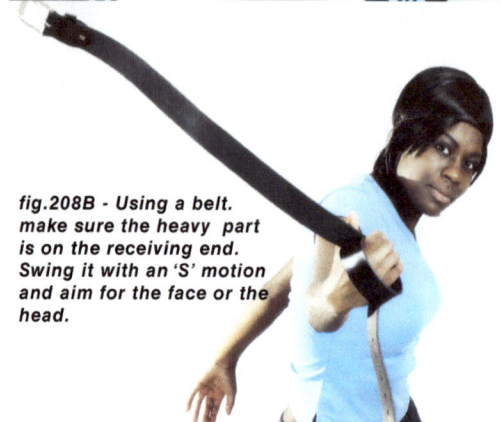

It is also very important to remember that in most countries the improper use of a very common object like an umbrella as a weapon can bear serious consequences if you go beyond what is considered by your local law the boundaries of self-defence and can get you into serious trouble.

Yet there are many ways you can use whatever is at hand in ways that until now has never occurred to you. Instead of thinking of striking type objects as weapons, I think it's better to consider them as a distracting maneuver to cause confusion in your attacker, throwing something for instance at his face and running to safety. It is quite useful if you go jogging for instance, to bring with you an insect repellent spray, apart from being useful for what is designed for, it is also very effective as an improvised pepper spray.

fig.206A - Aim at the throat or face.

fig.208B - Using a belt. make sure the heavy part is on the receiving end. Swing it with an 'S' motion and aim for the face or the head.

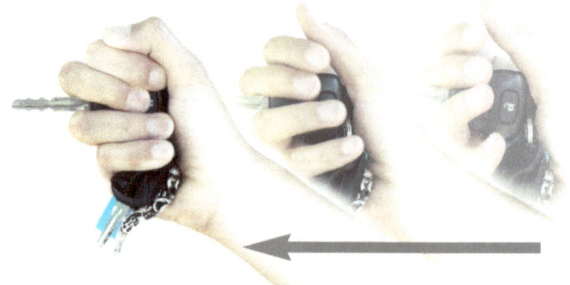

This type of defence is also very useful if attacked by a dog for instance: spraying insect repellent onto his nose or eyes will make him back off, more effectively than pepper spray since dogs do not have lachrymal glands, so they are not affected by it.

Surely you must have with you a bunch of coins normally, that if thrown effectively can be very devastating. You have to remember though that if you decide to use an object you have to make sure that it doesn't fall in your attacker's hand, and it can be counter productive if you use it without fully thinking it through.

Any self-defence action should always consist of a combination of moves, at least three, and always be conducted in a powerfully explosive manner with great determination.

If you find yourself using a chair like a shield (fig.206), for example to defend yourself in a bar from somebody lunging at you with a knife, it's very effective to use a chair as a shield, but at the same time you should kick and throw him, using the chair, to the ground. I have witnessed once in South America a woman defending herself from a pack of wild dogs using her bra as a sling to throw stones, the beasts scattered away in no time.

One of my favourite all-round defence-weapons is the ever common belt, especially one with a reasonably heavy buckle and made of thick leather, it can be used to keep an attacker away or even to tie him up if you manage to knock him out. The Japanese have taught chain swinging techniques since NINJUTSU times, using the MARIKIKUSARI, a chain with weighted ends (see GLOSSARY for more - page 198).

The same techniques can be applied to a belt. In an emergency you can use anything that surrounds you, including a very humble pencil to defend your own life.

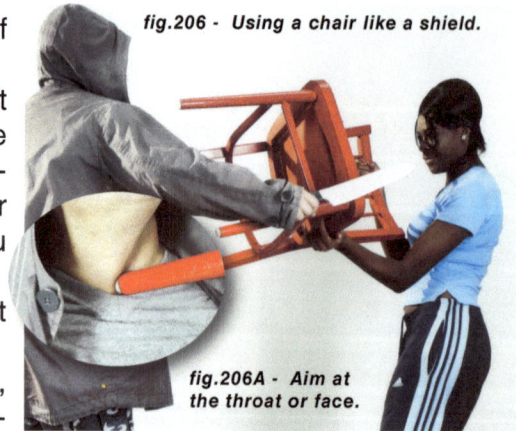

fig.207 - How to hold your car keys in your fist.

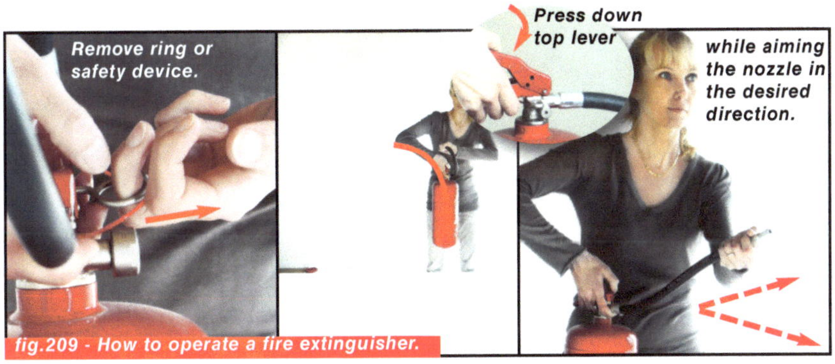

Press down
top lever

Remove ring or
safety device.

while aiming
the nozzle in
the desired
direction.

fig.209 - How to operate a fire extinguisher.

These days, a very common ready-made weapon that you can find everywhere, especially in public places is the ubiquitous fire extinguisher.

Any type of fire extinguisher will keep an attacker at bay or incapacitate him quite seriously; there are several types of fire extinguishers but they are mostly all activated in the same way (see fig.209).

There is a safety pin that needs to be pulled out and normally either a nozzle or a short pipe to direct the liquid, gas or powder, that needs to be detached, with a lever that needs to be pressed. Very common is the CO_2-type (an inert gas that has a freezing action) or the powder-type (often causing breathing difficulties and eye injuries) that work at a good distance.

LOOK AROUND, PLENTY AVAILABLE!

In a recent course I've done I was quite amazed that the majority of people have never used a fire extinguisher and wouldn't know how to use one even in an emergency, never mind as a form of defence. It's a good thing to know how it works, and not just for self-defence obviously, but also for the purpose it was designed for originally. I would also recommend keeping a small one in the car, there are some types designed specifically for that, and it might turn up being useful in more than one way. It is needless to remind you to always stay within the law, but you could use it to go to someone's rescue.

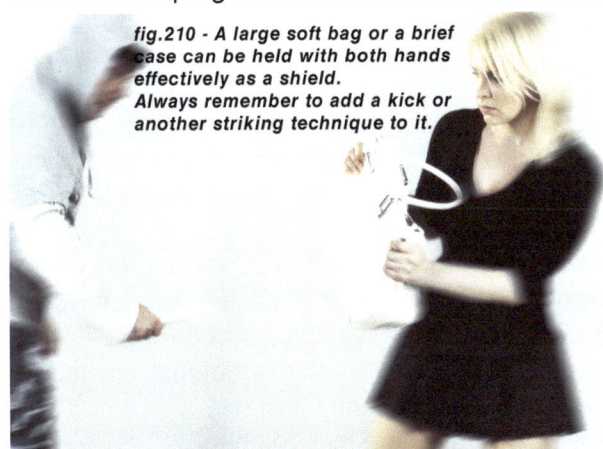

fig.210 - A large soft bag or a brief case can be held with both hands effectively as a shield. Always remember to add a kick or another striking technique to it.

Lastly, I wouldn't try to break a bottle to use the resulting sharp edges to defend yourself. Breaking a bottle might often cause you more harm than good.

Just hold it by the neck and use it like a short stick, and it's as effective. What you see in films doesn't apply in reality most of the time.

Shield-like objects can be very effective to block off attacks made with a blunt object, like a knife or a syringe. A large soft bag or a brief case can be held with both hands effectively (see fig.210) and always remember to add a kick or another striking technique to it.

You can use your jacket or coat to throw it onto the head of your attacker and blind him, for instance as a distracting technique, especially if he is facing you asking for money.

You can be more effective saying that he can take the whole jacket and throw it into his face, kicking him at the same time (see fig.211).

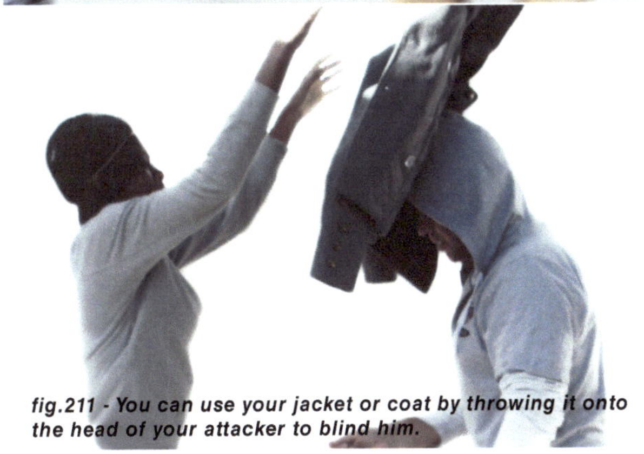

fig.211 - You can use your jacket or coat by throwing it onto the head of your attacker to blind him.

As a general rule, remember that depriving somebody of his capacity of sight means achieving superior control over your opponent.

IF YOUR ATTACKER CAN'T SEE HE CANNOT HARM YOU.

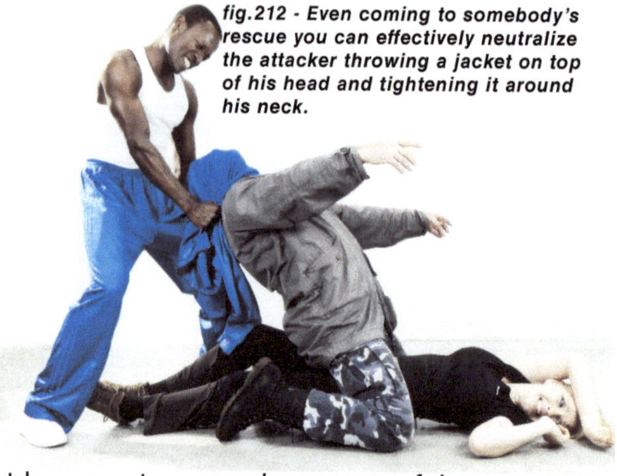

If you are often in the car make sure you keep a good torch in there, ideally within easy reach.

The classic medium size Maglite torch is also very useful to break the window if for instance you end up trapped in a canal full of water, as well as being very good if you need to defend yourself against someone.

fig.212 - Even coming to somebody's rescue you can effectively neutralize the attacker throwing a jacket on top of his head and tightening it around his neck.

Lastly, fixed objects like a lamppost, a wall, a post-box or a tree, can be very useful.

For instance you can use a wall to push from it and increase the power of your counter strike as well as using a lamppost to use as a fulcrum to bend your attacker's arm in a lever.

You can slam a door on his face, including the car door to his groin or knee, or use a tree between yourself and your attacker and keep circling to get out of his reach. If a dog attacks you, simply climbing on top of a car will put you in a safe spot, dogs are bad climbers and a car is very slippery. There is more advice on animal attacks in ANIMALS (page 160).

Generally speaking, if you are under attack, you can decide not to strike back but at least as you run try to find something that will offer you protection, including a lake or pond.

As we have discussed before, we might feel embarrassed about it but just consider how awful the alternative is if you don't do it.

Using everyday objects to great efficacy as a weapon is a Japanese skill, developed historically after a moratorium on edged weaponry was issued under the Satsuma Daimyo (= clan) after invading Okinawa in the 17th century, but that did not stop bandits attacking people, especially in the countryside. Farmers started looking into everyday objects and work tools to use them as weapons, without modifying them.

This created in time a series of disciplines that eventually made simple tools more effective as weapons than some of the so-called traditional weapons. For instance the NUNCHAKU was originally designed to beat rice, the TONFA (GLOSSARY - page 198) was a part of the mill, even a long scarf was used and practiced with to exploit its potential as an offensive or defensive weapon.

Using objects as in self-defence is a last resort if you feel that there is no other way to stop an attacker from hurting you, not just because of the damage that you can create, especially if you aim at his eyes, ears or soft tissues, but also because it can have serious legal consequences.

This is also why I would discourage anyone to carry on their person objects that can obviously in the eye of the Law become weapons including KUBOTANS (fig. 213), a highly effective tool developed by Takayuki Kubota in the '70s for police officers to restrain suspects without injury.

Generally speaking any blunt object is considered a weapon in most legislations, and unless you have a dispensation by the authority because of the type of work you do, for instance if you are a paramedic carrying scissors in your jacket, it is hard to justify to a Police offer why you are carrying a screwdriver in your pocket while going to a discotheque or meeting some friends at night and

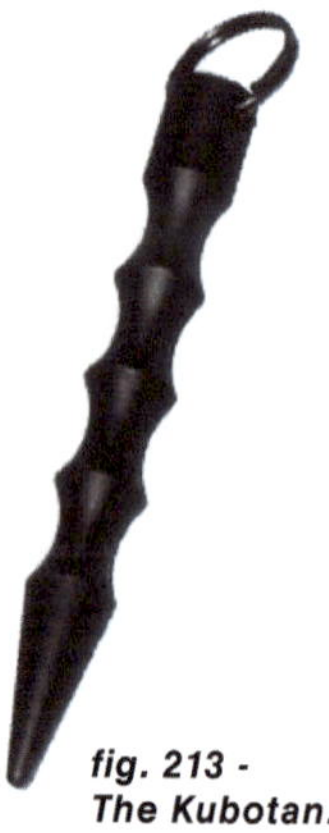

fig. 213 - The Kubotan.

135

remember that if you are carrying instruments or tools for work or sport reasons, most foreign countries' laws require that they are in the boot of your vehicle and not on your person or on the seats or floor.

CHECK YOUR LOCAL LAWS!

You should always check with your local Government bodies about the appropriate laws regarding this matter, not to get caught out while you go fishing with a spear gun that is considered in some countries completely illegal.

The same applies if you go on holiday and you have packed something in your suitcase that can, in the eyes of local Authorities, be considered a criminal offence.

Also if you carry something that cannot be justified for everyday use, such a stick to throw to your dog while you are out without the dog, or a baseball or cricket bat and you are not going to training or a match, it can cause you a lot of trouble.

In the United Kingdom the Criminal Justice Act 1988 (Offensive Weapons) Order 1988, regulates the prohibited weapons list and anything that can be considered an offensive weapon in the UK if you use it for that purpose.

I am quite against carrying objects that are designed for self-defence, even if some can be quite effective, such as the KUBOTAN, I am also against PEPPER SPRAYS and anything specifically designed to harm someone, including TASERS (see GLOSSARY - page 198).

CAUTION

In WEAPONS (page 198) we examine all these more in depth. I am happy to suggest you carry with you objects to secure your room while travelling, such as the ones indicated in fig.214.

fig.214 - These are some small objects that you should take with you when traveling for your personal safety.

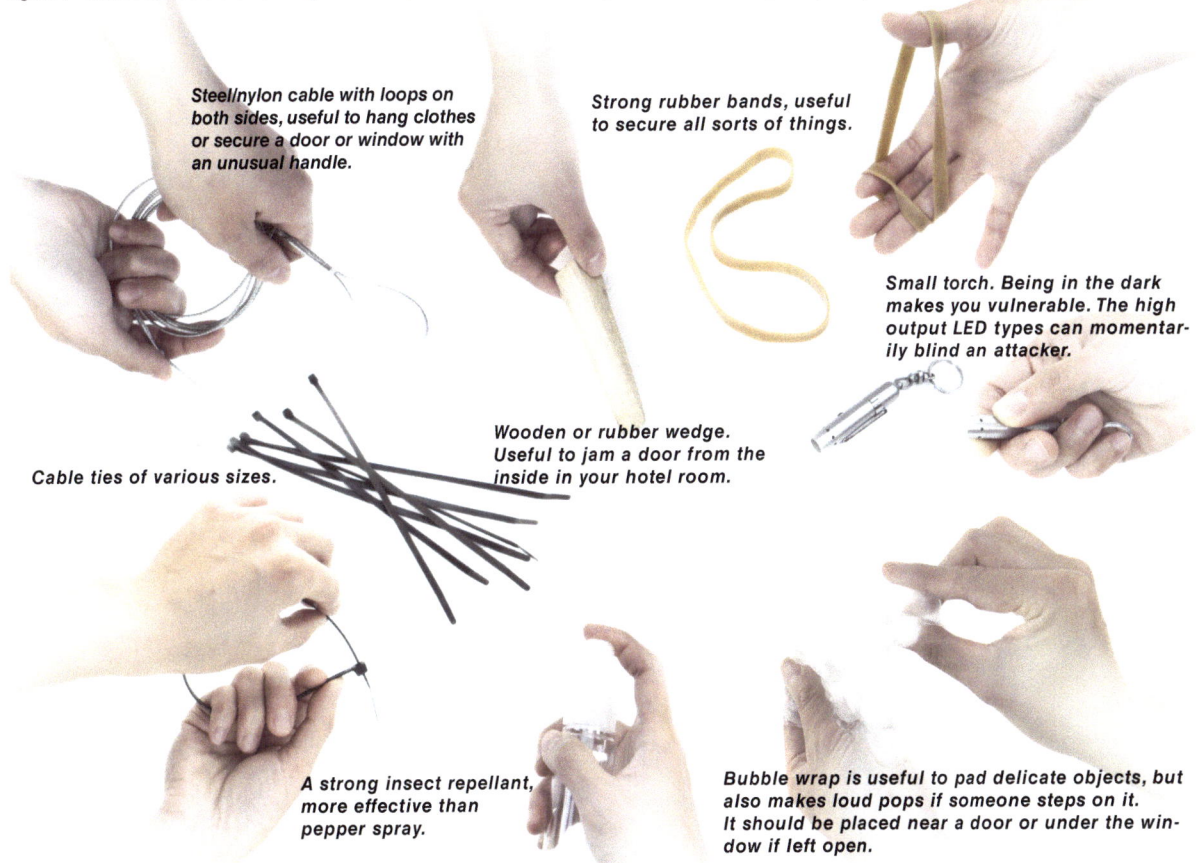

Steel/nylon cable with loops on both sides, useful to hang clothes or secure a door or window with an unusual handle.

Strong rubber bands, useful to secure all sorts of things.

Small torch. Being in the dark makes you vulnerable. The high output LED types can momentarily blind an attacker.

Cable ties of various sizes.

Wooden or rubber wedge. Useful to jam a door from the inside in your hotel room.

A strong insect repellant, more effective than pepper spray.

Bubble wrap is useful to pad delicate objects, but also makes loud pops if someone steps on it. It should be placed near a door or under the window if left open.

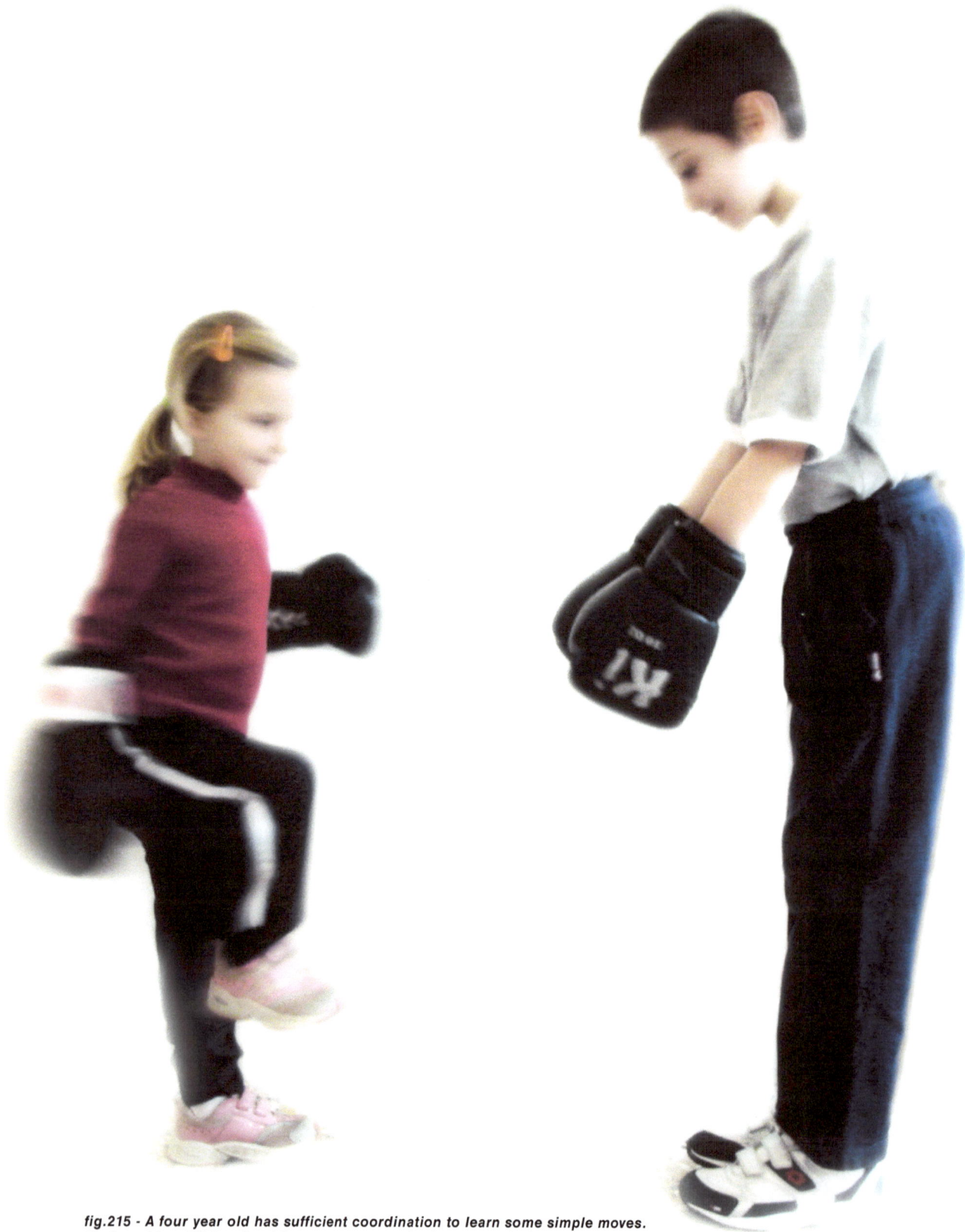

fig.215 - *A four year old has sufficient coordination to learn some simple moves. Having older children teaching younger ones is always a real plus.*

children

This is probably the most difficult subject of this entire book and it is very easy to fall into the absolute ridiculous or the plain over-kill when it comes to teaching children how to defend themselves. In discussing "children" we are talking about anyone between the age of four and thirteen years, both for practical reasons but also because from the age of four children already have developed certain skills that can help them to help themselves effectively.

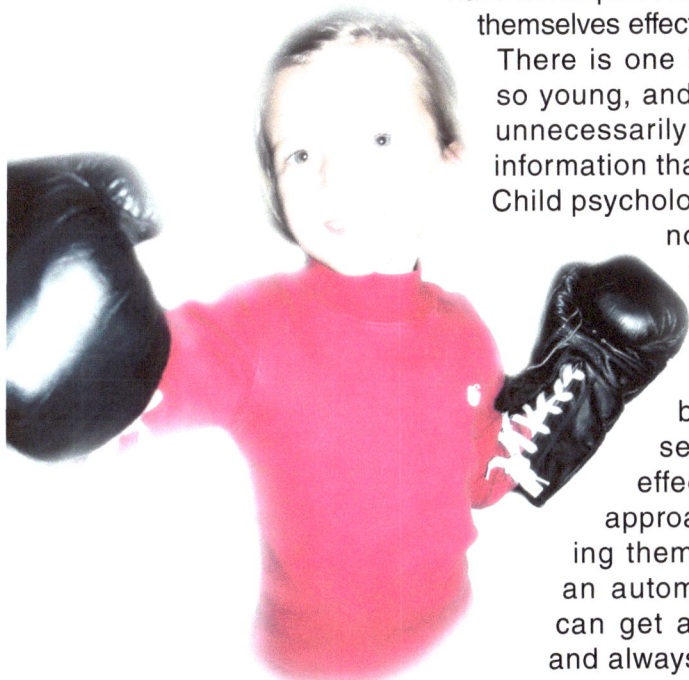

There is one big obstacle in teaching people so young, and that is that it might scare them unnecessarily or overfeed them with too much information that they cannot digest or that confuses them. Child psychology is vast and complicated and we will not enter this field, we will limit ourselves to basic, simple rules based on factual information and proven studies already widely available.

We would like to point out that it is possible to teach a four year old to free himself or to kick a grown-up where it hurts effectively, but that should be made with a lucid approach, it should always be fun for them, teaching them moves which are easy to apply in almost an automatic fashion. For instance, you can get a child to wear punching-gloves and always make it fun, having them hitting pads or part of your body, teaching them

fig.216 - Make it fun and make it ever changing.

coordination as well as not to be afraid to punch an adult. All the way through always keep a light-hearted approach, and don't burden them with any kind of information relating to self-defence, don't say things like "if somebody grabs you..." or "if you get attacked..." Instead say things like "I'm going to come and get you!" or "Big monkey grabbing you" or even better "Now hit me and run away as fast as you can." The emphasis should always be on the fun bit, an almost hide-and -seek spirit.

You obviously should not scare children unnecessarily, and should not do this by explaining to them what could potentially happen or why you are doing that.

That is all information that is not only upsetting but just boring to them.

SELF DEFENCE SHOULD BE TAUGHT TO CHILDREN IN A FUN WAY.

CAUTION

TEACH THEM NOT TO BE AFRAID TO HIT AN ADULT BUT DO NOT TELL THEM WHY.

⚠ **CAUTION** The main dilemma is teaching a child not to be rude if somebody says "Hello, little one, what's your name?" and at the same time teaching him or her not to talk to strangers. Ideally, children that young should never be left unsupervised, and I think it is wise to teach them some simple rules that they can understand easily and have fun practicing.

🚫 Simple rules: do not answer to strangers, do not accept lifts from strangers, and don't listen to what they say, even if they say mommy or daddy

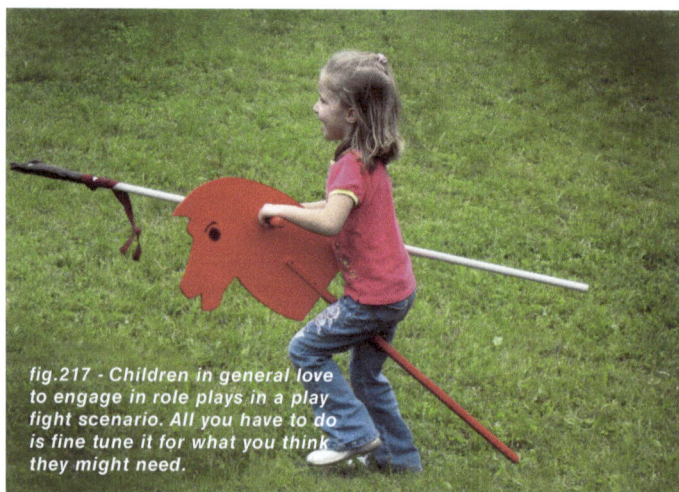

fig.217 - Children in general love to engage in role plays in a play fight scenario. All you have to do is fine tune it for what you think they might need.

told them to pick them up or that they should follow them for whatever reason.

IF ANYONE SAYS "DON'T TELL MUMMY", DO TELL MUM STRAIGHT AWAY. Tell them that the fact that a stranger knows their name is irrelevant (they might have read it on their schoolbag, or heard a teacher or a friend call their name). Tell them never to take shortcuts, and especially teach them, that the first thing to do if someone tells them (including relatives), not to tell mummy or daddy, actually means to tell mummy or daddy straight away. But it gets more complicated if you are thinking of teaching children to be totally self sufficient when it comes to defending themselves against someone who wants to harm them. Is it really possible?

We are firmly convinced famous phrases such as "It's only down the road" or "It only takes 5 minutes" are synonymous with trouble.

Do not let very young children go and shop by themselves, or walk down the road unsupervised. Are these exaggerated measures? Maybe, but you should talk to parents who had their children abducted or had an accident because of the 5-minutes blind spot. Once they reach 6 or 7 years of age you can explain things with a bit more detail, still being careful not to frighten them unnecessarily.

It is important that they don't fall for a sweet, charming look or a soothing voice.

Don't forget children tend to picture "baddies" as big, ominous, often wearing black clothing, talking with a scary voice, as seen in countless cartoons and films. Children's attackers often look like your next-door neighbour or grandparent.

As you can see, it's very complicated and you do not want to spoil their natural good nature or innocence but at the same time you want

🚫 them to be aware of danger.

Furthermore, you don't want to turn your child into someone that because he knows where to kick or punch, starts using it against school mates and friends with obviously bad consequences for his or her fellow pupils.

👆 If you are teaching them some moves say clearly they cannot try them with friends.

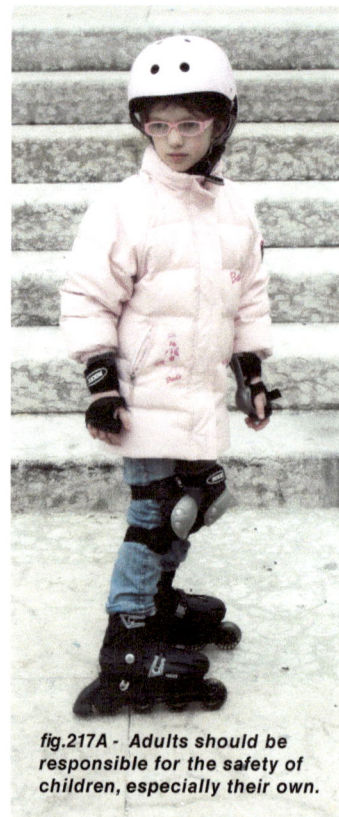

fig.217A - Adults should be responsible for the safety of children, especially their own.

Teaching specific scenarios to children is equally dangerous: the reason is if what happens to them doesn't fit that scenario, they will not recognise it as being dangerous.

For instance, if you give to your child as an example, a scenario of a man approaching from his car as they walk, offering a lift back home, what if it is a couple approaching, and a woman asking.

As you can see, it's impossible to guess every scenario, and it's better to stick to simple principles.

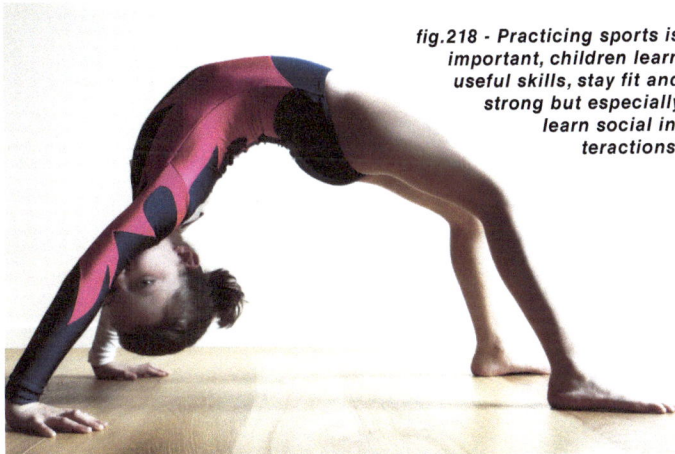

fig.218 - Practicing sports is important, children learn useful skills, stay fit and strong but especially learn social interactions.

Do not accept any lifts from any strangers, independently from what they are or what they look like, or what they say, man or woman, old or young, boy or girl, uniform or dog collar and teach them to not let them come near them.

CHILDREN CAN EASILY BE DISTRACTED BY GADGETS.

Children can be quite easily get distracted by a fancy car, shiny toy or tempting ice cream and lately, mobile phones, high tech gadgets, videogames and obviously money.

Some paedophiles have been using puppies or small dogs to get the children close to them.

Remember, try to teach your children the simple rule that nothing in life is given free without something wanted in return: if you want to teach some simple moves to your children, concentrate on kicks, aimed at the shin. The reason is that children cannot punch effectively, and they cannot reach an adult's face.

That's why teaching them to kick is highly effective. If appropriate, you can teach them to bite the hand that grabs them, and always point out that they should run screaming for help.

Most people would come to a child's rescue if he/she were screaming for help.

As we can see, it is really up to us to protect children, and it is naive to think you can teach a child effectively to fend off an attack from an adult.

Teaching children to defend themselves is a constant balance between making them aware of dangers without being alarmist. You can start explaining to children that they do have rights, and they have the right to refuse to do things if they feel it's wrong.

Don't forget that children are taught to respect authority, especially from adults and older people, without questioning it.

It's up to us to find the balance, so they can discriminate between good and bad. You should also explain to children, especially your own, never to have any secrets, especially when told to do so by adults.

Do not patronise children and equally important, don't let them think that they will not be believed when they come and tell you things. Children, some in particular, have fervently creative minds and love stories, some lie a lot as part of growing up. Sometimes they embellish or exaggerate what happened, but all in all you should always listen carefully and watch with particular attention the way they tell you things, the mood they are in saying it.

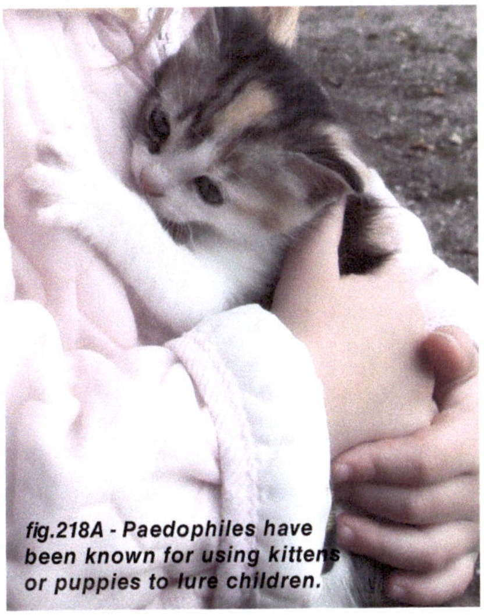

fig.218A - Paedophiles have been known for using kittens or puppies to lure children.

If a child comes and tells you about strange attentions that he got from another adult, including a relative of yours, it would be better to take it very seriously.

Do not force your child to go and kiss a stranger as a welcome, and explain that kissing and hugging is a very special thing. Tell your children that they should never talk to strangers, it might sound rude but it is worth considering that a well-meaning adult wouldn't really talk to a minor, unless thinking the child needs help.

Do tell them that it is fine if they do not answer back to a stranger, and that you are not going to get upset with them

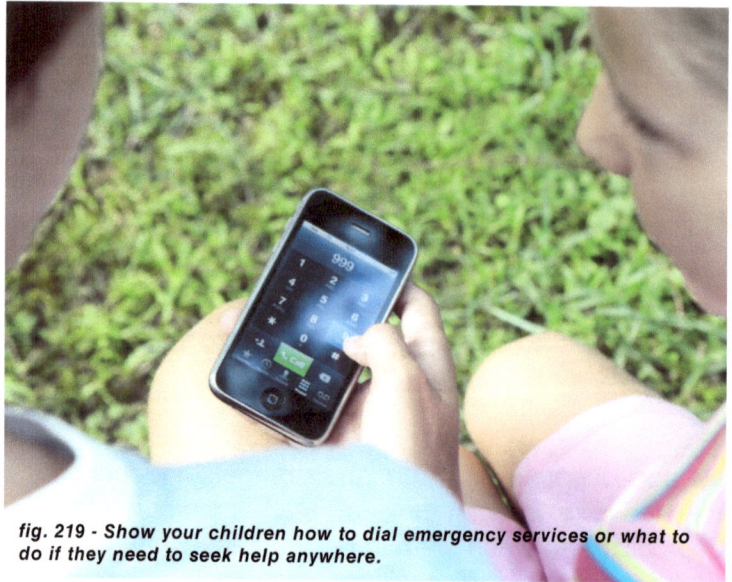

fig. 219 - Show your children how to dial emergency services or what to do if they need to seek help anywhere.

because of that, and at the same time that you do want to know if a stranger approaches them.

It is also wise, to teach your child how to call the emergency services.

There have been cases of children calling an ambulance to rescue their parent prevented doing so themselves by a serious accident.

Finally, the number one rule is children should always be in the company of some other children or adults, ideally more than one.

If by any chance you find yourself in a situation where you see a child in trouble, maybe looking lost or on his own, and you do want to intervene, please consider the following: your action might scare the child or make people think you are trying to take him/her away, independently by your good intentions.

It is best if you also ask somebody else to help you as well, tell them to stay with you and the child and to call the police while you are trying to reassure the child.

fig.220 - When reassuring children come down to their height or lower.

Do not take the child away from where you have found them unless there is an immediate danger (oncoming traffic for instance) but in any case, stay near the spot where you find him (or her). Chances are that the child's parents are nearby, maybe looking for him/her at that precise moment quite frantic.

At all times, keep a calm appearance and reassure the child that you are trying to help. You might witness a toddler being pulled forcefully by an adult, and see him crying desperately. If you are in doubt that you are witnessing an abduction, call the police anyway. I have once experienced such a case, a big man carrying a child about 5 years old who was obviously in distress, so I decided to confront the man, asking him to stop and asked the child if he knew that man.

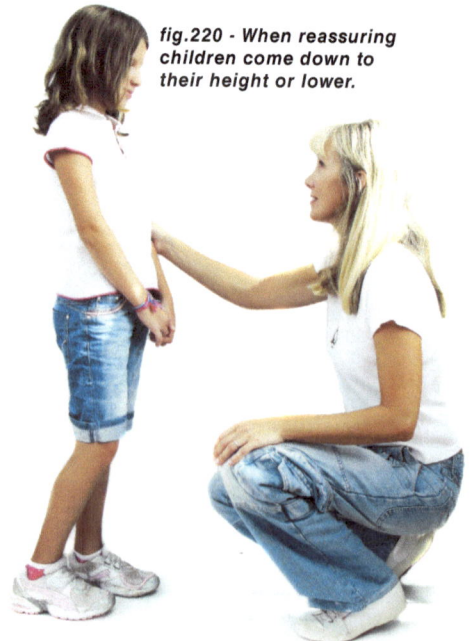

The guy became quite aggressive, telling me to mind my own business, but I calmly replied that if he was the father or a relative he should appreciate my concern.

I kept asking the child the same question until I got a satisfactory answer.

At that moment a police car pulled up, who had been called by an equally concerned passer-by. The man turned out to be the child's uncle, and the child was crying because he didn't want to go back home.

The man saw sense in what I had done and thanked me for confronting him.

I remember after the very high profile case in the United Kingdom of a small child being abducted and killed by two young boys, reading in the papers that a woman saw the boys taking the child with them, thought there was something odd about it but decided not to intervene.

She now has to live with the horrendous consequences of her inaction for the rest of her entire life. It's up to you to decide what to do. I would suggest if in doubt, call the police.

One of the most common questions that are raised during courses is what type of activity or exercise children can take up to build confidence and in order to learn self-defence.

 I have no doubt that probably the best way to build character and make a child more assertive and confident is by doing Judo practice.

Children can start as young as five years old and it is great fun as well as good to learn simple techniques that can prove quite useful. We'll see in INTERNET (page 152) what can be done to keep children safe while they use a computer to go onto the Internet.

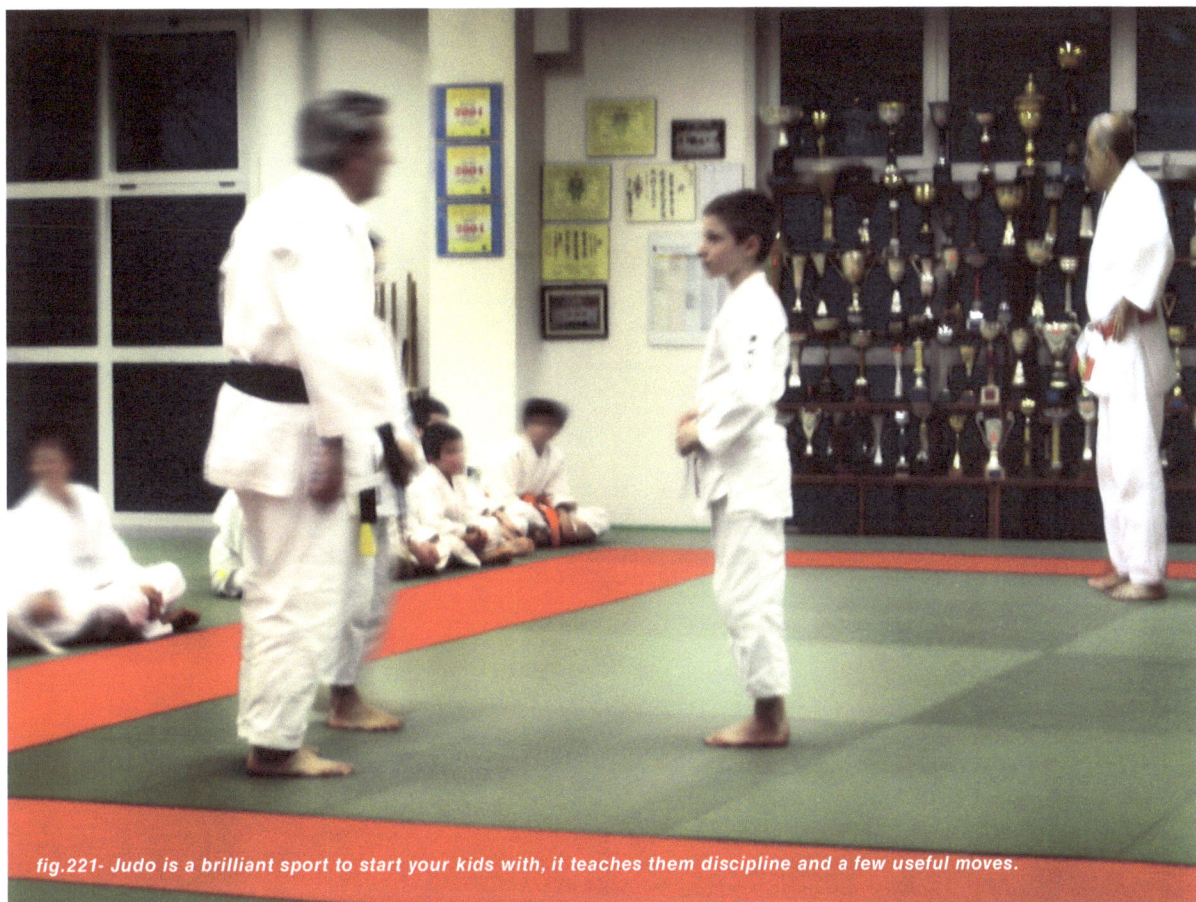

fig.221- Judo is a brilliant sport to start your kids with, it teaches them discipline and a few useful moves.

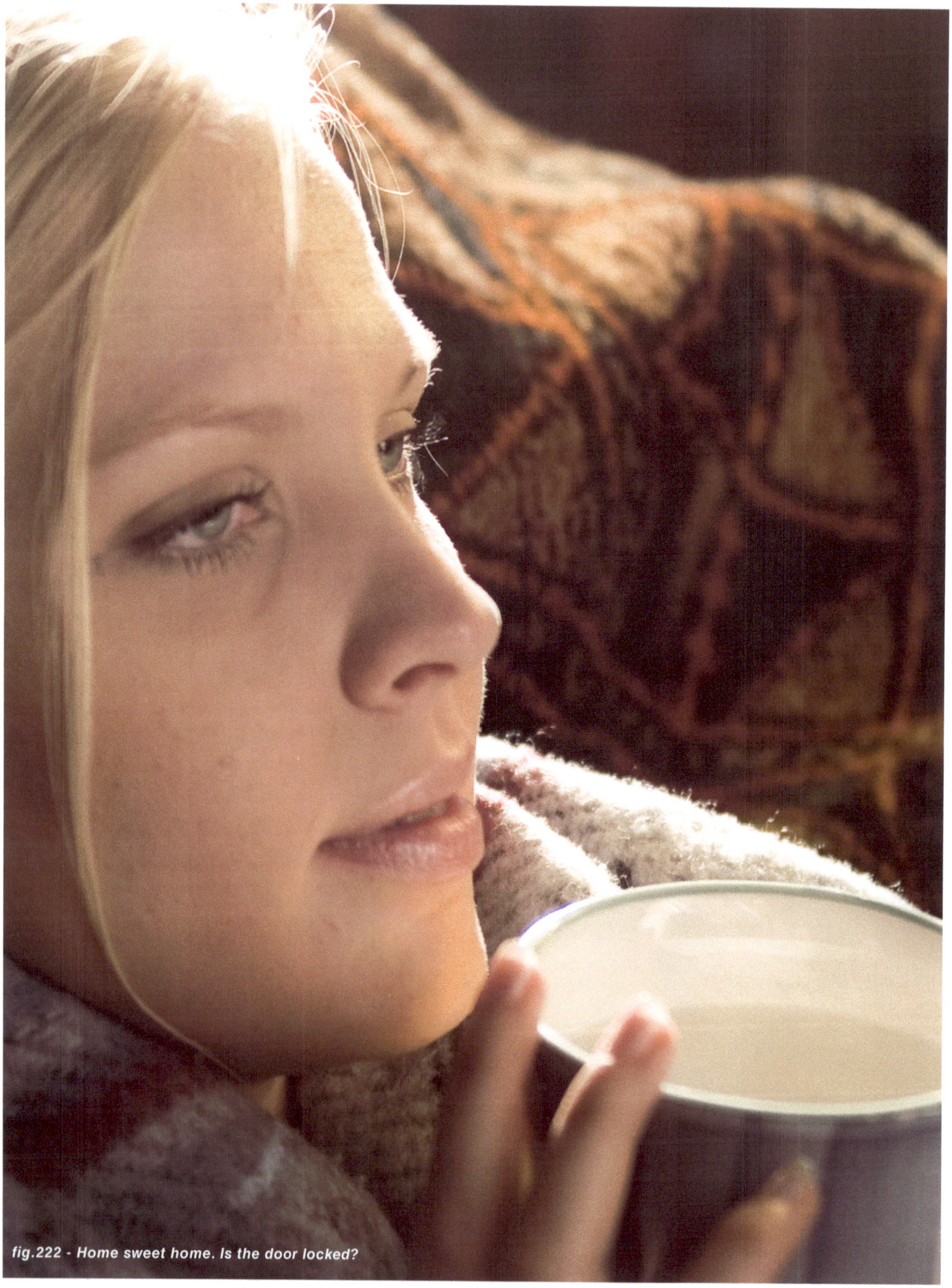

fig.222 - Home sweet home. Is the door locked?

It is quite amazing how people go to extraordinary lengths to secure their car or the own person but are very casual when it comes to securing their home.

Burglaries occur every minute in most countries; it is, after all, the most common crime. It is quite rarely carried out by professional criminals these days because it's considered low profit and high risk.

BURGLARIES ARE MOSTLY IMPROVISED BY PETTY CRIMINALS.

This means that you can secure your home cheaply and effectively. In fig.229 we will show you the vulnerable areas of an average house or flat. Often enough burglaries are carried out without forced entry, a window was left open or the back/patio door was unlocked.

It is wise to use security deadlocks that can only be opened with a key, on both windows and doors. Even if burglars succeed in breaking the glass, they still have to climb through the broken glass, with the risk of cutting themselves or making lots of noise any way.

Installing a burglar alarm is mostly a visible deterrent, and you shouldn't rely on it too much, unless you are connected to a private security company or to the police.

How many times have you heard a siren going off, and how many times have you ever be bothered to check what was going on?

The most vulnerable areas are back-doors and back windows, away from view. Install, or have installed, a light with a sensor to illuminate the rear-garden or the rear-entry of your property.

Fit a door safety chain and a wide-angle peephole at the right height on your front door. To check potential weaknesses in your home stand outside and think about what you would do if you lost your keys and were locked out?

Would you climb up the porch to the first floor window, would you climb up the drainpipe, and so on? If you go out at night, or are away on holiday, install timer switches on some lights, ideally in a random pattern, and you can install a switch on a radio as well, positioned in one of the rooms on the back.

LIGHTS AND SOUND GIVE THE PERCEPTION THAT THE HOUSE IS OCCUPIED.

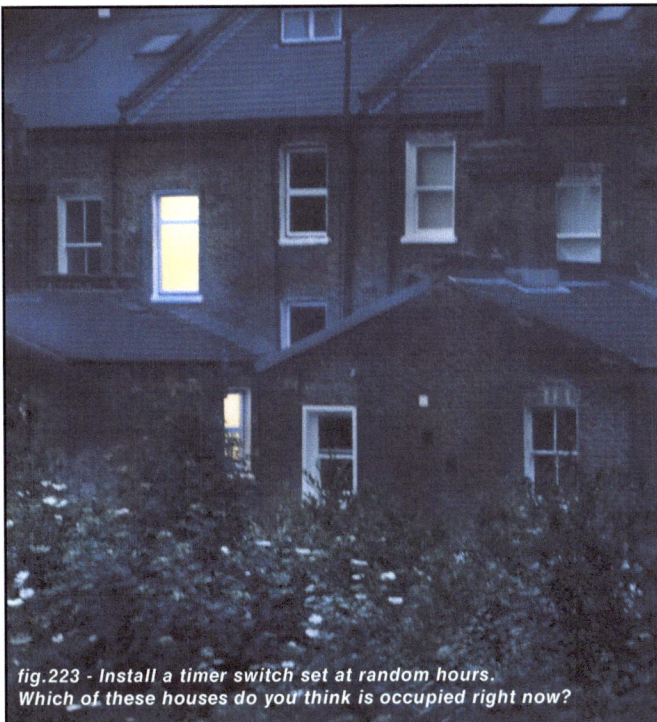

fig.223 - Install a timer switch set at random hours.
Which of these houses do you think is occupied right now?

Choose a radio channel known for a lot of discussions or chats, with little or no music; it will make burglars believe there are people talking. Make sure that your garage is properly locked; especially if it has another door for entering the house.

IF YOUR BAG GETS STOLEN MAKE SURE YOU CHANGE YOUR MAIN DOOR LOCK

Do not put your name or address on your keys, and if your keys get stolen with your bag or to-gether with some documents or anything with your address on it, quickly change all locks before you re-ceive unwanted visitors. If you live in a flat by yourself and you are female, do not put your full name on the doorbell, and omit Mrs. or Miss at the front.

If you moved into a previously owned flat or house it is wise to change all the main door locks.

You do not know who else has the keys to your home.

If you sell your home make sure that you do not show around potential buyers on your own, it has happened that people posing as potential buyers ended up raping and killing the occupant. It is better if you go through a reputable Agency and let them deal with it. In some countries you can

fig.224 - What does your name on the entry-phone or doorbell tell criminals?

ask the police to send you a crime prevention officer from the local police station for further advice. This is common sense but there are other measures that you should take and some other less ob-vious things to be considered to avoid your house becoming a target to criminals.

If you go away for some time, ask a friend or a neighbour to keep an eye on the house.

IF YOU GO AWAY FOR A WHILE MAKE SURE THE HOUSE DOESN'T LOOK ABANDONED.

Suspend regular deliveries of your mail, or have it redirected or picked up regularly. Also be aware that calling unauthorised car services to pick you up to take you to the airport, will make them aware that you are going to be away. Ask them to pick you up outside your next-door neighbour's house, pretending you live there. It might seem to you overkill but without "pointing fingers" at taxi drivers they might be talking to a friend or someone and the wrong people will know that you are going on hol-iday or leaving your house unattended for some time.

We'll see in more detail about identity theft in INTERNET but let's take a few precautionary steps even at home to avoid being a victim of this crime that basically uses your personal details for illicit gain in many different ways.

You should shred any letters you have received from the bank, electricity bills, gas statement and any other utility bills. There are some really cheap shredders available nowadays.

If you don't want to shred them you can also burn the documents before disposing of them.

There have been reports of criminals trawling through people's rubbish to access confidential information and using it to either create bank accounts in your name or purchase goods that then will be debited to you without your knowledge, the so called iden-tity theft. (we will discuss this more in INTERNET page 152).

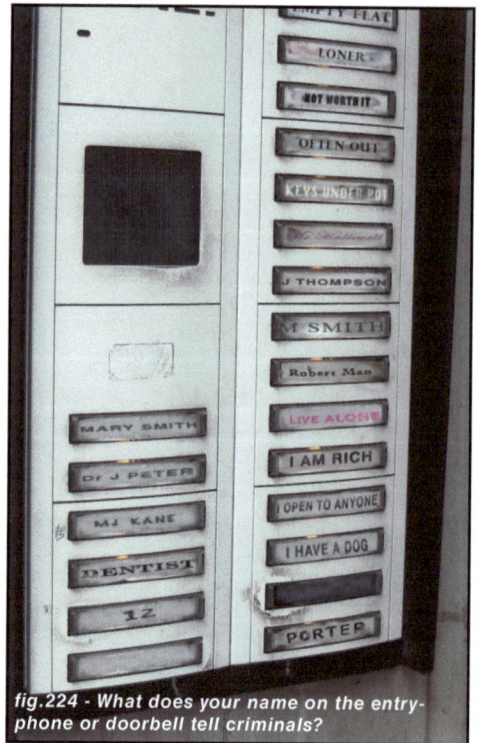

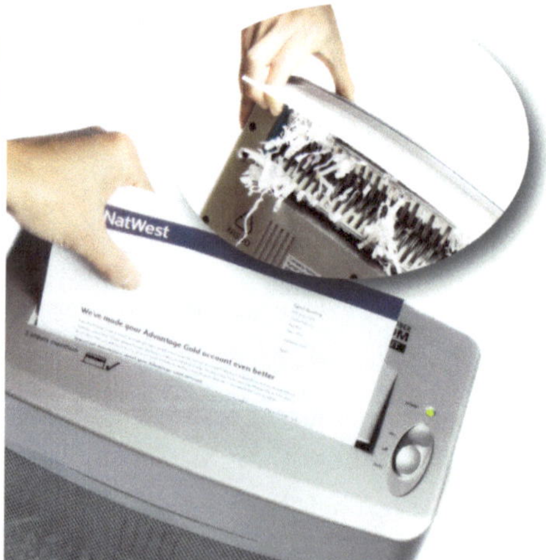

fig.225 - A shredder is a very useful tool, especially the cross cutting type shown here.

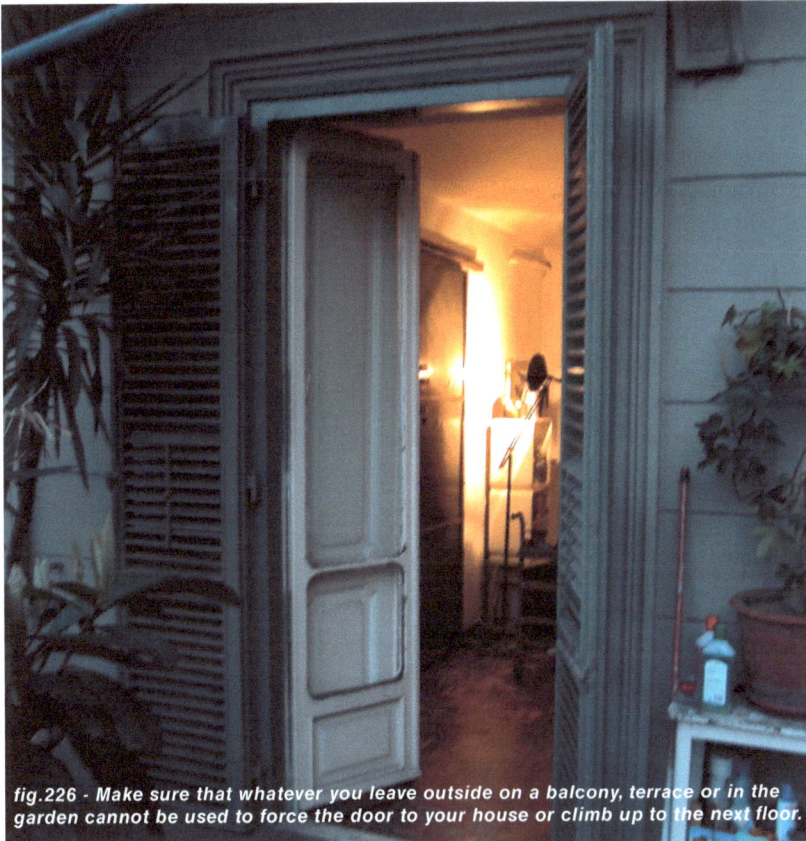

fig.226 - *Make sure that whatever you leave outside on a balcony, terrace or in the garden cannot be used to force the door to your house or climb up to the next floor.*

So whatever information ending up in your rubbish which can potentially reveal personal details, including medical records as well, should be carefully disposed of, in a way that they cannot be put together again.

Expired credit card or debit cards should be cut up into several pieces, especially along the magnetic strip and the microchip, and then binned in different places or on separate occasions.

The best way to store precious items such as jewellery or expensive electronic items is to place them in a hidden place in the house.

Look around your house and see if there is any niche or part of the furniture that can be used to safely hide your precious stuff and remember that a jewellery box next to your bed is very handy but if you leave your house every day to go to work, you really shouldn't leave the box in view, especially if some of the items have a sentimental value to you.

If you have a garden make sure you fit some good lighting and even if you don't own a dog you can always put a "Beware of the Dog" sign on the gate.

Don't leave tools lying around that can be used to force windows or doors open.

Hide or secure ladders that can give access to first or second floors, and check if any tree is near enough to the house to allow entry to floors above.

You can also make good use of some anti-climbing paint on parts of your property that a fit burglar could climb on and gain access to your house, drain pipes, climbers, even security grills can offer anchor points for that.

What should you do if someone breaks into your house at night? If you are sure this is what is happening and you live in a two-storey house, lock yourself in your room and make noise to let the intruder know that you are awake and dial the emergency service number straight away, speaking very loudly. If your flat is one floor and the intruder is far enough away, lock yourself into the room you are in (as a habit keep keys in the lock inside the room) and call the police.

Even if you don't have a phone in the room or with you, pretend that you are calling them anyway. Say very loudly something like "Hello, police. This is (your address). Please come immediately. There is an intruder in my house."

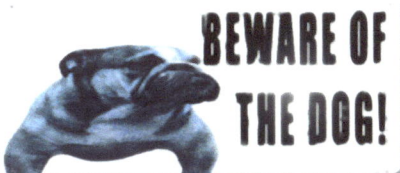

BEWARE OF THE DOG!

If you are woken up by the intruder within your room, rummaging through your drawers for instance, resist from getting up and screaming if you can.

Just move slightly and make a light noise that alone should be enough to make him leave.

If unfortunately, you scream, and he attacks you, use your sheets or duvet as a shield and throw anything within reach at him, a lamp or book and scream your heart out.

If he tries to silence you, see the other techniques described on this book (GROUNDWORK page 82) depending on how he attacks you. If you succeed in your defence, do not try to restrain him, let him run away, don't block his exit route. If you find an intruder during the daytime, for instance, when you come out of the bathroom or the kitchen, and someone has broken in, retreat to where you came from and lock yourself in. (see SCENARIOS page 214).

DON'T BLOCK AN EXIT ROUTE TO A BURGLAR.

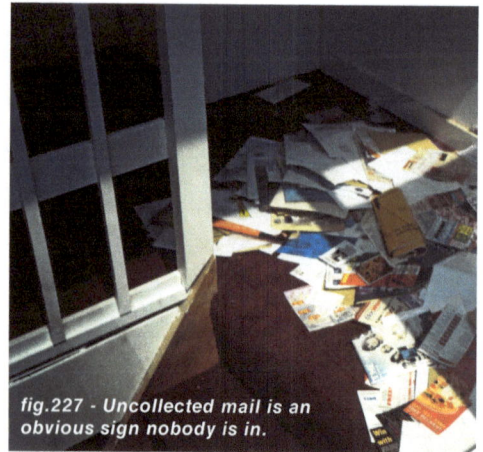

fig.227 - Uncollected mail is an obvious sign nobody is in.

If he attacks you use whatever is around you (see also OBJECTS page 132) against him and apply the techniques shown throughout the book, depending upon his action.

If you come back home and you have a feeling that someone has broken in or you see the door being forced open, don't go inside, they might still be inside, best if you call the police or a neighbour but in any case make sure someone is with you before you walk into your house.

It's always a good idea, even if nothing has been taken, to report it to the police. It helps to let them have an idea of what the situation is in your area and enables them to tackle it better.

Remember that unfortunately, once somebody has broken into your house, chances are he'll come by again in a matter of a couple of weeks.

He knows that you will replace the goods with brand new ones and he knows your house as well as your habits. Make sure the house is made secure throughout, not just where he came through the first time.

To protect your home it is important to understand who the average burglar is and when they operate, not just how.

The majority of home burglaries are carried out by young males under 25, during the daytime when most people are away at work or school.

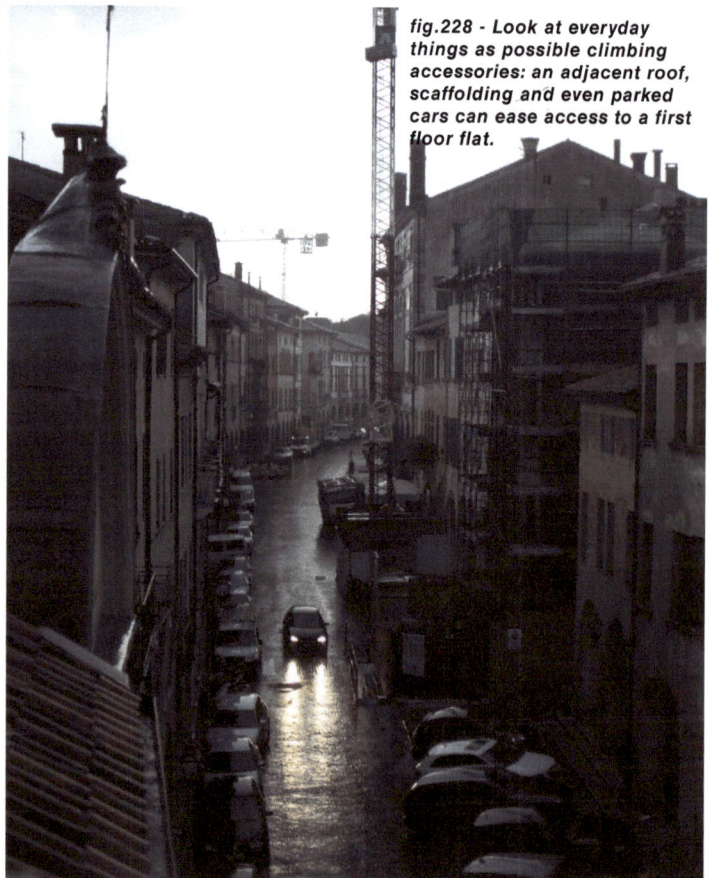

fig.228 - Look at everyday things as possible climbing accessories: an adjacent roof, scaffolding and even parked cars can ease access to a first floor flat.

The most sought after items are anything of maximum value that can quickly be converted into cash, such as jewellery, electronic goods and so on and burglars normally **EARLY AFTERNOON IN HOT DAYS IS THE HIGH RISK TIME.** choose the target that offers the easiest access, the greatest amount of cover, and the best escape routes. Summer and hot months normally see the peak of burglars' activity. Favourite points of entry are the front, back, or garage doors.

The garage door is usually the weakest point of entry followed by the back door that also provides the most cover. Remember to lock your car even if parked inside the garage or garden.

It is wise to install proper locking devices (see HELP page 246) on all doors, including sliding patio doors. Remember that unfortunately some back doors can be opened with a firm kick to them and you should make sure that a proper dead bolt heavy-duty lock is properly fitted.

Also it is quite a good idea to attach adhesive labels onto the window glass warning that an alarm has been installed (even if it's not true) and fit a fake alarm box outside.

Of course if you can you should consider having a proper burglar alarm fitted by a qualified and proven company. Some alarm systems can be connected to either a security firm or the Police.

Windows are particularly vulnerable, especially windows in the back of the house or hidden from the main street. Make sure that if you leave the window open for ventilation it is blocked so it cannot be open more than 6 inches.

Also make sure that you befriend some neighbours, especially the one opposite you, so you can look out for each other when away and report anything suspicious to the police.

Once you know them well enough you might consider trusting them with spare keys, avoiding leaving a spare set around your main door, one of the first place burglars look, such as flower pots, doormats and so on.

Your neighbour can even check on your mail and remove obvious signs that nobody is in.

You should also consider having good lights fitted outside your property, maybe motion activated, to light the patio or front steps.

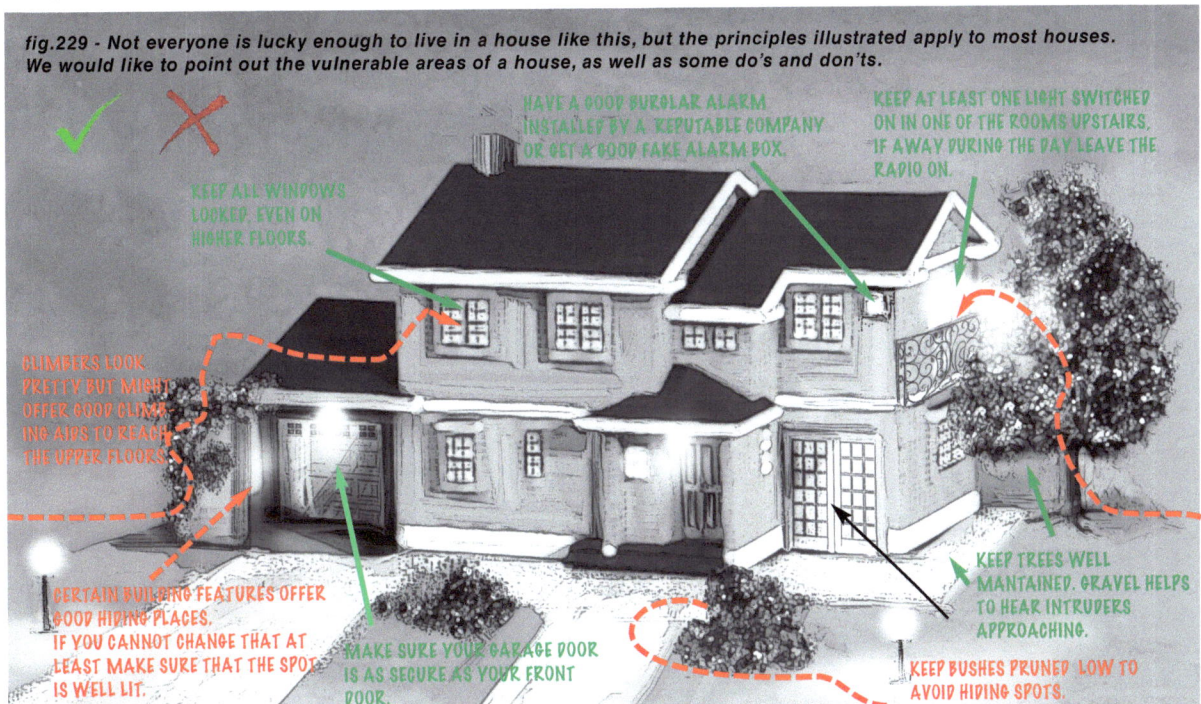

fig.229 - Not everyone is lucky enough to live in a house like this, but the principles illustrated apply to most houses. We would like to point out the vulnerable areas of a house, as well as some do's and don'ts.

Indoors it is good to install some timers to control lamps next to front and back windows, as well as a radio tuned to a programme with a lot of talking, to give the impression that people are inside chatting away and timers are very cheap and truly effective. You should also consider creating a secret place to store valuables such as passports or jewellery, even a safe is a good investment to keep your valuables safe, and nowadays safes come in all shape and sizes and are quite affordable.

A hidden safe, also called a diversion safe, is an everyday object that hides a valuable: they come in all types and sizes, beer cans, fizzy drinks, books, but I would encourage building your own, or use the hollow cavity of an object (old lamp for instance) as a safe place.

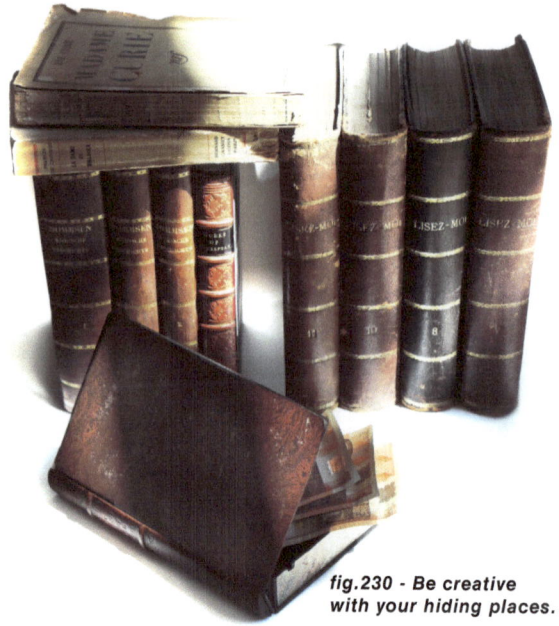

fig.230 - Be creative with your hiding places.

TAKE PHOTOS OF ALL YOUR VALUABLES. Avoid using objects that can be themselves targets, for instance a HI-FI speaker.

Identify your most precious items, including a bicycle; with your postcode or driving licence number, it helps the authorities to find the rightful owner as well as securing a conviction when people are found in possession of your belongings without justification. It is also a good idea to take photographs of all your valuables and store them with a scan of every document/card that you keep in your wallet, it makes things easier in case you are burgled, to show your insurance company and also to claim the items in case the Police notifiy that stolen goods have been seized.

Once you have given a good look at your house from the outside, identifying potential weak spots, it is useful for you to know that there are some organised or professional burglars who "mark" houses as good targets, to come back at a later date to steal or to signal to fellow burglars a good target. In fig.232 (opposite) you can see some commonly used symbols that appear as scribbles or stickers on doorbells, entry phones or other outside elements of a property to identify it as a good or bad target.

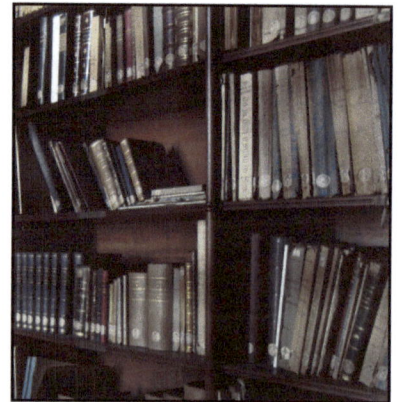

Other tricks to mark a property as a target are shoes left on the driveway to indicate that the house is easy to enter, or innocent looking rubbish such as a green crumpled up paper.

It is best to keep everything around your property tidy and remove any graffiti or litter immediately.

A more dangerous situation when at home is the so called "home invasion", either smashing through the front door or tricking the occupants to open the main door pretending to be bringing a delivery or that they are a utilities reader and even impersonating police officers or other authorities.

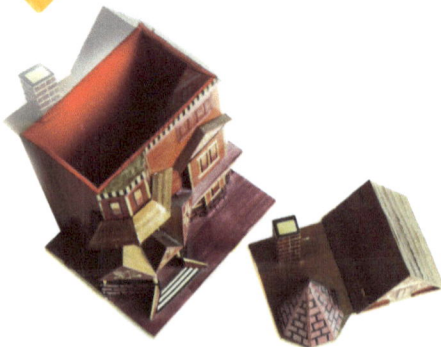

fig. 231- Perfect hiding place?

◇	ABANDONED HOUSE	△	WOMAN ALONE
X	GOOD TARGET	😐	PEOPLE WILLING TO GIVE MONEY
O o O o	EXTREMELY GOOD	///	JUST BURGLED
Q	LEAVE ALONE-FRIENDS.	○	POINTLESS TRYING
—	DOG INSIDE	⊗	NOT INTERESTING
▱▱▱	DOG	⊻	OWNERS GIVING-WORK-LEAVE ALONE
⋆	HIGH RISK	Ⅲ	AVOID AREA
N	NIGHT TIME IDEAL FOR ENTRY	⊰⊱	POLICE OFFICER
A M	AFTERNOON IDEAL FOR ENTRY	D	SUNDAY IDEAL FOR ENTRY
⊏	WEALTHY	M	MORNING IDEAL FOR ENTRY
⊗	NOTHING OF VALUE	Oℜ	BURGLAR ALARM
+o XX	POLICE ACTIVE-AVOID		

fig.232 - Some symbols used by burglars to identify a target. They are normally scribbled on the wall or as small stickers next to the doorbell or door of residences but also shops or factories.

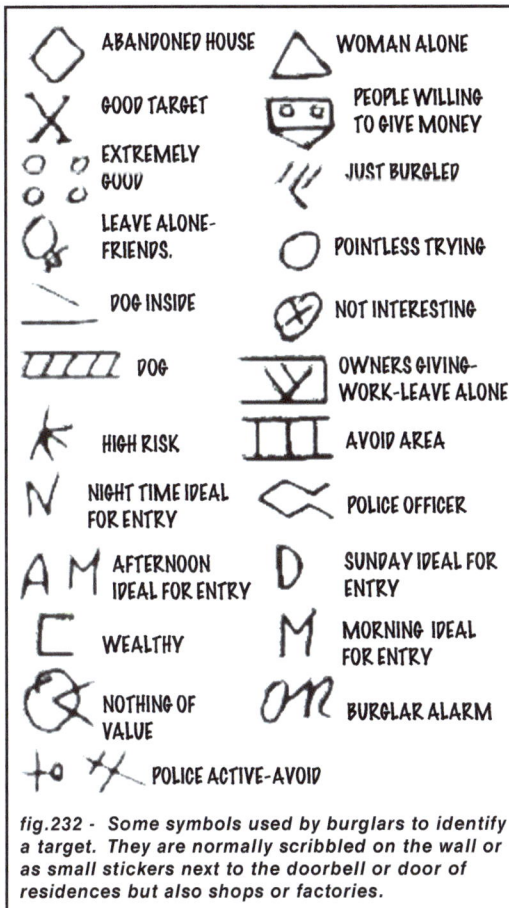

Once the door is opened the robbers often tie up the occupants, ransack the house and unfortunately use violence even forcing one of the family members to follow them to an ATM machine to withdraw money.

It can happen at any time of day or night, mostly towards the end of the day though.

Be suspicious of any stranger calling and teach all member of your family never to open the door to anyone. Some "tricks" consist of even crashing into your car parked in the driveway to make you open the front door. Be wary.

Preventing measures are the same ones to prevent burglaries: solid doors and locks and do not leave back doors or garage doors opened or weak.

BE WARY OF STRANGERS CALLING ON YOUR DOORSTEP.

Some homeowners have safe or "panic" rooms in their house, a room with a very strong door and a telephone in it. However just keeping a spare mobile phone, always on charge, in a room easy to retreat to, can be a good safety measure. At night keep your curtains drawn, especially if living at street level, you shouldn't really display your contents to passers by with a criminal intent. And lastly, remember that there are special occasions that can make your home more vulnerable, such as a party or Christmas for instance. If you organise a party for your birthday or your daughter's for instance try and avoid having it at home if it means more than ten people, the loud music and people going in and out of the house attracts the type of people that you would not welcome.

It is difficult to keep an eye on those things in these circumstances; you are too busy having a good time. It is better to hire a venue such as a restaurant or other venue and celebrate the occasion away from home. The periods of the year normally dedicated to spending and holidays tend to attract criminals. Ask yourself if the Christmas decorations and pile of boxes with the expensive Japanese TV logo on it are advertising the wrong message to people that might have a better look at what you have bought as presents or prey on the Christmas spirit to gain entry to your property. Do not forget that there have been also cases of burglars targeting houses when the family was out at a wedding or a funeral, therefore if you know that many people will know about that event ask someone to come and stay for the day while you are away or make sure you have put some extra or proper safety measures to avoid being burgled.

Some burglars check the local paper to see about family functions such as a wedding or a funeral, and they visit the home while people are out celebrating. Ask someone to keep an eye on the property or to stay there for the duration, you can always return the favour.

The general purpose of all these measures should mostly be to make your home a hard target, most burglars prefer a soft target, and they want to be in and out in the least possible time.

Whatever makes this difficult or makes it appear like it's going to be too much hassle will work as a deterrent and burglars will move on to the next easier available target.

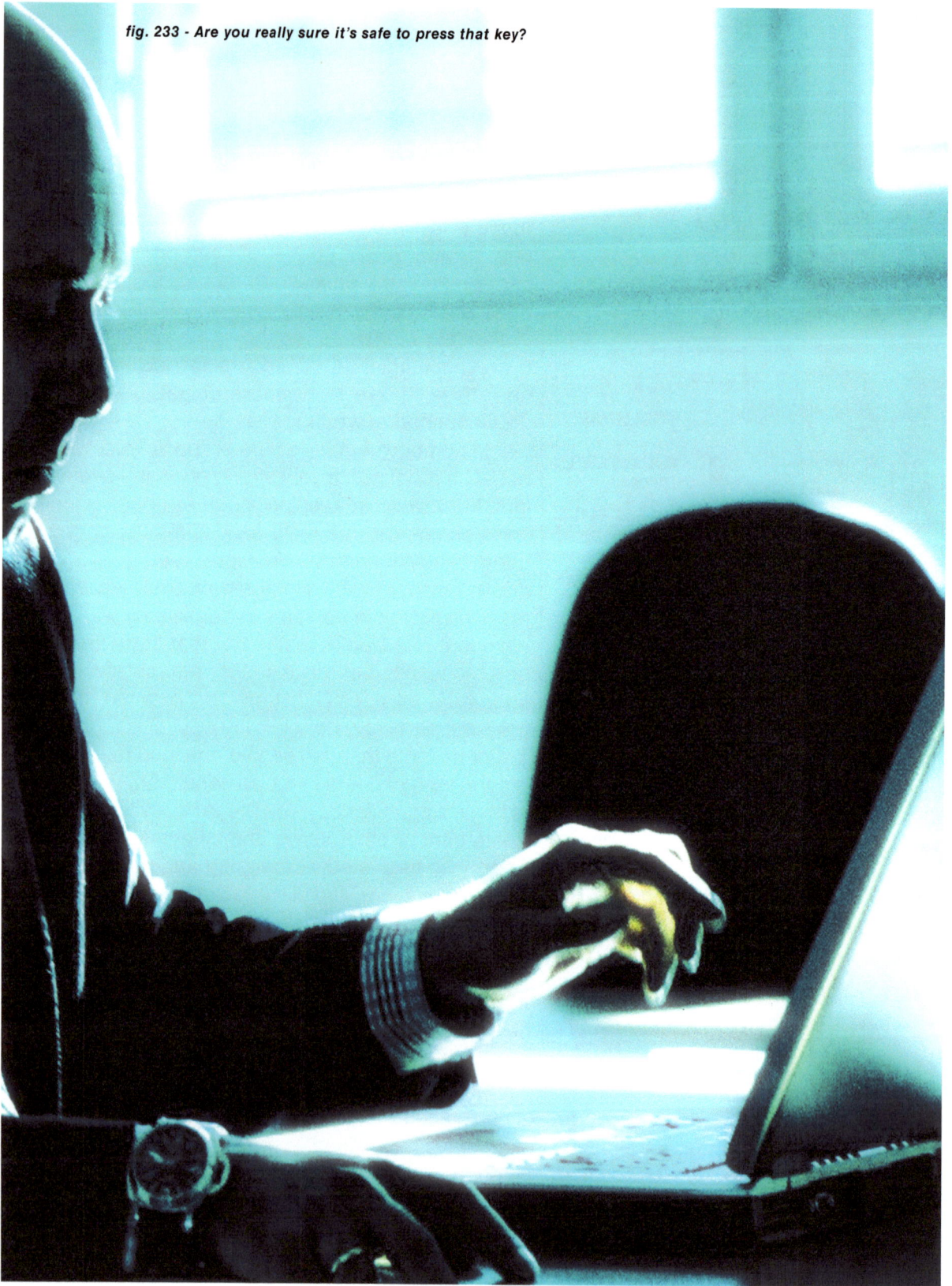

fig. 233 - Are you really sure it's safe to press that key?

This chapter has been written in collaboration with Sascha Beyer, IT security expert.

We always worry about the real world, sometimes unnecessarily so.

However, looking at recent crime statistics you'll be surprised to discover that one the most lucrative and safest crimes committed at present is Internet fraud.

I hear you wondering why bother to discuss "virtual" crime in a self-defence manual, but believe us, the damage these scammers do is very physical, and the more people know about some simple defensive measures the merrier.

VIRTUAL CRIME CAUSES PHYSICAL AND VERY REAL DAMAGE.

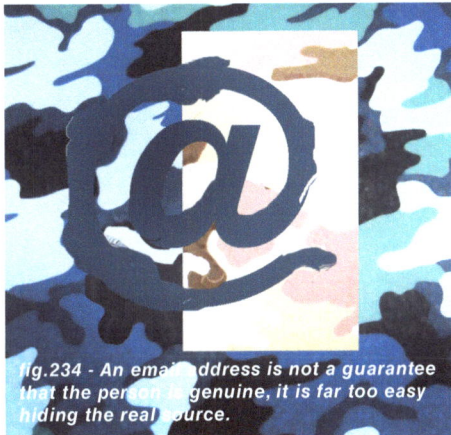

There are lots of reasons why internet fraud is on the rise and this is not the place to discuss why, what we want to point out is what we can do to avoid being hurt in the cyber world.

People subjected to online frauds have committed suicide or took it out on their families or colleagues physically.

Even more abominable is when children are being lured through online chats to meet paedophiles posing as children. There are fundamentally two types of scams on the net: the first one is someone contacting you posing as your bank or an auction site such as Ebay, and secondly someone posing as somebody else, for instance getting your child to believe the criminal is also a teenager when in fact he's a dirty old man to say the least.

So, what are the telltale signs?

fig.234 - An email address is not a guarantee that the person is genuine, it is far too easy hiding the real source.

Let's have a look. Is someone contacting you to transfer millions of dollars into your bank account? Is anyone paying you to cash cheques and sending you money? Have you met a pen pal or possible date through a site and she's desperate for money? Has a dying person contacted you asking you to sort out lots of money she wants to leave to charity? Have you recently sold an item and the buyer is suggesting you accept a payment larger than the original amount?

Well, wakey,wakey! It's a scam! The old saying nobody gives you anything for free also works in the cyber world: if it's too good to be true, it is. If somebody tells you that you won the lottery, ask yourself when did you buy the ticket? And isn't it surprising that your bank contacts you without remembering your exact name as well as basic English grammar?

This is called "phishing" and has brought misery to a lot of people and institutions.

Phishing works like this: you receive an e-mail that claims to be from a known company, Ebay, NatWest, Lloyds, whatever, in any case a recognised institution. It might offer you buyer's protection or asks you to re-enter your account details for security reasons or threatens closure of your account if you don't take immediate action.

Think again: even if presenting all the bells and whistles such as the logos and graphics is your bank really so mean and unprofessional not to contact you in a more secure way?

DO NOT UPDATE BANK DETAILS OVER THE INTER-NET IF ASKED TO DO SO.

Clicking on the link that is asking you to update your details is asking for trouble. If in doubt, call your bank or e-mail them through their official website and see what they say. Other tricks by seasoned fraudsters include the classic cheque over-pay-ment where a buyer or employer or possible tenant will send you a cheque of higher value than the money agreed, and then asks to send the surplus money to a third party, for example to pay for shipping, money transfer or whatever other reason.

CAUTION

The cheque will eventually clear into your bank only to be refused weeks later. And do you have any idea what is going to happen next?

At that point the bank will take the full amount written on the cheque from your account, conse-quentially you lose your goods and your money. Is it too good to be true? Of course it is.

The same applies if you are buying an item online and the seller tells you that before they ship the item into your country there are some fees such as import duty or carnet, or similar stuff.

Do not pay such a fee. You'll never get the product, and any money that you paid for fees is also gone. This type of fraud is also targeting people offering services such as photographers.

The potential client will contact the photographer wanting a wedding photo shoot.

Money is agreed without fuss, maybe even plane tickets arranged (they can be cancelled at little cost). The problem is that they send you too much. They ask if you can return the difference please by Western Union. You do, then days later their cheque bounces.

An increasingly clever scam is setting up fake escrow sites. The way it works is that a buyer or a seller sug-gests using an escrow service to complete the transaction making it "safer". They will recommend a rep-utable escrow service that even if it looks totally proper is almost cer-tainly a fake, and you'll never see your money or your product ever again. If you want to use escrow services, do your own research and get in touch with a reputable com-pany (see HELP page 246)

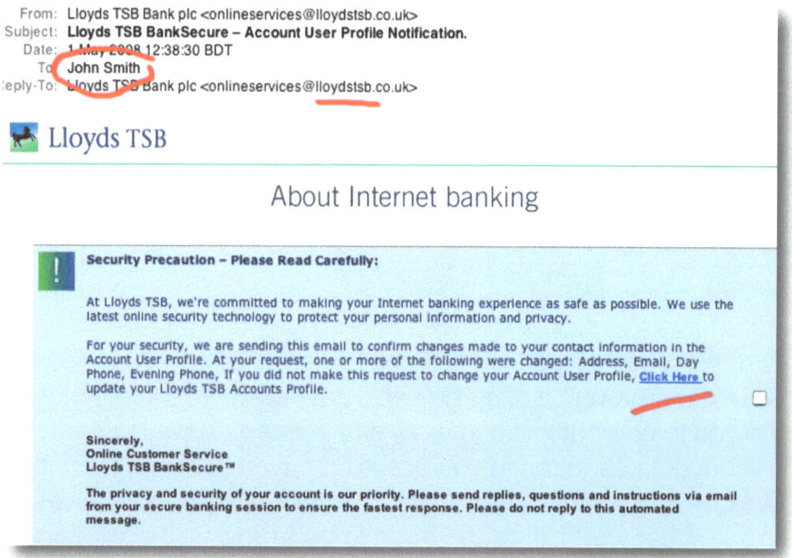

Another scam is when someone con-tacts you through the internet suggesting that you can make a lot of money working from home. For instance, suggesting that you can make nice money just stuffing envelopes. What they omit to tell you is that to do that you need to sell that system to others. It's called a pyramid or Ponzi scheme and it is actually outlawed in many countries. You should be wary of anyone offering you an amazing job opportunity to make money quick; it just doesn't work like that in real life does it? Then the letter from Ubungu Ubangi (or similarly exotic sounding name), son of the uncle of the vice-president of some African country who unfortunately died in a plane crash and by sheer chance finds you, yes you, a God - believing reputable person they want to trust with the billions of dollars witting in a dormant account that nobody knows about.

fig.235 - A sophisticated example of an email posing as LLOYDS bank. As you can see everything looks good, except that a "proper" Bank would NEVER ask you to submit your details in this way. If you are still not sure call your bank, but without using the contact details within the email , just call the number on your statement or past correspondence which you are absolutely sure of.

From: Lloyds TSB Bank plc <onlineservices@lloydstsb.co.uk>
Subject: Lloyds TSB BankSecure – Account User Profile Notification.
Date: 1 May 2008 12:38:30 BDT
To: John Smith
Reply-To: Lloyds TSB Bank plc <onlineservices@lloydstsb.co.uk>

Lloyds TSB

About Internet banking

Security Precaution – Please Read Carefully:

At Lloyds TSB, we're committed to making your Internet banking experience as safe as possible. We use the latest online security technology to protect your personal information and privacy.

For your security, we are sending this email to confirm changes made to your contact information in the Account User Profile. At your request, one or more of the following were changed: Address, Email, Day Phone, Evening Phone, If you did not make this request to change your Account User Profile, Click Here to update your Lloyds TSB Accounts Profile.

Sincerely,
Online Customer Service
Lloyds TSB BankSecure™

The privacy and security of your account is our priority. Please send replies, questions and instructions via email from your secure banking session to ensure the fastest response. Please do not reply to this automated message.

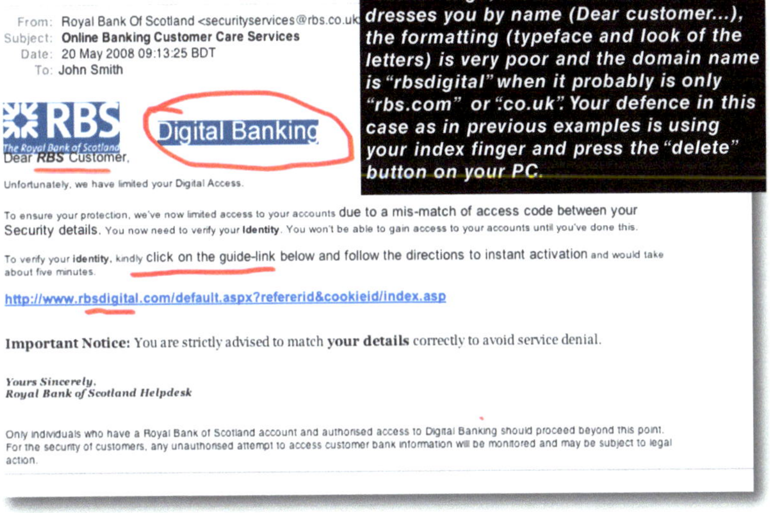

fig.236- A less sophisticated email trying to "phish" your details. Note the crude "cutout" logo, the fact that it does not addresses you by name (Dear customer...), the formatting (typeface and look of the letters) is very poor and the domain name is "rbsdigital" when it probably is only "rbs.com" or ".co.uk". Your defence in this case as in previous examples is using your index finger and press the "delete" button on your PC.

From: Royal Bank Of Scotland <securityservices@rbs.co.uk>
Subject: Online Banking Customer Care Services
Date: 20 May 2008 09:13:25 BDT
To: John Smith

RBS
The Royal Bank of Scotland

Digital Banking

Dear RBS Customer,

Unfortunately, we have limited your Digital Access.

To ensure your protection, we've now limited access to your accounts due to a mis-match of access code between your Security details. You now need to verify your Identity. You won't be able to gain access to your accounts until you've done this.

To verify your **identity**, kindly click on the guide-link below and follow the directions to instant activation and would take about five minutes.

http://www.rbsdigital.com/default.aspx?refererid&cookieid/index.asp

Important Notice: You are strictly advised to match **your details** correctly to avoid service denial.

Yours Sincerely,
Royal Bank of Scotland Helpdesk

Only individuals who have a Royal Bank of Scotland account and authorised access to Digital Banking should proceed beyond this point. For the security of customers, any unauthorised attempt to access customer bank information will be monitored and may be subject to legal action.

Yeah, right, more likely it is a so called "419" scam.

The "419 scam" (see also GLOSSARY page 198) is one of the most successful frauds on the net, and it's shocking how many people still believe that somebody out of the blue would find out about you and trust you with millions of dollars, just like that.

If you want to learn more about this type of scam there are plenty of websites that will give you all the information you need (See HELP page 246).

Needless to say you should not answer and the best action is to press the delete button.

If you are a pet lover you will probably be contacted by someone who has a pet that he needs to ship from a country overseas and because it's a rare breed, he needs your help, such as booking seats on a plane. Dog breeds such as Yorkshire Terriers, Chihuahuas, and other exotic breeds are mostly used to attract your interest.

Don't be fooled by the pictures accompanying these e-mails, they are obviously fakes. In short, why would you trust somebody on the net with money if you wouldn't trust somebody approaching you on the street with the same proposal, only because they seemed legitimate? Think again. The main principle should be to behave as if you are walking down the street, even an impressive website can be a clever design by someone who is just good with the computer. If in doubt, call the company and talk to a real person.

WHY TRUSTING SOMEONE ON THE NET BUT NOT SOMEONE IN THE STREET?

The rules that would apply in the real world apply more so in the virtual world and common sense should prevail: if it's too good to be true, it is, if it smells badly, it is rotting. So, let's sum up some general tips on fraud schemes:

IT TAKES VERY LITTLE KNOWLEDGE TO CREATE IMPRESSIVE WEBSITES.

1) Don't be fooled by appearances: remember that there are plenty of easily obtainable and cheap software to create a website that looks as if it represents a company or institution with hundreds of employees. Just because it is out there does not mean it actually exists. Go by word of mouth if shopping online or do a quick search on GOOGLE typing the company's name together with the word "bad" and see what comes up. Also try to find out if there is a real address. And check that it corresponds to a real company (GOOGLING street view can help) or phone up a local nearby business or even a nearby Police station.

2) Avoid at all cost giving out personal details online. If you receive an email message asking for any personal details, such as bank details, address, passport or anything else, it is almost certainly a scam. Once scammers have your personal details, they can do a lot of harm.

3) An email address even if legitimate does not mean it is: there are plenty of ways to set up a proper email address such as your bank's onto something that has nothing to do with it. Therefore what comes up on your computer as: security@yourbank.com in fact can well be youarescammed@fraudsters.com

4) Anyone asking you for advance fees or offering to pay you more for goods you are selling, and asking to send the difference by Western Union for instance, is definitely a scam.

Let's now talk about passwords: technically speaking you must use a password that has all of the following elements, length, strength and duration.

APPEARANCES CAN BE DECEPTIVE IS A RULE ON THE INTERNET, NOT AN EXCEPTION.

Length of your password should be more than 8 characters, the strength of your password means that it should be a combination of at least three of the following four elements: uppercase, lowercase, numbers and special characters.

fig.237 - This is a classic email where the scammer pretends to be a relative of a deceased rich man, often using the names of people truly deceased in an accident. This type of scam is called "419".

For example: "Self$dEfenx£e52" responds to all of these elements. Avoid using your mother's maiden name, birth date, phone number or just a series of consecutive numbers as your password. It is safe enough to use your car registration or somebody's birthday or anniversary.

Remember that every password can get cracked; it's just a matter of time, so change it regularly, once a month would be ideal. You can make up a password using a pass phrase: "Iwas21in1985". Do not use words that are in common use, or easily found in a dictionary, they are easy targets for hacking attacks, up to 50,000 words a second can be processed by a password cracker software, and if you feel clever because you are using a foreign word think again: dictionary files for any language are publicly available, even African dialects or dead languages.

There are some websites that offer a strength test for passwords, such as http://howsecureis-

MAKE A STRONG PASSWORD, CONSIDER IT AS A LOCK TO YOUR FRONT DOOR.

mypassword.net/. A more serious security issue is identity theft. It is bad enough that someone lures you into paying something, worse still is if someone poses as you on the web, doing nasty things. This can be achieved with relative ease, stealing your identity, hijacking your PC using "bots" (see GLOSSARY page 198)) and distributing child porn from your pc. If you are prosecuted you will discover that all the evidence your pc, your IP address (GLOSSARY page 198) etc. is yours and the fact that you haven't been at home for months does not matter in the least to a Judge or a Jury.

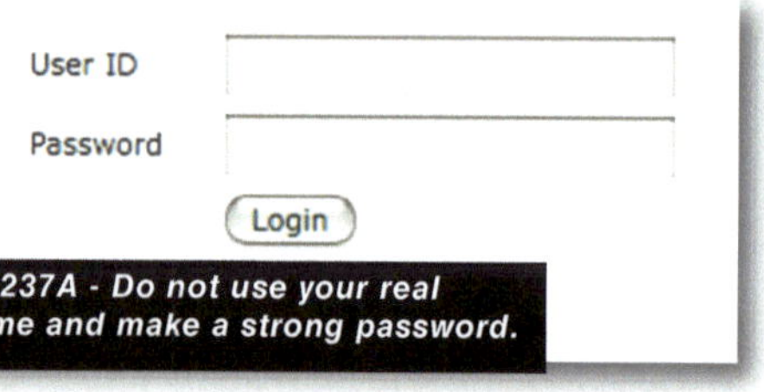

fig.237A - Do not use your real name and make a strong password.

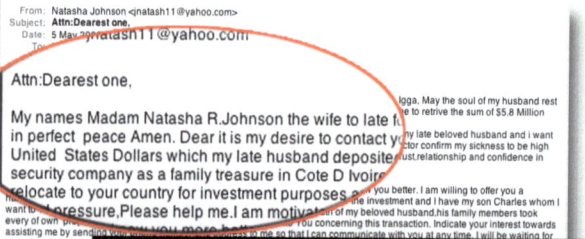

Now you understand why safeguarding your personal information with a safe password is absolutely fundamental.

It is quite shocking that people are very weary about giving away personal information to strangers or they don't even want their home telephone number to appear in the phone book, but then publish all their personal information everywhere on the web (Facebook etc.)? With data mining techniques it is easy to collect all your personal information, no matter how far it is distributed on the net. One person caught recently was using false identities (three different ones). It took three days until they chained them together and got him arrested.

The cyber investigator even knew his school and had a picture of his class, all information found through the internet, without hacking into any PC, just clever surfing methods.

Normally victims of identity theft don't realize that their identity has been stolen until is quite late but there are some simple steps to take to check if this has happened.

Utilities, bills or credit card statements arrive very late or do not arrive at all. Strange transactions appear on your credit card statement. Companies such as mobile phone providers suddenly contact you about your account or a service that you haven't asked for.

Credit cards or store cards are suddenly refused when trying to buy goods, meaning somebody else is asking for credit on your behalf a long way past an acceptable threshold.

fig.238 - Tedious but safer if any online form is filled in manually and not automatically by your computer.

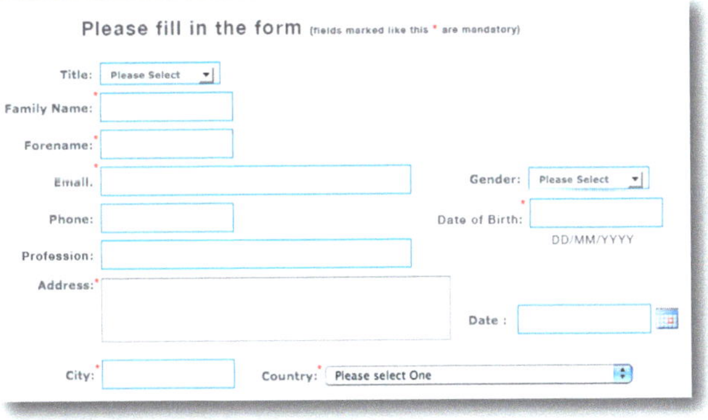

Please fill in the form (fields marked like this * are mandatory)

Title: Please Select
Family Name:
Forename:
Email.   Gender: Please Select
Phone: Date of Birth:
                                DD/MM/YYYY
Profession:
Address:
                                Date :
City: Country: Please select One

To avoid being a victim of identity fraud you should follow these simple suggestions. Make sure that your internet browser on your computer is not set up in your preferences to automatically fill out a form when you go onto a website to fill out an online order or other operation requiring your details.

It is a pain to fill in every time, but somebody can hack your computer and access all the information at hand. If you go onto a website, including your bank make sure that you check the website URL accurately, it is very easy to be fooled by "nameofyourbank_Security.com" when in fact the correct URL is "nameofyourbank.com" and nothing else. If you are not sure it is your bank phone them up on their usual number or check if some recent letters exchanged.

When it comes to credit cards make sure that you know which number to call in case you either lose your card or a new card that you have ordered hasn't arrived.

Also sign and activate recently ordered cards immediately.

As we have said before make sure that before disposing of all documents both at home and in the office they should be shredded, crosscutting or confetti style are quite safe.

Stay on top of your billing mail and bank statements; make sure that you always check your bills as soon as they arrive especially from credit cards. If anything is strange or you are not sure of something, contact your credit card company immediately.

Make sure you are careful when in a public, giving access codes and other personal information as you are calling the bank while on the bus, train or taxi. Anyone could hear all the passwords and security questions answered and it doesn't take much to understand what is what.

If you move house make sure you don't leave anything about your previous activity as rubbish behind, squatters might get hold of it or even the new tenants might find some of your personal information very useful to obtain things fraudulently. You can use a mail forwarding service to avoid your post still going to your old address. Also make sure that if you

KEEP YOUR PC SAFE SO YOU WILL NOT HAVE TO PROVE IT WAS NOT YOU.

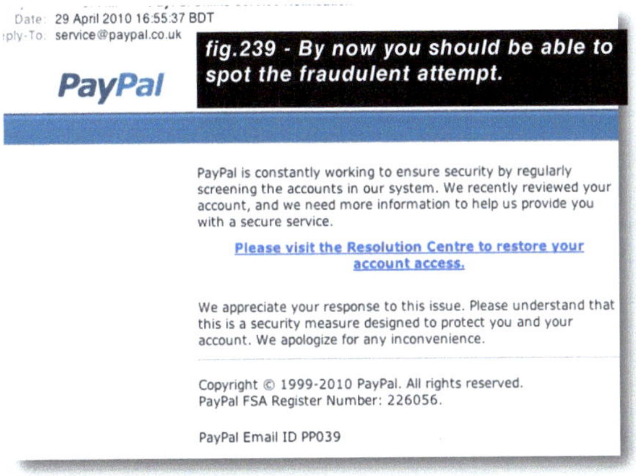

dispose of your personal computer you erase all data on the old hard drive completely.

Normally reformatting the drive should be enough but in case you're not sure smash the hard drive to bits or drop it in water. Be careful not to put any personal information on portable pen drives or portable hard drives, if you have no choice make sure they are encrypted.

A lot of the most common word processing software allows encrypting documents with a password. If you have a feeling that somebody has used your name or your personal details to get a credit card or a loan or buying goods contact your bank or credit card company and cancel all cards

Date: 29 April 2010 16:55:37 BDT
ply-To: service@paypal.co.uk

PayPal

fig.239 - By now you should be able to spot the fraudulent attempt.

PayPal is constantly working to ensure security by regularly screening the accounts in our system. We recently reviewed your account, and we need more information to help us provide you with a secure service.

Please visit the Resolution Centre to restore your account access.

We appreciate your response to this issue. Please understand that this is a security measure designed to protect you and your account. We apologize for any inconvenience.

Copyright © 1999-2010 PayPal. All rights reserved.
PayPal FSA Register Number: 226056.

PayPal Email ID PP039

explaining what happened. You can also contact the CREDIT CHECKING AGENCY (see HELP page 246), and the local police station to obtain a crime reference number and make sure you keep a record of all letters sent to credit cards and creditors such as utilities companies such as electricity, telephone gas etc. informing them you have been a victim of identity theft.

Opening Mail Attachment

⚠ Opening: document.doc

WARNING: Web pages, executables, and other attachments may contain viruses or scripts that can be harmful to your computer. It is important to be certain that this file is from a trustworthy source.

What would you like to do with this file?

○ Open it
○ Save it to disk

[OK]   [Cancel]

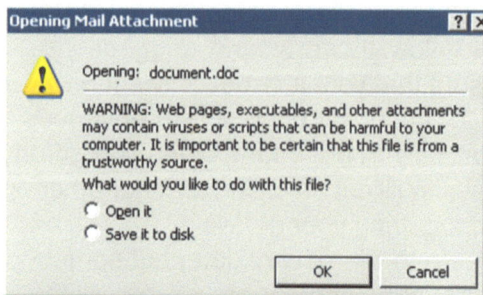

fig.240 - Can you trust who is sending you the attachment? Did they really send it?

REAL WORLD RULES SHOULD BE APPLIED TO THE CYBER WORLD AS WELL.

You can also contact CIFAS (page 246), the United Kingdom fraud prevention service, and sign for protective registration; this will help because they carry out additional checks if anyone applies for anything in your name.

And now let's talk about viruses and other nasty cyber creatures.

More and more often you hear of new viruses and worms and Trojan Horse programs that spread or can be sent by e-mail and can do a lot of damage to your computer. In order for a virus to be able to attack it needs some kind of access to the PC. This can be the Internet, USB stick, CD-ROMS etc.

In every file that needs to be executed, e.g. *.exe or *.com there can be a hidden virus, even text documents of the type *.doc or tables of the type *.xls can be contaminated. It is estimated that there are now more than 200,000 harmful programs in circulation. So how can we protect ourselves?

These are the basic steps to take in addition to what we discussed earlier:

CAUTION

1) Install an Anti-virus programme and an anti-spy-ware programme and keep them constantly updated, be careful opening attachments received by email.

2) Set up a personal firewall and update it frequently. If this is configured correctly it will protect you from all sorts of dangers from the Internet as well as preventing data that has been obtained without your knowledge being sent to an attacker if your PC is infected.

3) Always take great care of all usernames and passwords that you have.

Try to change them frequently; do not use the same for everything.

4) Be careful when opening e-mail attachments. Harmful programs are often distributed via attachments. If in doubt, ask the sender of the e-mail if the attachments are really from him.

Set up your e-mail program in a way that attachments do not get opened automatically.

In general, do not open e-mails from unknown senders.

5) Be careful when downloading web pages or programs from the internet, make sure that the source is trustworthy, and update your Anti-virus programme regularly.

6) Only give out personal information where really necessary. Online fraudsters often approach individuals: data that they have managed to obtain before, e.g. your surfing habits or names from your personal surroundings are used to get your trust.

7) If you are using VoIP or WLAN then think about encoding your communication when transmitting confidential information, as your communication can be read or heard by third parties.

8) If in spite of all these security measures your PC gets infected lots of data previously saved on your PC can get lost. In order to minimise the damage, you should always create security copies of your files on CD-ROM/DVD or on an external hard drive.

Now let's also look into what you can do to keep your kids safe online.

The popularity of chat lines, blogs and social networking websites such as "Facebook" means more and more young and very young people spend time in front of the computer surfing or chatting, and most of them have no idea how dangerous is in there.

It is worth pointing out that the same rules that applies in the real world apply in cyberspace, and while sites such as Facebook or Myspace are doing all they can to make it a safe and enjoyable experience, there are some simple rules that people, especially if young, should follow just as they normally would in the real world.

Keep all personal details to an absolute minimum, use a pseudonym or nickname if possible, not your real name. Absolutely do not publish phone numbers, no names, no school names and just keep that personal information to yourself or hidden behind that front page.

You can check the security settings that you most certainly have access to when you join these websites. Also check the website's security page, where they tell you what to do and not to do, and ensure it is kept up to date. Another very important way to keep your children safe is to make sure that you can see what they are doing on the computer, position the monitor in their room in a way that just entering the room in a casual way you can see what is happening on the screen. It gets more difficult when they are unruly and curious teenagers but if you feel bad about spying on their privacy remember that unscrupulous people are out there with some seriously sick intentions.

MAKE SURE YOU CAN SEE YOUR CHILDREN's PC EASILY.

Initially use and surf the internet together with your children, have a chat about potential risks and explain a few things that we have discussed and be aware that some websites offering free on-line games are run by paedophiles. By all means you should set the internet browser with safe parameters (they all provide parental control of some degrees) and you should also create a user account specific for them with their own password (that you obviously know) and limiting in your computer system certain functions and privileges, such as having an administrator password to install new programs, or not giving access to parts of the system.

It is worth remembering that no programme or security settings are as effective as a parent supervising, and that does not mean hovering constantly behind them, as they play with their favourite videogame or surf online to research material for a school project.

However it's the chat-rooms, blogs and social network sites that you have to monitor, make sure you have full access to all their communications online, and do not tell them off if they swear or exchange the odd rude photo, keep their confidence and intervene only when there's something REALLY serious. Things can be difficult because teenagers learn quicker and more when it comes to technology, but don't be intimidated by their knowledge and ask the help of a friend who is a computer buff in case you are at loss.

If you suspect there is something wrong going on, such as a self declared teenager chatting with your son or daughter in a way that makes you uncomfortable, seriously uncomfortable, talk to a friend or a relative for a second opinion and then contact the authorities.

The Internet is one of the greatest inventions ever; it does make our life more informed and fun, offering almost endless possibilities, including job search and social networking. But at the same time it is a constantly ever changing ever adapting world that is almost impossible to police, and there are a lot of criminals using it to profit from it causing grief and damage to honest people. Some of the advice you have read in this will probably be obsolete by the time we publish it, but remember the main principles that can keep you and your loved ones safe independently from the quickly evolving technology.

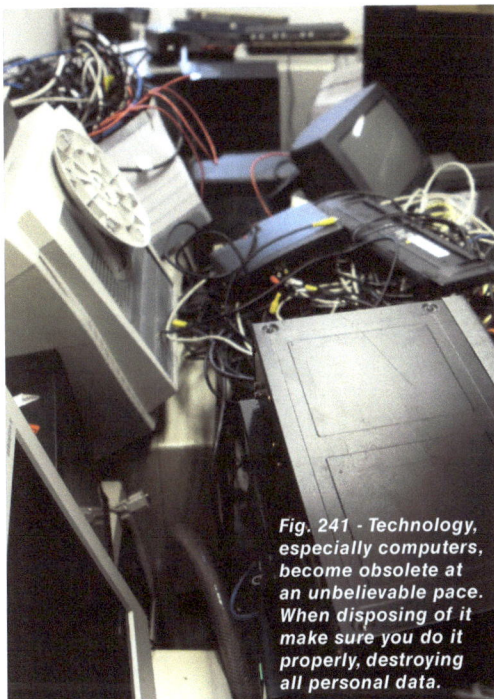

Fig. 241 - Technology, especially computers, become obsolete at an unbelievable pace. When disposing of it make sure you do it properly, destroying all personal data.

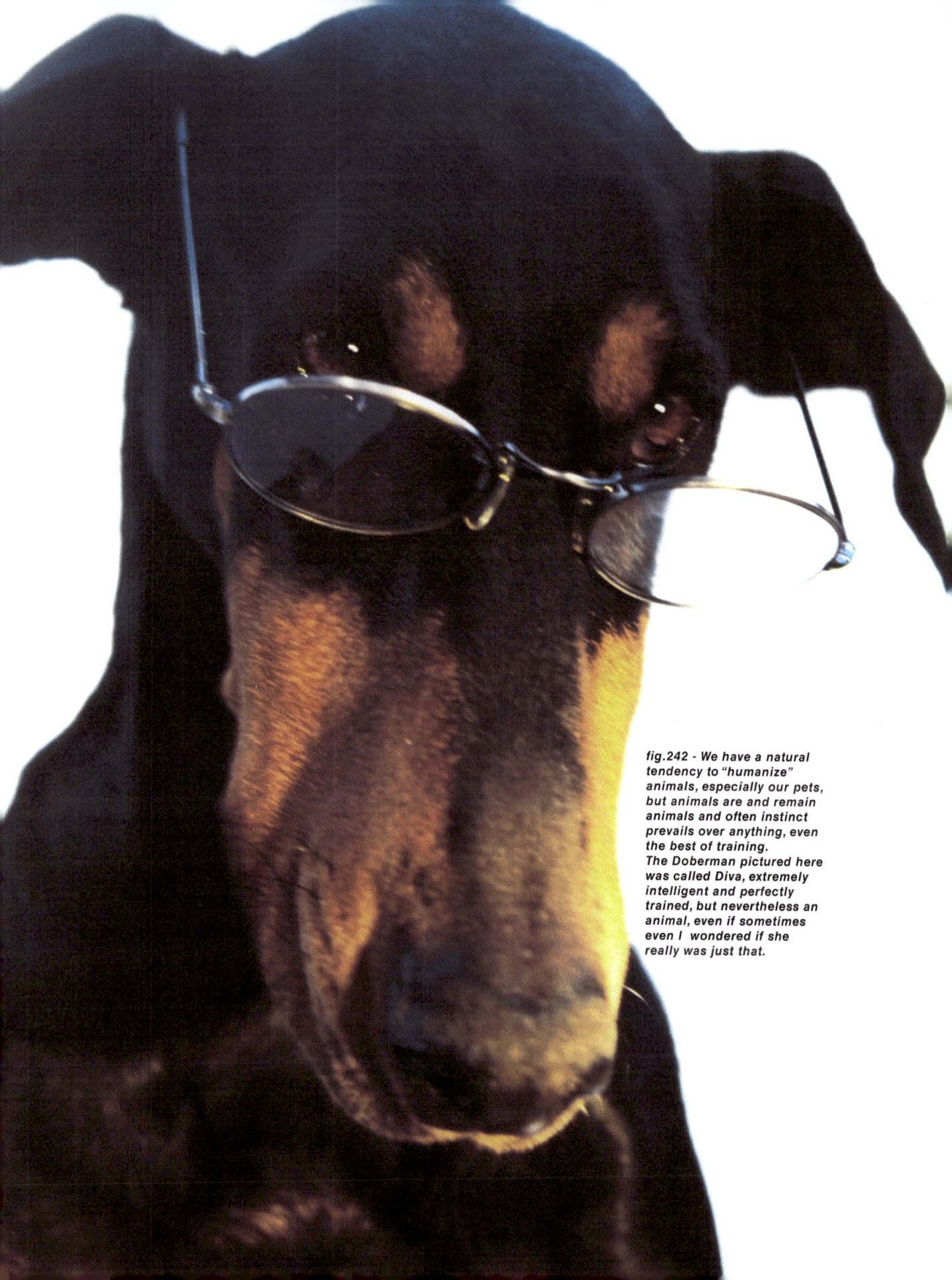

fig.242 - We have a natural tendency to "humanize" animals, especially our pets, but animals are and remain animals and often instinct prevails over anything, even the best of training.
The Doberman pictured here was called Diva, extremely intelligent and perfectly trained, but nevertheless an animal, even if sometimes even I wondered if she really was just that.

how to defend yourself if attacked by
animals

ATTACKS BY ANIMALS EVEN WITHIN A CITY ARE QUITE COMMON.

If you think men are unpredictable, especially when attacking somebody, think again, in fact, the opposite is true, with the obvious exception of somebody under the influence of drugs or alcohol, or because of mental illness.

When it comes to animals most zoologists will agree, animal attacks are quite unpredictable, but at the same time you should be able to be prepared.

If you live in a city you probably will be smiling, wondering how much harm you can get from wild creatures. But if you go jogging in the nearby park regularly, you probably have experienced how it feels to suddenly see a dog bolting from under nearby bushes growling as you run past, or even being attacked by one. Even if you are the city type you might still decide to take a stroll in the countryside and cross a fenced field and meet face to face with a bull.

We had a few requests of giving some advice on what to do in case an animal decides to have a go at you; we are not going to explore possible attacks by every single creature.

The chances that you come across a cobra are slim unless you are often travelling off the beaten track in exotic countries. However, we'll give some general advice, including about snakes.

If you are carelessly crossing a field and suddenly notice the large bull that roams the space your best course of action is to back away making yourself small, and without losing sight of the animal (but don't make eye contact), try to go over the fence or wall as quickly as possible.

Bulls can run faster and swerve faster than us, and they are totally unpredictable, they will charge with no warning and no matter whether you wear red or not, anything bright will attract their attention.

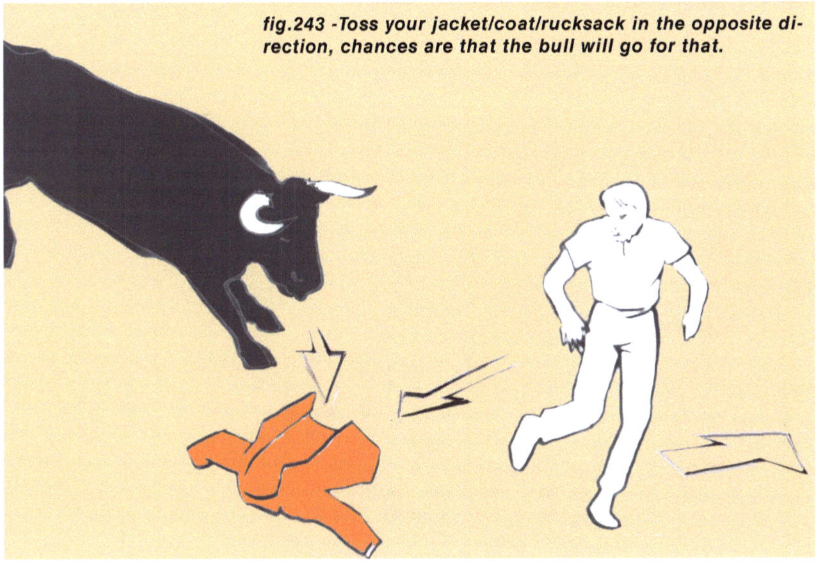

fig.243 -Toss your jacket/coat/rucksack in the opposite direction, chances are that the bull will go for that.

Therefore remove anything on you that is too bright, yellow, pink etc., doing so quite slowly and as discreetly as possible.

If you are too far away from safety, take off your jacket, coat or jumper in any case and be ready to toss it in the opposite direction of where you are running and hope the bull will go for that (see fig.243).

If you are with somebody slower than you, God forbid a child for instance, make him or her run in a different direction and attract the bull towards you waving and shouting.

If everything fails go to the ground and pretend you are dead, it has worked with quite a few animals, including bears.

A CALM, FIRM TONE CAN WORK MIRACLES WITH AN AGGRESSIVE DOG.

Probably the most common animal that you should learn how to handle is the dog and if you are ever attacked by a dog, or more than one, make sure you don't end up on the ground.

If the dog comes towards you in a menacing way try to talk in a firm tone, hoping that it had some training and will respond to a calm, firm voice. However most of the time that is not enough and there are few simple actions you can take that can be an absolute lifesaver.

Protect your forearm, wrapping something around it such as a jacket or jumper and throw anything you can, e.g. stones or coins at it.

If nevertheless it bites you in the arm don't tear or pull the arm away, do the opposite. Push back towards the rear of the dog's throat, it will weaken the grip and provoke the gagging reflexes and he might let go. If the dog has a collar grab it and twist it to choke the animal and do not let go until someone comes to help or the dog loses

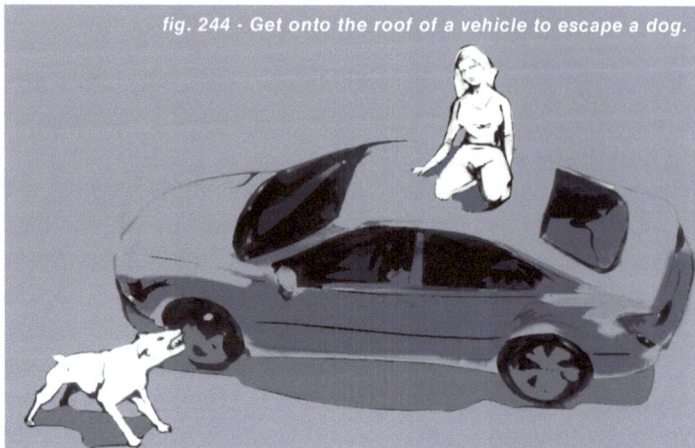

fig. 244 - Get onto the roof of a vehicle to escape a dog.

consciousness. Remember that there are many different types of dogs; the majority will back off if you stand your ground, but some will attack and will be quite resilient to any of these techniques. It is also worth remembering that hitting the dog might increase the ferocity of the attack.

If you fall to the ground, possibly under the dog's weight, wrap your legs around its ribs and squeeze, extending your legs out, with a scissor-move as strong as you can.

With your free arm, hit hard or even bite the dog's nose. This works against wolves as well. With these types of animals, including big cats, such as leopards or tigers, it also works to appear much bigger than you are. For instance, holding the folds of your coat or jacket open, almost like wings, they will perceive you are being able to increase your size at will.

If jogging in a park, remember that you can jump into a nearby lake/fountain or pond if chased by a dog, lots of animals, including bulls, don't like water too much.

If you come across someone that is being attacked by a dog the best thing is to grab the collar and twist as if it is a tourniquet. Do not let go of the dog once you have decided to proceed like this, otherwise the dog will turn and attack you. Another technique in case the dog has no collar is to grab hold at the rear on its groin and lift the dog up so all its weight is on the front legs.

This technique requires a confident and firm grasp, and can be quite dangerous if the dog manages to twist his body and bite your arm. Also you can use something to pass around the dog's neck and twist into a choke, something like a belt or a bag strap.

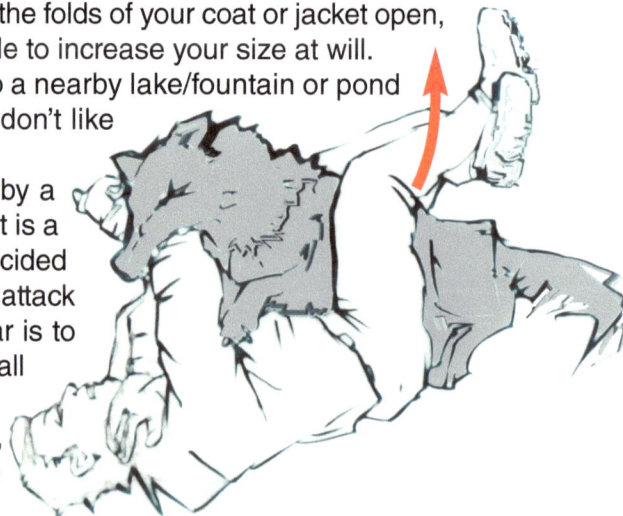

fig.245 - Wrap your legs around the wolf/dog ribs and squeeze, extending your legs out, with a scissor-move. Protect your throat with your other arm.

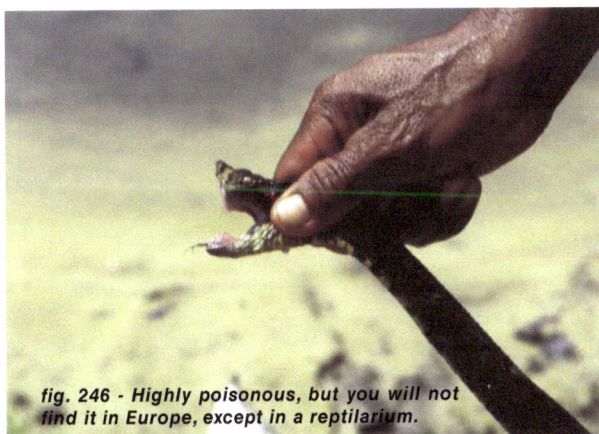

fig. 246 - Highly poisonous, but you will not find it in Europe, except in a reptilarium.

And since we've mentioned the lake, remember that swans, especially when with cygnets can be extremely aggressive, and their wings can easily break one of your limbs, or they can give you a nasty bite. Throwing something at them or splashing water or making yourself big, might work. In the unlikely event that you come across a viper or a snake, move away slowly; don't make sudden movements, keeping an eye on it.

If you have something like a rucksack, a bag or a stick try and put it between you and the snake, so that if it launches to bite, he'll bite whatever you put forward, keep your face and neck well away. In general with most animals that are displaying aggressive behaviour the best defence is a slow retreat; don't run but slowly back away, avoiding eye contact, keeping an eye on the animal position and behaviour.

Slow movements are the best; don't wave your arms, it is normally perceived by most animals as aggressive behaviour. Most animals might feign an attack, just to scare you, and standing your ground will possibly make them retreat. Running away unless you are definitely able to reach a safety point, such as inside a car should be avoided and also shouting or screaming is normally not a good idea. Animals don't understand what we are screaming about and they perceive the loud sound of our voice as aggressive behaviour. If you ever observed documentaries about animals confronting each other you probably noticed that rarely will such attacks end up with serious consequences, unless one of them is on a hunt. Most of the time what the animal looks for is submission of his opponent achieved with minimum blood spilled and minimum effort.

A gorilla would charge, stop, beat his chest, show his fangs and jump up and down, a bird would rough his feathers, trying to make himself big and so on, the moment the opponent shows submission the winner leaves, content with his success.

Obviously, even a simple nudge by an animal often translates into serious harm to a human and we often do not know what behaviour we should display to show submission.

I really cannot see many people keen to roll on their back offering their neck to a dog attacking. Nevertheless we can avoid some behaviour and gestures that most animals, big and small, will take as an aggressive response. Staring at the eyes is a big no-no, gesticulating and stepping forward is bad, and so is running, believe it or not: it is best to walk away slowly, keeping your eyes down, without ever losing sight of the animal at the same time.

OFTEN JUST WALKING AWAY CALMLY CAN STOP ANIMAL ATTACKS.

It should work with most animal threats. With some animals, such as horses or even dogs, trying to put an obstacle such as a tree or a car between you and the animal can help. In desperate cases the most vulnerable point of most animals is their eyes, or their nose, even a bull will probably have a ring on his nose, and if you unfortunately end up at such a close distance, grab the ring and pull down with all your strength.

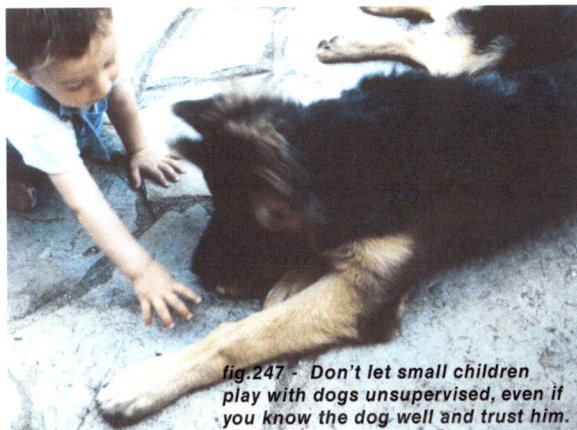

fig.247 - Don't let small children play with dogs unsupervised, even if you know the dog well and trust him.

That is what it's there for, to control the beast.

Obviously, as ever, our best advice is always prevention.

If you walk in the countryside, be informed of what animals you might encounter. Use some sensible precautions, such as do not walk too close to horses or cows, since even a sudden movement might scare them and they might trample you.

Animals in general don't want to attack you but if they do, it is because you are invading their territory where they are protecting their cubs nearby, or because they are sick. Even animals that might seem friendly, such as dolphins for instance, can turn very aggressive if a cub is amongst them.

So behave accordingly. If you respect animals they will respect you in return, but in looking at smaller creatures in the animal kingdom that we'll notice that the dangers can be greater.

BEWARE OF THE SMALL CREATURE, THEY CAN CAUSE GREATER HARM. If you end up in the Amazon forest for instance you will receive advice from the locals that it is normally the smallest tiniest creatures that can create the biggest damage. The Irukandji jellyfish is only 2.5 centimetres in diameter, but can cause death to humans within days.

fig. 248 - Poisonous.

fig. 249 - Non poisonous.

In Europe there aren't many poisonous animals, the odd viper and a few spiders that most of the time will give you a nasty bite but nothing more. The European scorpions are as dangerous as a wasp, and not as common, they are found in old buildings, near the roof or where it is warm and moist.

Normally snakes have two types of poisons: one is neurotoxins that normally paralyse your muscles including your heart and respiratory system, and this type of poison is the most dangerous. The other kind of poison, called digestive toxins, normally causes only tissue damage, and you'll be glad to know that some snakes have venoms that combine both effects.

Normally avoiding being bitten is a good precaution if threading in snake or scorpion territory, to wear high boots and long trousers, thick at the calves.

Always carry a long stick, to tap the ground in front of you or fend off an attack at safe distance. As you walk make some noises, and if by any chance a snake bites your boot or other garment without actually succeeding to penetrate your skin, make sure that you carefully inspect the area later, including the inside of your boots, since a snake's broken tooth still carries enough poison to harm you. Obviously try to keep boots and clothes off the floor at night and shake them well in the morning before putting them on in case unwanted visitors have taken up residence in them.

Anti venoms can be a good thing to have with you but make sure your doctor knows about it in case you may by allergic to the toxins, it might cause you more damage than the poison itself.

It is also important to remember that a snake will not necessarily inject the area that was bitten with enough poison to seriously harm you.

NEVER BLOCK AN ESCAPE ROUTE, HOWEVER SMALL THE ANIMAL IS. Always remember that snakes and other creatures have no intention of harming you, they are just defending themselves because you startled them or invaded their territory in the first place.

If you startle an animal in an enclosed space, either a hut or room, make sure that you do not stand on the line of exit, blocking its escape route.

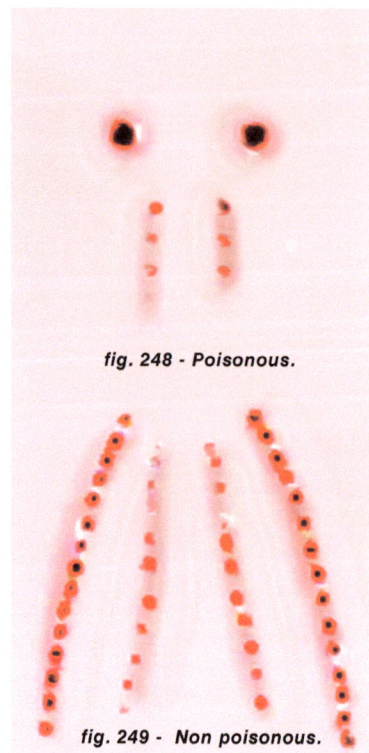

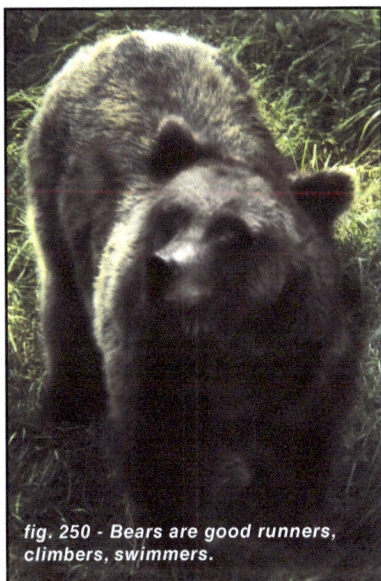

fig. 250 - Bears are good runners, climbers, swimmers.

In the event it attacks you and you're blocking the only exit route, step aside as quickly as possible and allow the animal to get out, the poor thing is probably more scared than you are.

In case you're waking up and an animal is curiously investigating what are you doing in your tent, try not to scream but if you can try to regain your composure as quickly as possible and don't throw anything to the animal.

If you wake up and you can control yourself move slowly and make soft sounds, the majority of animals including bears as soon as they realise that you are alive will back away and quickly make way to the nearest exit. Try to avoid facing the animal frontally, since most animals especially bears will take that as a challenge, always keep to their side. However if you are in a shelter and the animal enters aggressively with the intention to attack your either because he's hungry and want to get some food, fight with everything you've got, animals do not

ANIMALS WITH SHORT LEGS CAN RUN EXTREMELY FAST.

CAUTION

like to fight in a close environment and as soon as it realises that you are putting up a good fight it will probably leave looking for an easier prey.

The areas that you should aim for are the eyes, nose, and ears: hit them with a stabbing motion and keep hitting without stopping.

Bears especially can be extremely dangerous, and sounds like yawning or chattering teeth will make them start pacing nervously; it usually means they are about to attack you.

Don't be fooled by the fact that bears have short legs, in fact they can run extremely fast, much faster than you can, they also extremely good climbers so trying to get up the tree quickly is not really an option. Don't run but stay and make yourself as big as possible opening your jacket and remember that often they bluff charges to see what you are made of.

If the attack is real throw yourself to the ground protecting your neck, spread your legs and stay put: this is taken by most bears as an act of surrender and it has worked in the past.

They may still sniff you or pat you but unless it starts mauling you do not react, stay still. Even after the bear is gone do not move until you are absolutely sure the bear has definitely left the areaIf you get up too soon you will be attacked again more

AN INJURED ANIMAL IS VERY DANGEROUS.

viciously than ever.

Animals that might look cute can actually be quite vicious: donkeys or squirrels can give us very nasty bites, and often without apparent reason.

Remember also that injured animals can be extremely dangerous and if you're going to their rescue you should approach them with caution, wearing protective gear, most importantly keeping out of the way especially your face and wearing thick gloves. In any case you are always better to keep your distance from all large animals, even if they have no intention of attacking as they can still injure you with a sudden move or they can step on your foot.

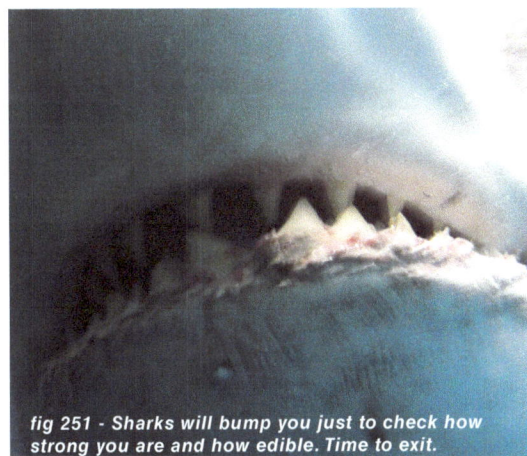

fig 251 - Sharks will bump you just to check how strong you are and how edible. Time to exit.

If you sense that an animal is about to attack you remember that the majority of animals, including birds will go for your eyes or your face and some for your throat. It is therefore important that you try to protect this area of your body more than anything else. If you can, put something around your arm such as your jacket or coat, anything that will pad your arm, and (!) offer it to the animal. They normally go for the part of your body that protrudes the most.

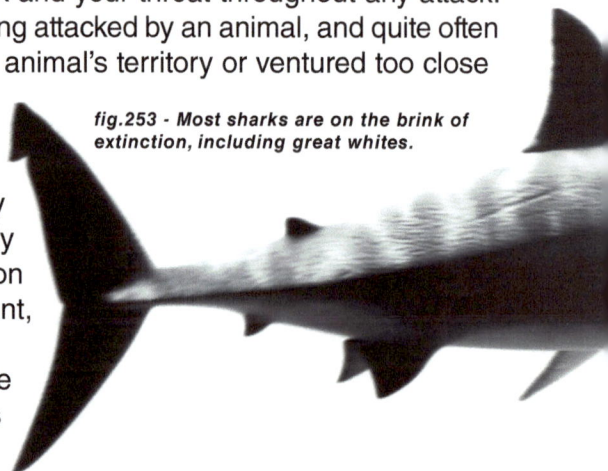

fig.252 - Roll onto the side at the last minute.

As a general rule always remember for that the majority of animals as soon as they realise that you are human they will stay well clear. Given the chance, back away into a shadow area or in a dark area slowly without losing sight of the animal, but try not to make eye contact.

Try to back away in a subtle manner where possible. If possible get a stone or similar ready to throw out at the animal just in case.

An animal such as a dog continuously moving towards you in a ring, with all the hair standing on its back, almost certainly is about to attack you.

Don't turn your back on it and don't run, instead try to open your jacket to make yourself as big as you can and throw stones or whatever comes to hand, including a mobile phone or shoes at it. This has worked in the past, but it may also provoke an attack.

Non-predatory animals such as cows, bulls and buffalos react in a completely different way if you throw something at them, quite often they will charge you if you do so.

In the case that a defensive animal charges, run for cover or to anything that will keep you out of its reach or behind something hard and large such as a car, wall, tree or a big rock.

If there is nothing you can take cover behind as you run throw something in the opposite direction for instance your jacket, your hat, rucksack, even your shirt is enough to distract and make them change direction, as we have seen already with bulls.

If all that fails, roll onto your side at the last minute and then repeat when the animal charges again. If you get onto the ground go for the nose and hit as hard as you can. As for humans the most sensitive part of an animal is the sensory organs, always make sure that you are protecting your neck and your throat throughout any attack. You should ask yourself why is someone being attacked by an animal, and quite often it is because the person trespassed on the animal's territory or ventured too close

PROTECT YOUR NECK IF YOU ARE BEING ATTACKED.

to the cubs. This is why it is a good idea to leave the area if you are in the wild and you have been the subject of a false attack or you can see animals being nervous about your presence, then you know you really shouldn't be there in the first place; move away calmly without losing sight of the animal in question. The reason can also be because you carry something that they want, most of the time food or because they can sense blood.

fig.253 - Most sharks are on the brink of extinction, including great whites.

(!) It's worth reminding ourselves that animals are quite spooked by loud noises and quite often making noises is enough to keep animals at a safe distance.

Inevitably talking about animal attacks one question that always pops up is the one about sharks. In the unlikely event that you find yourself in shark infested waters, keep away from blood and vomit or leftovers from food. Do not dangle hands or feet over the side and if you go into the water enter in the quietest possible way without jumping in and splashing about.
Clothing or objects or anything highly reflective attracts their attention, and quite often sharks bump into you just to check you out. Stay calm and continue swimming slowly without making any sudden movement. If you are definitely going to be attacked always face-out towards a shark and kick out and try to stab the eyes with anything you have.
There have been reports of people screaming in the water and sharks swimming away, you can also try that I'm sure you'll be in the mood for it, in any case the chances that you will be attacked by a shark are very slim, therefore swim at sea without worrying too much, there are more people killed by bees than killed by sharks worldwide every year.
As we said before animals shy away from humans, the most fearsome predators, and it is worth remembering that animals will attack only if cornered, surprised or with their young.
Very rarely animals attack if unprovoked.
Because we normally fear what we do not know or understand, or we tend to disrespect what or who we consider inferior, here are some amazing feats some animals, big and small, can do that can put humans to shame.
- Starfish can regenerate themselves and have no brain.
A human brain is composed of 75% water, the tooth is the only part of the human body that can't repair itself but we cannot regenerate.

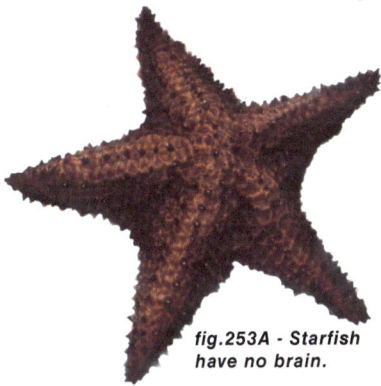

fig.253A - Starfish have no brain.

- Ants are able to lift fifty times their own weight and if intoxicated they always fall on their right side. The strongest muscle in the human body is the tongue, if intoxicated we tend to fall forwards.
- Mosquitoes can hear other mosquitoes flying more than one hundred metres away, even in very noisy or windy conditions. We can hear someone's normal tone voice in good weather conditions at a maximum of 50 meters away.
- A spider's silk line is only .001-.004 mm thick but is about five times stronger than steel and twice as strong as Kevlar, pound for pound, and it can stretch thirty percent longer than its original length. One human hair is much thicker and can only support 3kg.
- Cats can see six times better than humans, dogs see better in the dark.
-Catfish are real connoisseurs having more than 27,000 taste buds.
Humans have about 9,000 taste buds, three times less.
- A flea can jump a distance equal to 350 times the length of its body, the equivalent of a man jumping the length of a football pitch.
- A decapitated cockroach survives 9 days.
- The woodpecker, even if beating their beaks like a jackhammer, does not suffer from headaches. Mother nature has provided a spongy bone that softens the blows impact.
- A sheep can recognise the faces of 50 other sheep and more than 10 different human faces.
- Humans are the only animals that cry tears and blush.

ANIMALS SHOULD BE RESPECTED.

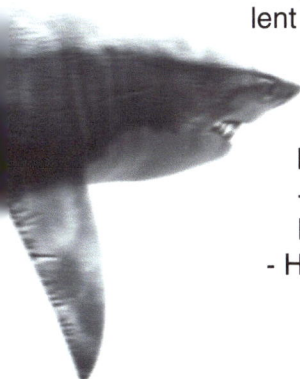

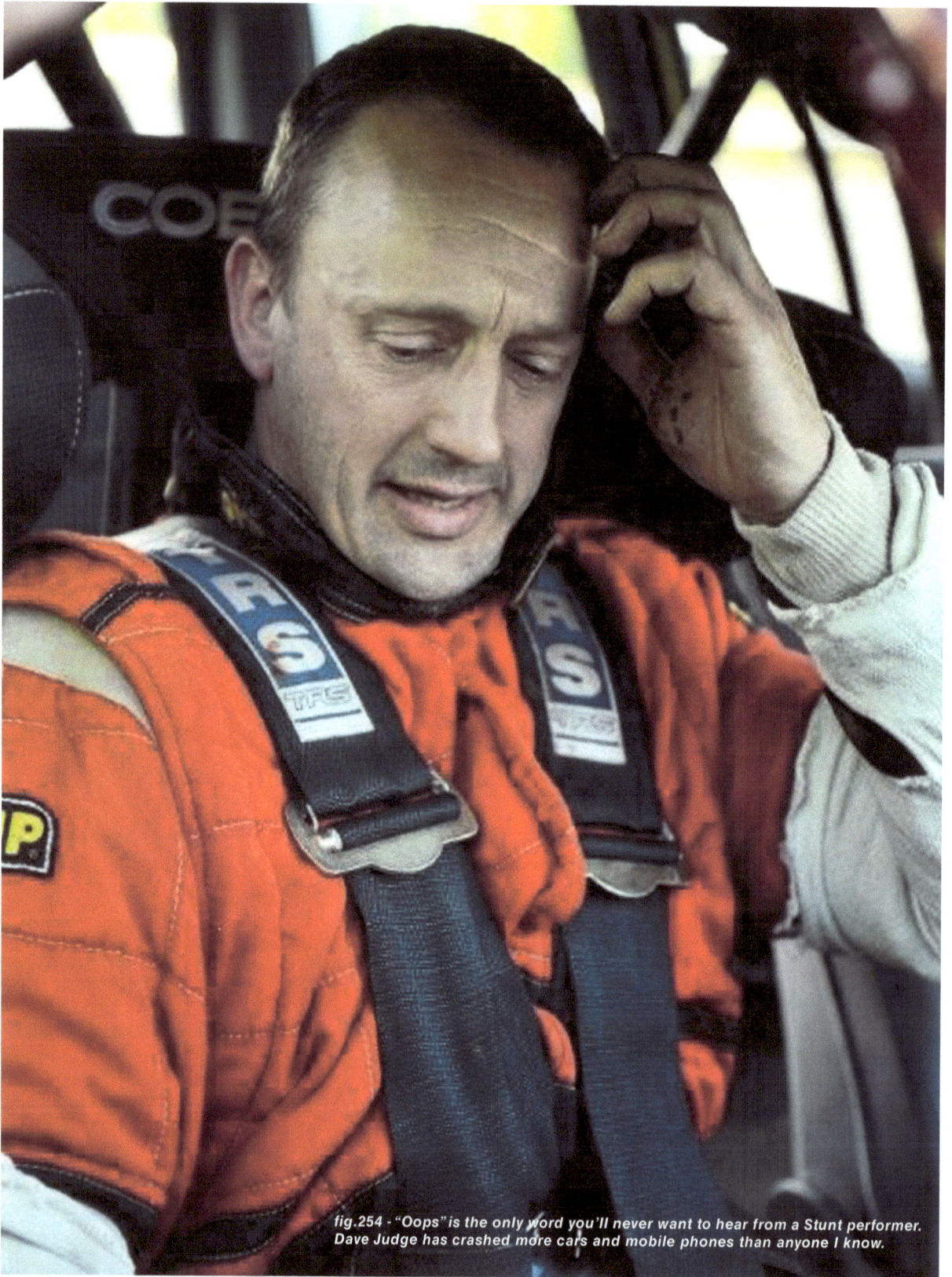

fig.254 - "Oops" is the only word you'll never want to hear from a Stunt performer. Dave Judge has crashed more cars and mobile phones than anyone I know.

cars

by Stunt Coordinator Dave Judge

We live in a society in which the car represents a primary tool in both our work and in our socialising activities.

Cars are not only a fundamental means of transportation but often a hobby and indeed sometimes a status symbol and hence a great deal of our time is attached to the use of the motor vehicle.

WE SPEND A LOT OF TIME IN OUR CAR: SPEND TIME LEARNING HOW TO BE SAFE IN IT.

It therefore comes as no surprise that most people at sometime in their lives will become involved in a dangerous situation while at the wheel of their vehicle.

Situations may even occur in which their safety or even survival may depend on appropriate action or application of basic manoeuvring skills.

I work as a stunt co-ordinator and performer, my work often means being involved in car chases, and high and low speed controlled maneuvers and violent crashes.

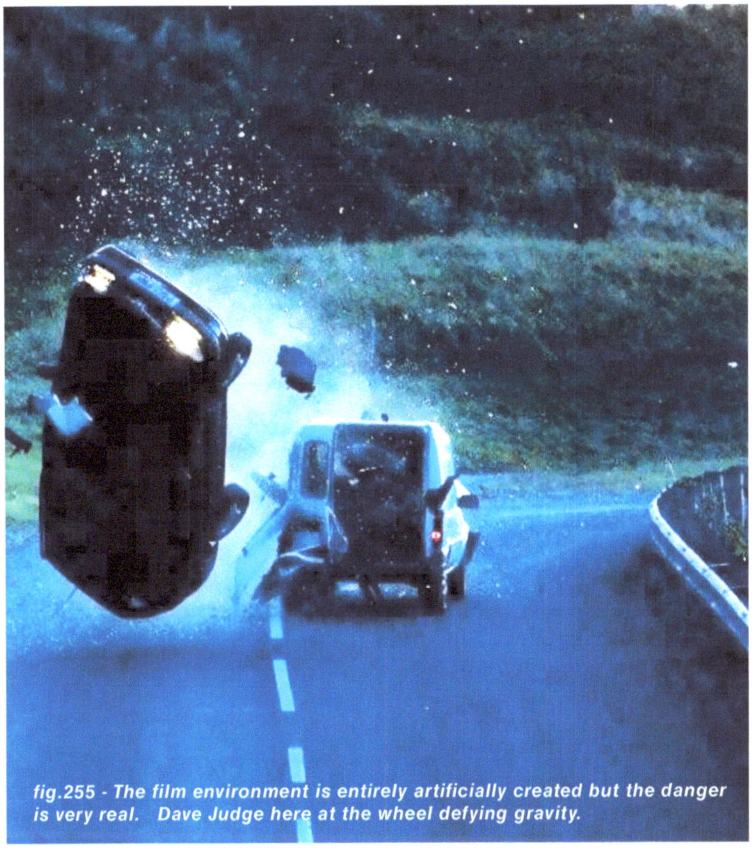

fig.255 - The film environment is entirely artificially created but the danger is very real. Dave Judge here at the wheel defying gravity.

While the film environment is entirely artificially created, my survival (and that of the camera crew) often depends on the application of specific skills, know-how and being prepared to react and indeed be proactive to all kinds of situations and scenarios.

Under certain circumstances a little knowledge can be just as useful as finely honed manoeuvring skills and techniques that I might employ. The following sections explore likely and also unlikely yet entirely feasible scenarios, which anyone may find themselves in, together with a few straightforward and also some more advanced maneuvers that may just save the day.

Before we go on to advanced evasive driving skills let's consider some more likely, everyday circumstances that might present themselves.

168

Low speed traction loss is generally caused by very poor surface conditions and possibly heightened by poor or inappropriate tyre tread. Ever found yourself driving on wet grass, soft ground, snow or ice and slowly losing speed as the engine revs increase?

Once friction is lost, i.e. the tires are turning at a higher speed than the road speed, it can be very difficult to recover grip.

IF THE ROAD IS SLIPPERY AVOID SHARP TURNS OR SUDDEN ACCELERATIONS.

In such very slippery conditions, run the highest gear possible that will not cause stalling, at least second gear if travelling very slowly.

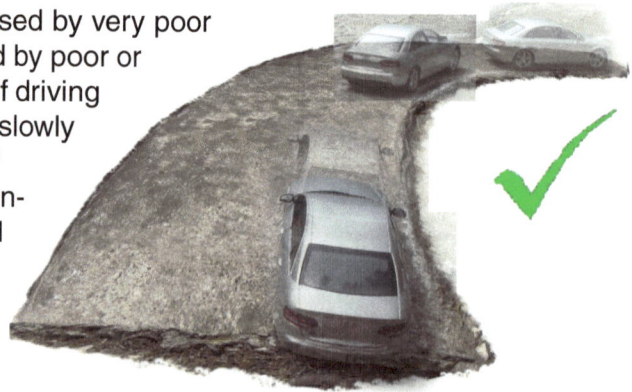

fig.256 - *Stay well away from cambers or slopes as these will have a drastic effect on your state of traction and forward drive. Turn smoothly and steadily, always aware of road conditions, especially if wet.*

Try to avoid sharp turns or hard accelerations and just keep a controlled steady forwards momentum. Stay well away from cambers or slopes, as these will have a drastic effect on your state of traction and forward drive.

CAUTION Finding yourself stationary and the wheels spinning, stop immediately as spinning the wheels while stationary will simply dig a hole that will be even harder to escape from.

Firstly try reversing away from the point you have run out of traction, try a different route, have another run up. If reversing is also unsuccessful you may need to find a way of increasing the grip between surface and tyre. (fig.256)

Look for loose stones or sand that you can throw under the wheels (not while they are moving of course) to increase the grip of the surface.

Finding yourself in a self made hole through wheel spin or a natural hollow, you will often find the wheel will drive partly out of the hollow but then slip backwards.

It is possible to maximise on this effect by careful use of the clutch and accelerator.

Drive forward until grip is lost entirely, depress the clutch and let the wheel roll back into the hollow, it may even roll back past its settling point and back up the other side. (fig.257)

Carefully time the clutch to release and reapply forward drive as the car has rolled back to its furthermost point. You now have a slightly better run up. Continuing to clutch and re-apply drive at the correct moment will rock the car backwards and forwards with increasing amplitude bringing you nearer and nearer the point when you can escape the hollow.

High-speed traction loss can of course have far more devastating effects. Cars across the range behave in many different ways under different circumstances when losing grip at speed. Loss of traction may be just to the front wheels (known as understeer), just to the rear wheels (over-steer) or to both, if you have really over-cooked it.

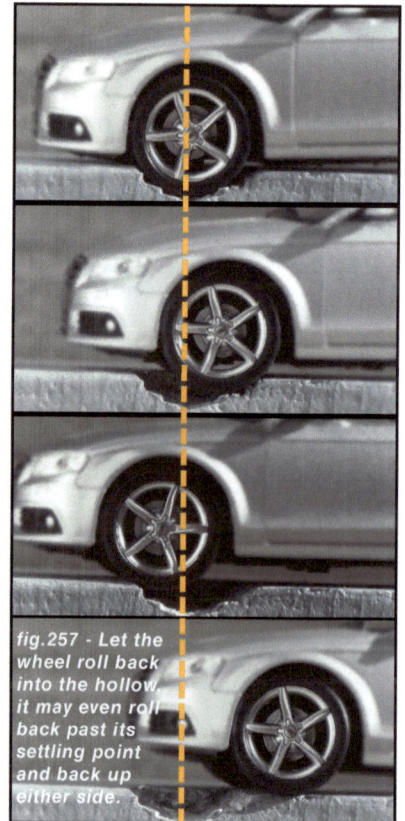

fig.257 - *Let the wheel roll back into the hollow, it may even roll past its settling point and back up either side.*

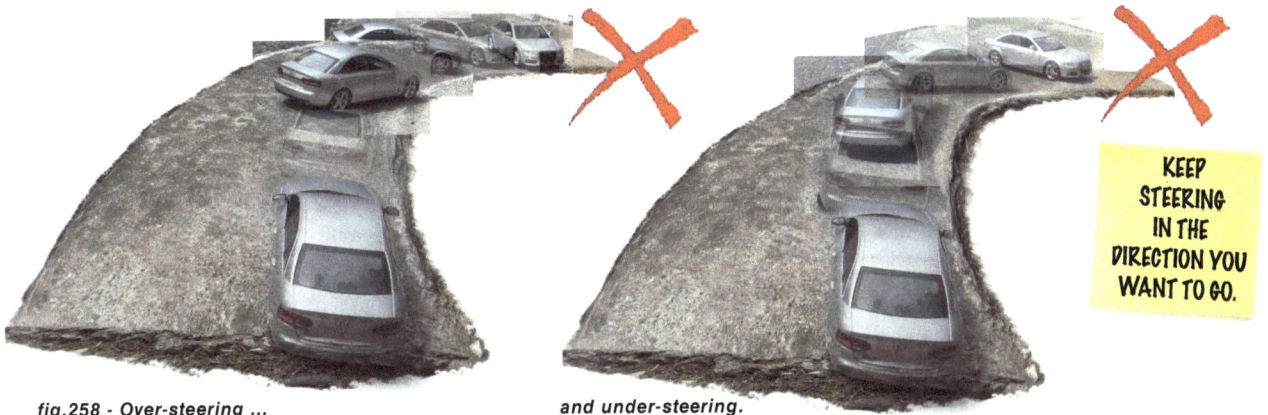

fig.258 - Over-steering ...

and under-steering.

KEEP STEERING IN THE DIRECTION YOU WANT TO GO.

To look at specific examples of car handling would be information overload.
However there are some tips I can share that can be priceless.

The simple rules are to steer in the direction you wish to go irrespective of which direction the vehicle is pointing while attempting controlled braking.

If steering is non responsive (the car continues to go in an unwanted direction), turning the steering wheel further will not help, you need to reduce your speed effectively.

Stamping hard on the brakes will probably be equally useless; this will simply encourage the slide and prevent regaining control. Gentle steering action and medium breaking, even repeatedly coming on and off the brakes, will give you a far higher likely-hood of regaining control.

In the event of over-steer (the rear end of the car slides outwards, again steer in the direction you wish to go.

If travelling over 25mph when severe over-steer occurs you will almost certainly experience what is known in the business as a 'tank slapper' (a phrase evolved from the motorcycle racing circuits where the bike slides and grips repeatedly, violently 'slapping' the legs of the rider straddling the machine). So the rear end of the vehicle is sliding sideways but suddenly gets grip, corrects quite violently and then slides out in the opposite direction, quite often with greater ferocity than the first slide.

A HIGH SPEED SLIDE IS OFTEN THE RESULT OF MISJUDGING SPEED.

Be ready for this and try to react to it.

Ultimately it may well get the better of you but hopefully by then you will have brushed off at least some of your speed and the conclusion of this total control loss will be proportionally less severe.

To find yourself in a high-speed slide will generally be the cause of misjudgement of speed relative to road conditions.

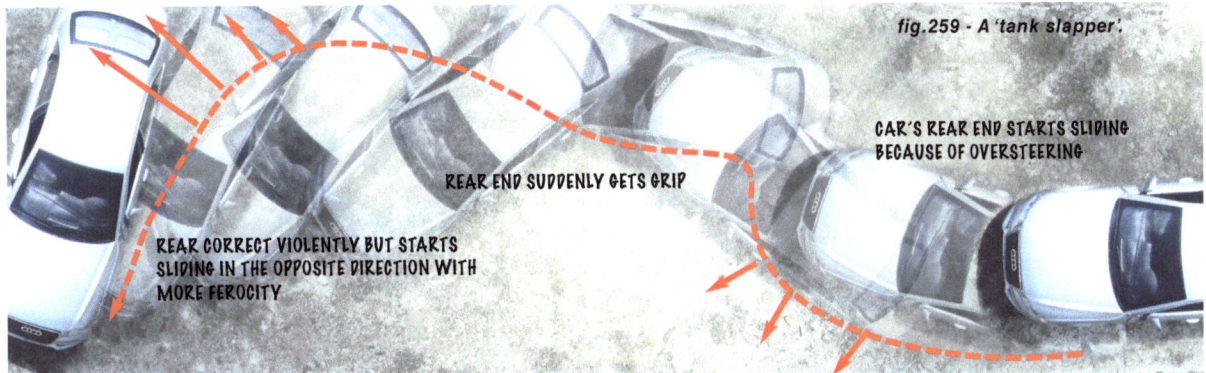

fig.259 - A 'tank slapper'.

CAR'S REAR END STARTS SLIDING BECAUSE OF OVERSTEERING

REAR END SUDDENLY GETS GRIP

REAR CORRECT VIOLENTLY BUT STARTS SLIDING IN THE OPPOSITE DIRECTION WITH MORE FEROCITY

Yes, oil spillages on the road or a sudden tyre deflation can be unexpected and contributory to incident and accident but in both cases if you are driving within the realms of sensibility both should be entirely manageable.

In the event you find yourself inevitably about to crash, there are still rules to follow.

As a youngster I was a keen motocross (a.k.a scrambling) competitor.

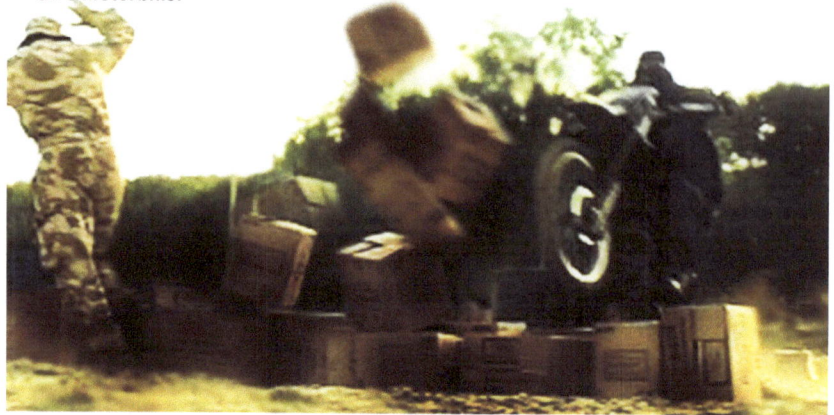

fig.260 - Focus on your escape route if you find yourself out of control or amongst others that are out of control. Here Dave Judge finding an escape route on a motorbike.

Brian Wade was five times British motocross champion in his day and ran a motocross training school that I attended early in my racing career.

IF OUT OF CONTROL OR AMONGST OTHERS OUT OF CONTROL FOCUS ON YOUR ESCAPE ROUTE.

I remember one piece of advice that has benefited me tremendously on many occasions both on and off the race track, both for cars and astride motorcycles:

"If you find yourself out of control or amongst others ho are out of control, focus on your escape route". Look for your escape, whether it is the gap between two trees (or lamp posts) or the space of road between two spinning vehicles". (fig.260)

He added " Accidents involving drunken drivers so often end in a head on impact with say a tree, hit square in the middle of the grill.

Of course they focused on the tree rather than the escape gap". If an impact is inevitable but nevertheless given some elements of control, you may still have options – better to hit a parked stationary car than an oncoming vehicle - better to crash through a fence rather than hit a tree. Remember steer in the direction you wish to go and use controlled, not heavy, breaking.

In much of the civilised world it is unlikely that you will ever find yourself having to make a hasty retreat from armed gang intent on establishing ownership of your vehicle (having worked in countries such as South Africa though, this does become a more realistic possibility).

It is unlikely you will ever need to use your vehicle as an escape tool. However, danger presents itself in many forms and should it do so, in most cases where evasive reaction becomes a necessity; the best way out is probably the way you just came in.

SPEED REVERSING BACK FROM WHERE YOU CAME FROM IS OFTEN THE BEST OPTION.

Speed reversing may well be the quickest means of putting a little distance between you and the danger in front of you.

Having made the decision to reverse away from the danger it is likely that the position of the front wheels are still such that you can simply reverse on exactly the same path you arrived on without much steering adjustment – certainly for the first few metres in any case.

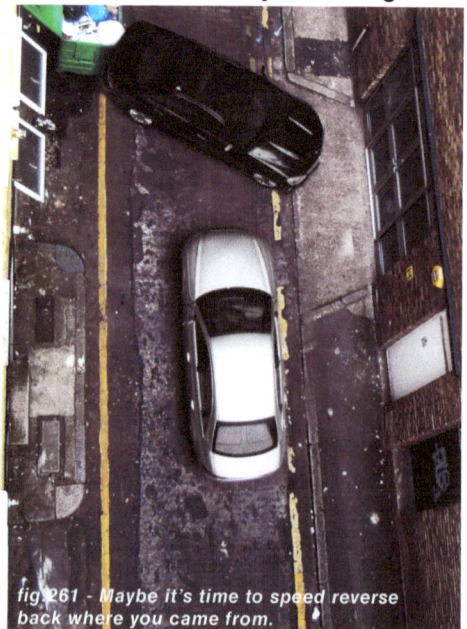

fig.261 - Maybe it's time to speed reverse back where you came from.

Engage reverse and then grip the back or top of the passenger side seat twisting your body so that you have good vision backwards down the centre of the vehicle.

This will also help stabilise yourself.

If your vehicle does not have through car vision such as in the case of a van with a solid bulkhead, then you should lean out of the driver side window instead. (fig.262)

Using just mirrors requires a great deal of skill and is highly dangerous.

Having accelerated away down your line of arrival it is only a short

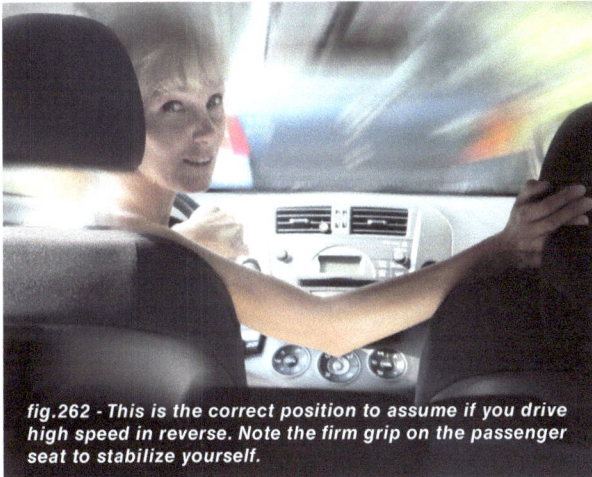

fig.262 - This is the correct position to assume if you drive high speed in reverse. Note the firm grip on the passenger seat to stabilize yourself.

matter of time before you will have to make adjustments, i.e. steer the car.

This is where problems and difficulties will become apparent: a vehicle behaves very differently when driven in reverse especially at speed.

The handling and road holding changes, the steering and suspension geometry means that the car will corner very differently indeed and appear more sensitive.

Loss of control will occur far quicker because of these very different handling characteristics.

If reversing in a fairly straight line, significant speed can be achieved up to 30mph in most vehicles. The secret is to make only very small adjustments to change the direction of the car, quickly return the steering wheel to its neutral positioning after making any correction and then re-evaluate if your correction is ok or needs further correction or counter adjustment.

Given the opportunity to practice this, you will find that over-correction is the biggest and easiest mistake made.

Warning; a car will refuse to take a corner at speed in reverse. (fig.263)

The front end will simply wash out and you will be left having to recover a spin or have a collision. For this reason and of course the limitations of speed and difficulty in manoeuvring in reverse, at some point pretty quickly, you will need to get the car going conventionally forwards. Having hopefully created a little time and distance to turn the car around you can now start looking for an appropriate forward drive escape route.

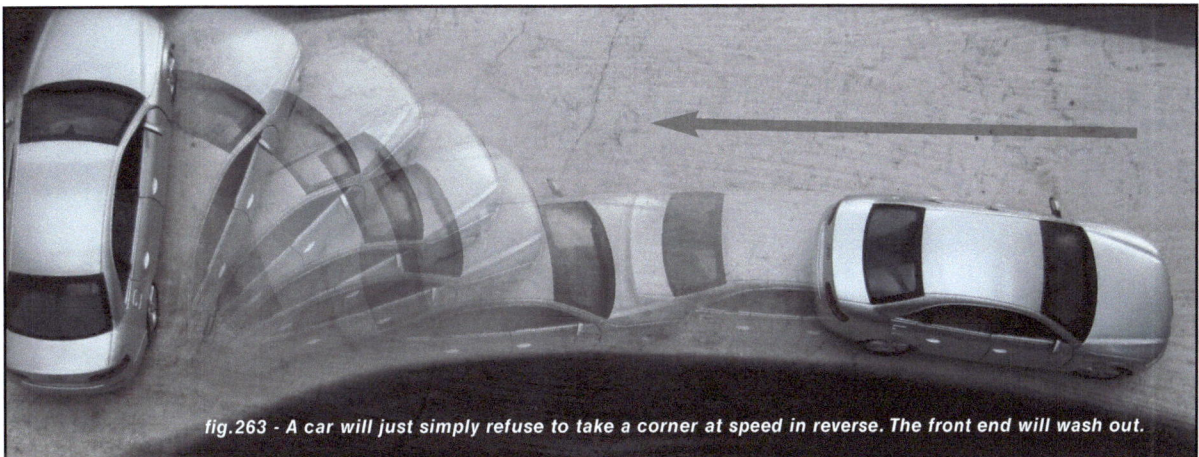

fig.263 - A car will just simply refuse to take a corner at speed in reverse. The front end will wash out.

fig.264 - Three points or "J" turn becoming reverse spin.

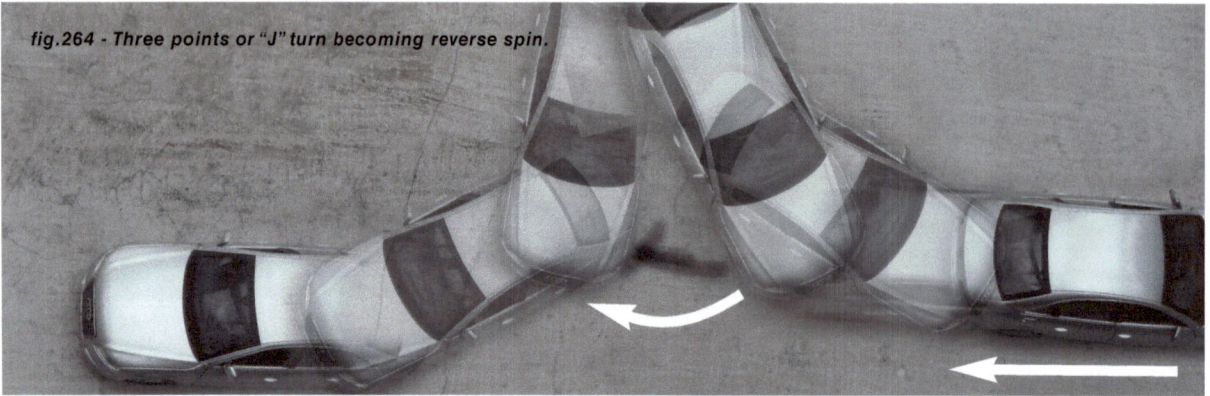

⚠ Pick your moment, try not to rush too much and make your escape accordingly.

⚠ Try to avoid rushing your gear change. It is here you may completely undo the advantage you have by selecting third rather than first gear and stalling the engine.

⚠ Automatic gearboxes are a real godsend in these scenarios.

Should circumstances demand that you need to turn the car 180 degrees, then the most conventional method is the three point turn or "J" turn which most people will be familiar with. (fig.264) Given time to practice however, this maneuver can be developed into something far more effective: the reverse spin. I mentioned earlier how the front end of a car will wash out if turning sharply at speed in reverse. In the case of a reverse spin this is used to our advantage.

Choosing the right moment with sufficient speed and road width we can sharply turn the steering wheel, which will initiate a fast turn. (See fig.264)

YOU CAN USE THE WASH OUT TO YOUR ADVANTAGE IF YOU KNOW HOW.

As the vehicle approaches 90 degrees in the direction of travel the front wheels will start to wash out and loose grip.

Depress the clutch and stamp hard on the foot brake and the wheels will continue to slide allowing the vehicle to continue its rotation.

If speed and technique are correct the vehicle will rotate 180 degrees leaving you facing in the direction you need to make your escape.

Engage first gear and go.

With lots of time to rehearse this maneuver, the action can become so tuned that the use of the footbrake becomes unnecessary and the gear change between reverse and first gear can be made during the spin, allowing the whole maneuver becoming one smooth, almost ballet-like action with hardly any loss of speed.

An easier option to the reverse spin is the handbrake turn. This is a means of rotating the car quickly through

⚠ 180 degrees but relies on forward momentum to generate the spin. (fig.265)

This means if you feel you are driving into a possible situation you need to commit to making this maneuver before too much forward speed is lost.

fig.265 - Handbrake turn.

ACTUAL PATH

INTENDED PATH

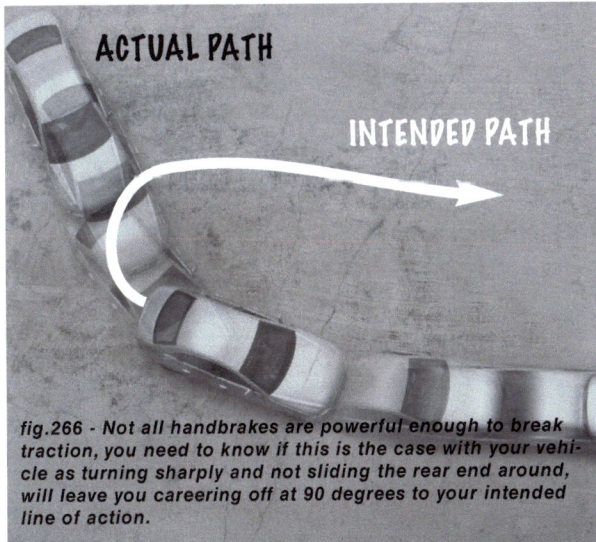

fig.266 - Not all handbrakes are powerful enough to break traction, you need to know if this is the case with your vehicle as turning sharply and not sliding the rear end around, will leave you careering off at 90 degrees to your intended line of action.

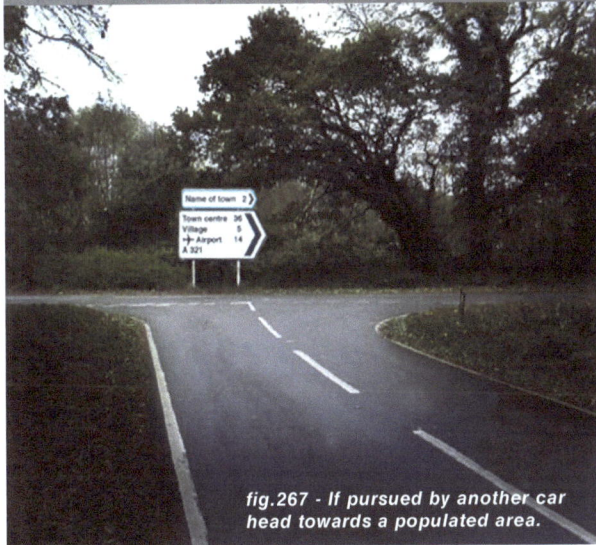

fig.267 - If pursued by another car head towards a populated area.

With a minimum of 15mph, turn the wheel sharply and as the car starts to corner hard, pull up the handbrake sharply. (fig.266)

THE HANDBRAKE TURN IS AN EASIER OPTION IF TRAVELLING AT 15MPH MINIMUM SPEED.

This will lock the rear wheels and cause them to slide around, leaving the car facing in the opposite direction.

Generally speaking you should depress the clutch before using the handbrake to avoid stalling the engine, essential for rear wheel drive cars.

More powerful front wheel drive cars are able to increase the effectiveness of this maneuver by driving hard when the hand brake is applied but of course stalling the engine at this stage almost defeats the object of attempting this escape maneuver in the first place.

Warning: not all handbrakes are powerful enough to break traction, you need to know this is advance about your vehicle **CAUTION** as turning sharply and not sliding the rear end around, will leave you careering off at 90 degrees to your intended line of action. (fig 266)

That would be embarrassing, to say the least.

In SCENARIOS (page 214) you will see references to road rage and attempted car jacking. The first course of action is one of verbal or psychological evasion and then departing the area ASAP.

IF PURSUED HEAD FOR A POPULATED AREA OR A BUSY ROAD.

Should this be ineffective and you find yourself being pursued by a person or another vehicle you need to head for a populated area where the situation can be far less likely to escalate in the eyes of the passing public. (fig.267)

Late at night or away from populated areas and with a persistent pursuer, you need to carefully consider your options.

A man on foot will easily be outrun by a vehicle or where speed is not an option a few hundred metres of foot chase will be enough to tire a pursuer and hopefully make him lose interest.

YOUR CAR IS A WEAPON, THINK SERIOUSLY OF THE CONSEQUENCES OF YOUR ACTIONS.

Only as a last resort, with no other options and only when you are sure you are in serious danger, should you consider using your car as a weapon.

Knocking a person down effectively without the intent to kill or seriously injure is a skill in itself. I have done it many times!

Your intended outcome should be to stun, concuss or at the very least let your pursuer know that you mean business. Maiming or killing should certainly not be your goal.

An impact in either reverse or forward drive should be approximately 20mph (30kmh).

YOUR CAR CAN BE A WEAPON TO KILL OR TO STUN.

Anything faster and you may seriously injure, possibly kill a person, anything much less may be ineffective.

As soon as you make impact (but definitely not before) hit the brakes hard.

This has the effect of firstly ejecting the attacker off your car, meaning he is going to receive a second hard impact on the ground but also helps to avoid running him over.

THE FRONT WINDSCREEN WILL NOT SMASH THROUGH BECAUSE IT IS LAMINATED.

In a forward impact it is likely the assailant will slide or roll over the bonnet and hit the windscreen, which will probably break. Don't worry - front windscreens (unlike rear) are laminated and will not smash through.

As a side note, should you find yourself on the receiving end of being hit by a car, remember the rules regarding falling outlined in FALLING (page 76)

KEEP ROLLING TO AVOID GOING UNDER THE CAR WHEELS.

You might also employ some of the techniques we use in the stunt industry when performing car knock downs. Avoid a hard impact with your legs on the front of the vehicle; try to roll onto the bonnet. (fig.270)

Use the windscreen to soften your impact. It is surprising how forgiving a windscreen can be if hit with the shoulders and / or back first.

We use it to great visual effect in performing this stunt.

If the car stops suddenly or alternatively you are thrown off the side of the vehicle, try and set up your landing for a roll and keep rolling at all costs to avoid going under the car wheels.

If you find that you are being pursued or attacked by another vehicle can be a dangerous affair for all involved.

AVOID A HIGH SPEED CHASE AT ALL COST!

You should look to avoid a high speed chase at all costs.

But if your pursuer is intent on stopping you and has demonstrated he is ready to impact your vehicle, then the best form of defence is attack.

The Parallel Immobilization Technique (PIT) is a maneuver developed by police authorities in the USA.

A minimum of 40mph (65kmh) is needed for this to be effective. (fig.268)

The maneuver requires you to get alongside the other vehicle and slightly behind.

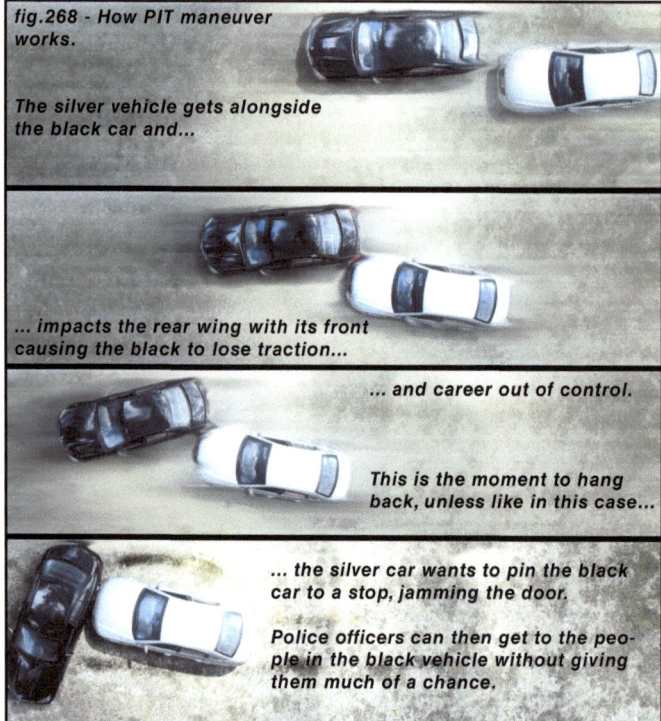

fig.268 - How PIT maneuver works.

The silver vehicle gets alongside the black car and...

... impacts the rear wing with its front causing the black to lose traction...

... and career out of control.

This is the moment to hang back, unless like in this case...

... the silver car wants to pin the black car to a stop, jamming the door.

Police officers can then get to the people in the black vehicle without giving them much of a chance.

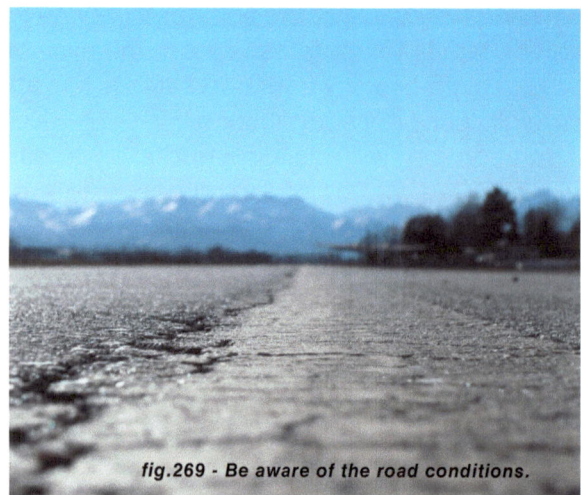

fig.269 - Be aware of the road conditions.

fig.270 - Hit the windscreen with your shoulders or with your back if you can, rolling over the bonnet.

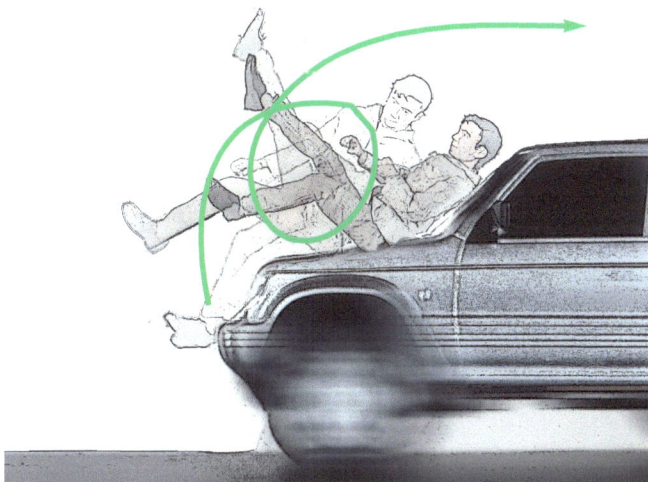

This might be achieved by fooling the pursuant into thinking they have beaten you into submission or simply out driven you.

> **BREAKING SUDDENLY AND LETTING THE PURSUING VEHICLE OVERTAKE YOU IS A GOOD SOLUTION.**

Alternatively, you may brake suddenly, making them overshoot past your vehicle. Then, using your front wing to side impact the rear wing of the other vehicle will cause their rear wheels to lose traction. (fig.268)

They will either spin off from this or possibly try to correct and then experience the 'tank slapper' we referred to earlier.

You of course, must hang back and avoid the vehicle and carnage as necessary.

Remember – focus on the escape route.

Side ramming the other vehicle into a stationary object can be just, if not more, effective.

Surprise is the key and of course once again you need to invite the other vehicle alongside yours. Choose your moment carefully as the other vehicle will be quick to react and counteract your efforts.

Steer your car suddenly and hard into the other vehicle and hold your course, directing the other vehicle into a collision with whatever obstacle you have chosen.

Do not stop the action until the moment the other vehicle hits the stationary object.

If you turn out early, the other vehicle will already be counteracting your efforts and will easily avert the impact.

> **CAR EVASION TECHNIQUES ARE HIGHLY DANGEROUS TO YOURSELF AND OTHERS.**

As is the theme of this book as a whole, physical reaction, or in our case evasive or dynamic driving maneuvers, should be a last resort.

Without hours of practice on a test track, you will not master the techniques I have discussed and this means that the moment you commit to making a tactical maneuver, you and your car will become a deadly weapon to anyone in the near vicinity, this includes yourself.

It often amuses me to see drivers cocooned in their air conditioned noise insulated vehicles speeding along with no more care than as if they were sat at home watching television.

Being in a position to be able to reflect on the experience of hitting water at 90 mph, rolling end-over-end at 50mph, or meeting a tree and making a dead stop from 30mph, I have enlightenment as to what a potentially dangerous environment you are truly in. Remember this.

Crash survival: when a car rolls over, surprisingly the impact as the car bounces is not incredibly hard and perfectly survivable (fig.271).

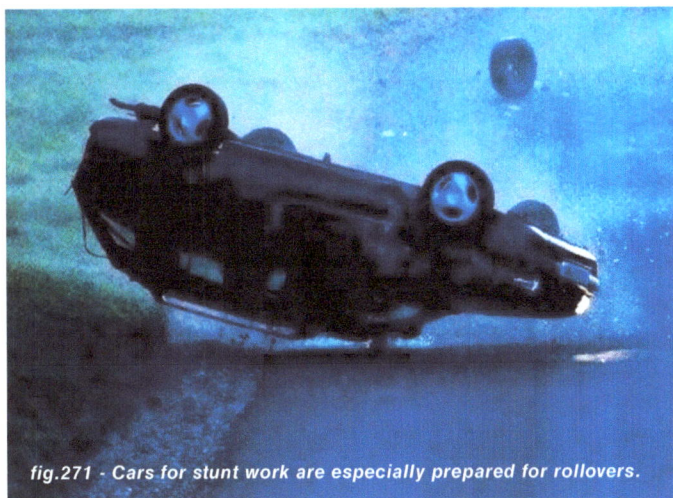

fig.271 - Cars for stunt work are especially prepared for rollovers.

What is important is that you protect your head from impact on the side of the car door and on the car roof.

In stunt rolls we have the luxury of helmet and helmet restraints, neck brace five-point harnessing (shown in fig. 254 on page 167) and of course a roll cage to help reinforce the strength of the car shell. In a conventional car you only have a single shoulder and lap belt. Try to favour your head towards the passenger seat and away from the door and roof.

In the early days of stunt work, car rolls would often be performed with the driver simply grabbing a rope tied around the passenger seat and pulling himself down onto it, thereby avoiding the crumpling roof or banging his head on the door side. By all means use the steering wheel to stabilise your-

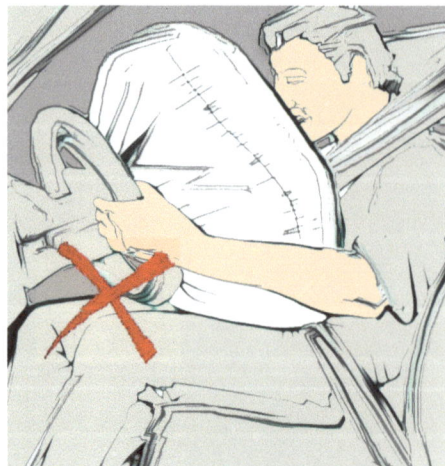

fig.272 - Don't forget the airbag, keep your arms well away.

self but do beware that at any time the car may come down on a wheel and send a massive force back through the steering mechanism causing the wheel to suddenly spin round. **CAUTION** This can result in wrist injuries. If you are unfortunate (stupid) enough to roll in a soft-top vehicle your chances of survival are greatly reduced.

You must either throw yourself hard onto the passenger seat and hold yourself into it or grab the steering wheel and use it to push yourself into the foot-well.

Be aware that the airbag could explode at any time; so try to leave room for that.

A similar approach should be taken in the case of driver side impacts as you slide into a stationary object or are hit by another car, your aim should be to push yourself away from the side of the car being hit.

Broken legs, hips and arms will all mend in time, the skull and brain is an entirely different affair. Head on collisions tend to be very severe as the car is decelerated at a very sudden rate.

Essentially part of your skeletal structure is restrained by the seat belt while your softer internals and free limbs want to carry on.

This puts tremendous strain on joints, and soft tissue throughout the body.

Tensing the core of your body will help hold everything together.

Do not put your hands up to protect your face, as the airbag if fitted will simply throw them into your face causing facial injury and probable broken arm or wrist.

A severe head on will certainly leave you with neck injury, often referred to as whiplash. In very heavy crashes the neck and spine can break which means if you are conscious do not turn your head sideways or move your neck in any way at all. Wait for the emergency services if you have any doubt whatsoever. I personally push my head hard into the headrest when I perform a head on collision. This can still tear the neck muscles but I find it reduces the degree of whip the head experiences, and for me that means less chance of spinal damage. After the crash there should be no immediate urgency to escape the vehicle unless you suspect a fire, in which case get out at all costs.

Otherwise take a moment to assess your predicament and what is happening around you.

fig.272A - Dave Judge is a very accomplished athlete in many disciplines.

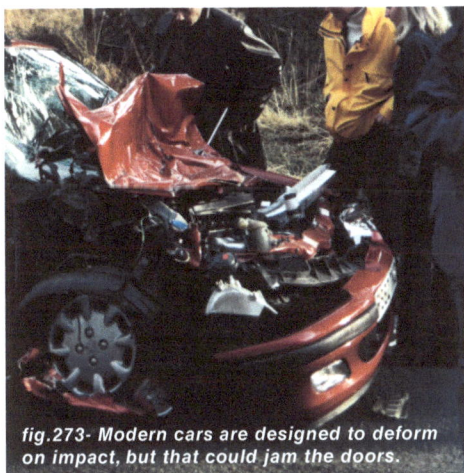
fig.273- Modern cars are designed to deform on impact, but that could jam the doors.

Crashes in motorway fog often result in multiple vehicles driving into the carnage.

Stay in your vehicle until sure there are no exterior dangers. If you suspect any injuries at all, stay absolutely still.

TO ESCAPE FROM A WRECK EXAMINE ALL OPTIONS AVAILABLE.

Your injuries may become compounded and possibly life threatening if you try to move.

Having chosen to make an escape from your wreck, it is possible that the chassis of the vehicle and panels may have deformed in the crash, it may be the case that some doors will not open. (fig.273)

Look at the options; does the passenger side door or the rear doors look undamaged?

Broken side door windows are an easy escape route as the glass will offer no resistance and as it is 'tempered' safety glass will not be too sharp.

Escape through the front windscreen can be difficult, as the laminate will make it impossible to break a hole. An escape through the front screen can only be achieved by kicking the entire laminated screen out of its seal – requiring a massive effort.

This is not the case with the rear window, which can often make a good escape route if all else fails.

A number of years ago I was travelling to the airport for an early morning flight to Moscow.

It was early late October and the first freezing night of the year. I was on the final stretch of motorway and running a little late when I hit a patch of ice and the rear end of the vehicle started to slide. I turned toward the direction of travel but the rear just kept coming round until I was facing the Armco and heading toward it.

fig.273A- Sometimes road conditions are treacherous without being obviously so.

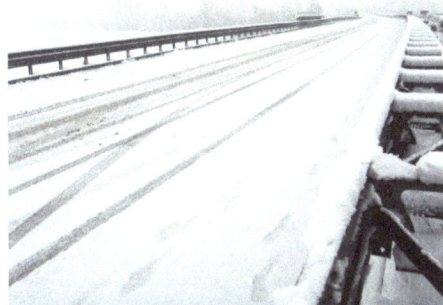

I reacted with a lightening change into reverse gear and a quick burst of backward drive to push me away from the Armco.

I then controlled the car into a high speed reverse, then dabbed the brakes and performed a reverse spin picking the traction back up as the car came out of its 360 degree spin.

My skill and experience got me out of that near disaster but more importantly it was my bad driving and poor appreciation of the road conditions that got me into it.

Safe driving.

Dave makes everything seem so easy and simple, and only a real pro can do that. He is truly the most talented stuntman I have ever met (and I have worked with many). His approach to car work has always been putting safety first and always finding the simplest of solutions for the most complicated of problems. This also is my approach to the entire Perfect Defence and this is why I asked him to explain how to defend yourself whilst driving a car, a space where we spend so much of our lives in and where so much can go wrong in so little time.

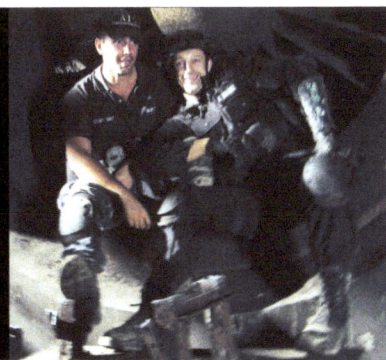

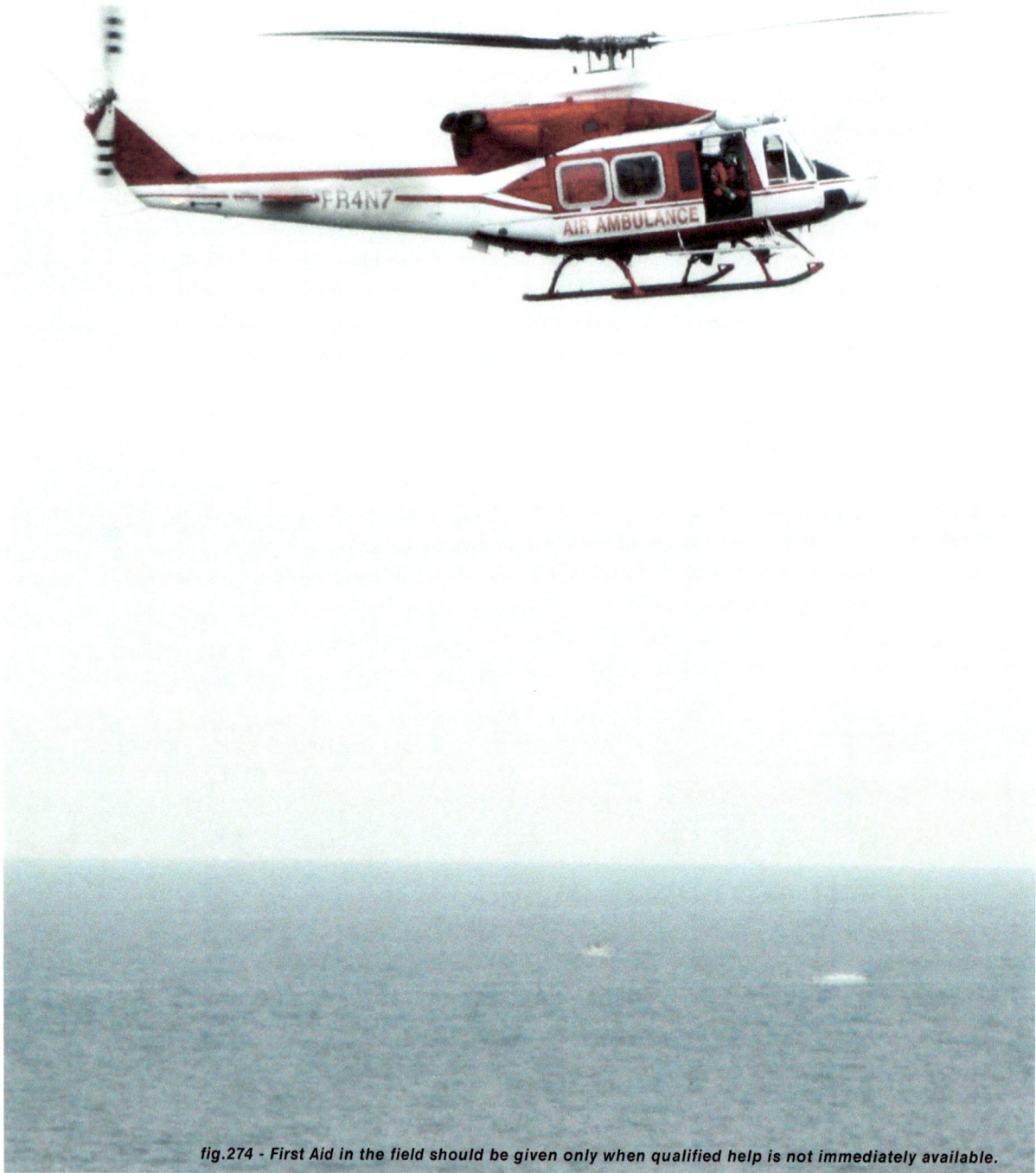

fig.274 - First Aid in the field should be given only when qualified help is not immediately available.

In this book we are giving some first aid references for general use.
The first rule is always to call qualified personnel, an ambulance or your local emergency number, and all the information you read hereafter are only intended to help you in case you find yourself far away from any medical care.

IT IS YOUR DUTY TO CALL FOR MEDICAL HELP OR TO GIVE FIRST AID EVEN TO SOMEONE WHO WAS TRYING TO HURT YOU.

It is important that you remember that all the self-defence techniques shown can cause severe injuries or even death, and that it is your fundamental duty to give medical care to anyone in need. This section of the workbook is important for several reasons.

You might find yourself in a violent situation and either yourself, people with you or people attacking you ending up injured. Even if you feel that you shouldn't help someone who tried to harm you, if his life is in danger as a result of your or his own actions, you still should call for medical help and give first aid. Furthermore, if you do end up getting hurt, even stabbed, knowing the following will give you enough information to understand what's happening in your body and help you to avoid doing the wrong thing (for instance removing a knife from the wound), or directing others trying to help you, so to avoid further harm. As we have seen knowing what to do will help you stay calm and survive. Stay calm, think before you act: panic is the real killer.

The guide that follows is not a complete first aid guide but only specific to the most common injuries occurring in the case of a violent attack, trauma injuries.

For simplicity we'll refer to the injured person as "patient".

The following information is only intended as a guide and is not a substitute for competent medical management of injuries. It is intended solely as a guide for medical stabilization by non-professionals in emergency situations where more qualified medical assistance is not available. First aid techniques are various, constantly changing and often subject to controversy. Remember that you are legally responsible for any negligent action you take, so do what you can while following the primary rule of medicine: do no harm. Do not perform any procedures you are unsure of, even if the result is death for the patient. Remember that once started it is illegal to discontinue treatment until: you are exhausted and unable to continue, help arrives or another rescuer takes over, the injured party recovers or dies. Your efforts will be protected under good Samaritan laws if: your efforts are done under the best intentions, your efforts are those that any reasonable human being would also do under identical circumstances, you have done no harm.

In an emergency situation follow these simple rules for medical treatment of others:

1. Be in **control of yourself** to be able to help others.
2. Always **assume the worst** until proven otherwise.
3. Do no treat anyone for anything **unless you are sure** that something must be done.

4. Do **not move anyone** who can safely be left unmoved.

5. Do not **unnecessarily endanger yourself** or assume the right to endanger others.

6. **Do not give medicines** or treatment when you are not sure of what to do.

7. If the injured person is conscious **say that you are not a doctor** but you will help as best as you can. Ask permission before performing any medical task.

8. Always sound **confident and calm** when dealing with an injured person.
Do not show fear, disgust or anger, and reassure the patient.

9. Always **assume the patient can get worse** so do not leave the scene just because symptoms have improved.

10 - **Stay calm** so you can think clearly. Only attempt rescue if safe to do so.

11 - Get the injured **out of immediate danger, only if necessary**.

12 - If more than one person is injured treat **first those with severe bleeding** (stop the bleeding), then those who are not breathing (perform CPR), those lying still (assess status), and those moving about.

Perform assessment in this order

CAUTION

(fig. 276) **Check for breathing.** If breathing not present give rescue breathing. **Check for pulse**. If no breathing do CPR. Stop blood loss with direct pressure.

fig.275 - Locate Adam's apple (A), then move fingers towards you and check for pulse here (B).

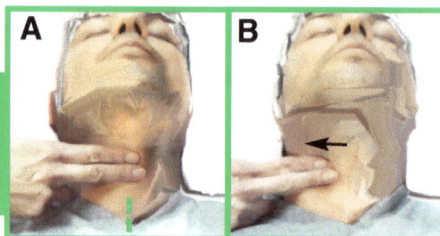

CHECK FOR BREATHING, PULSE, BLEEDING AND FRACTURES.

If the injured person is unconscious assume neck or spinal injury. **Stabilize the patient**. If the injured person is conscious do as follows: remove constricting clothing or jewelery near any injury, then starting from the head, check scalp for cuts and bruises, start at the back of the neck and work to the top of the head. Depressions or soft spots could indicate skull fracture. Blood or fluid draining from ears and nose could indicate skull fracture. Next **check the neck for lumps**, bruises or bony protrusions, which could indicate spinal injury. Check the back without moving the injured as you did for the neck. If lumps, bruises or bony protrusions present there is a possibility of spinal injury. **Check chest** for bruises and wounds, localize spasms or irregular movement during breathing. Feel carefully for signs of fracture; check the abdomen with gentle pressure for rigidity, pain or bleeding. Check pelvic area for fractures by pressing down on both sides of the pelvis at the same time. Pelvic fractures normally involve serious blood loss.

Check arms and legs for wounds, bruises or fractures. Ask the injured if he feels any pain localized anywhere. Check for pulse by sliding your hand from the chin down to the groove in the side of the neck (carotid). Alternatives are femoral and radial pulses (fig. 275).

WORK YOUR WAY DOWN FROM THE HEAD FINISHING WITH THE LEGS.

Check the pulse and look for signs of breathing for 5-10 seconds. If pulse present but no signs of breathing, give rescue breathing.
If no pulse and no breathing, initiate CPR.
Locate compression point positioning your hands, one on top of the other with interlocked fingers, two finger widths above the bottom of the breastbone (roughly nipples height). See fig.278 for positioning of hands. Keep your fingers OFF the chest, use only your palm.
Keep your arms straight, push downward, depressing breastbone 1 or 2 inches.

fig.275C - Position of hands.

Count as follows: "1 and 2 and 3 and 4 and..." going down on the number and up on "and".

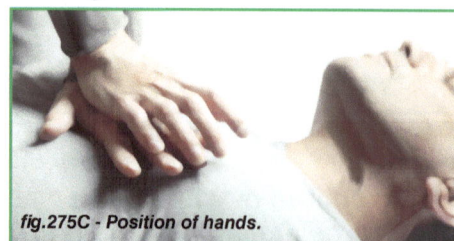

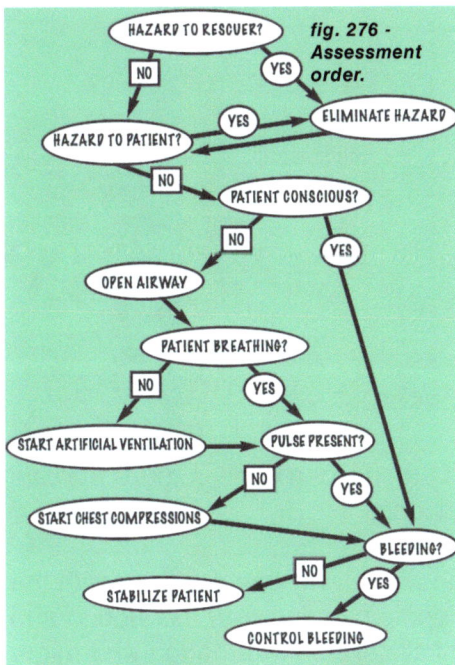

fig. 276 - Assessment order.

- HAZARD TO RESCUER? — NO / YES → ELIMINATE HAZARD
- HAZARD TO PATIENT? — YES → ELIMINATE HAZARD / NO
- PATIENT CONSCIOUS? — NO / YES
- OPEN AIRWAY
- PATIENT BREATHING? — NO / YES
- START ARTIFICIAL VENTILATION → PULSE PRESENT? — NO / YES
- START CHEST COMPRESSIONS → BLEEDING? — NO / YES
- STABILIZE PATIENT
- CONTROL BLEEDING

fig.277- Thrust the mouth open by gently applying pressure on the the chin or angles of the jaw.

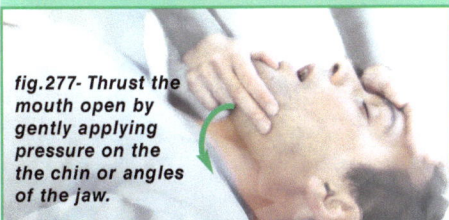

fig.278 - Pinch nose and seal mouth on mouth. Watch for rise and fall of person's chest.

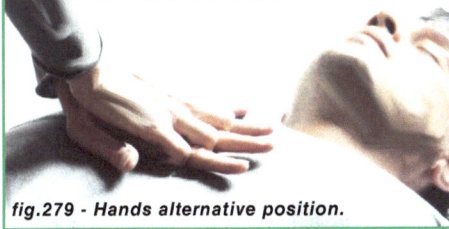

fig.278A - How to locate the compression point (top view).

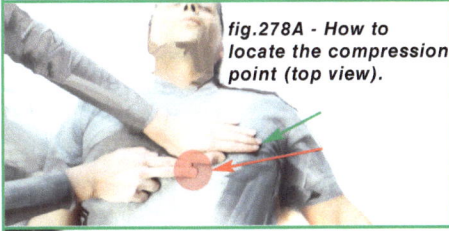

fig.279 - Hands alternative position.

Your arms should be locked and you should pivot up and down on your hip joint, keep your hands on your hands on the compression point at all time, your movement should be smooth and regular. (fig.278A) **Do 80-100 compressions per minute, 1-2 inches deep. Every 15 give two full breaths. Check for pulse after the first minute, then every 3 minutes afterwards.**

INJURY ASSESSMENT

80-100 CHEST COMPRESSIONS PER MINUTE, 2 INCHES DEEP, EVERY 15 GIVE 2 FULL BREATHS

Remove any foreign material from the injured person's mouth. To open the airway, tip the injured person's head back, supporting his neck from underneath, unless spine injuries are involved. If so, thrust the jaw upwards with upward pressure on the angles of the jaw. (fig.277) Look, listen and feel for **3-5 seconds** to see if the person is breathing.

Pinch injured person's nose closed and place your mouth over his mouth (if mouth severely injured seal mouth and blow through nose). Give **4 slow, full breaths, lasting 1 1/2 seconds** each to inflate lungs. If the air will not enter, repeat, if still not possible check for obstructions inside mouth or throat. Continue rescue breathing, **one full breath every 5 seconds**, allowing victim's lungs to deflate between breaths and remove your mouth from the injured person's mouth. (see fig. 285B)

RESCUE BREATHING

CAUTION

Take a new breath while the injured person breathes out. Watch for rise and fall of the injured person's chest as you breath, and listen to the return of natural breathing.

Do not over-breath air into the victim's lungs or it will enter the stomach. If accidentally done so, roll him gently onto his side and press down on his stomach to expel abdominal air. Then roll him back and continue rescue breathing.

Bleeding **fractures** need immediate attention, putting direct pressure to stop blood loss, covering the protruding bone with dressing.

Always compare the other side to judge severity of fractures. Fractures are characterized by

FRACTURES

the following: severe constant pain in the area of the fracture, especially during movement, a crack sound was heard when the break occurred, or grating sounds are heard afterwards during movement.

The natural shape of the area looks deformed and it cannot be moved without severe pain. Swelling and bruising present. Treatment should be as follows: treat for shock before looking at fractures, remove clothing or jewelery in the affected area. Do not try to push the bone back in place, stop the bleeding if present, applying pressure, elevate the area to reduce swelling.

RIB FRACTURES

Rib fractures are normally marked by sharp pains in the chest when moving or breathing. Internal bleeding might be present and possible pneumothorax.

If a rib has punctured the skin, listen to see if air is escaping from the hole, indicating chest puncture. In this case, act fast. Cover the wound with anything, even your hand, to seal the leak. If you delay, the injured person might suffocate. Place a seal over the puncture wound, anything airtight, like plastic. If safe to do so (no head or neck injury), roll the patient onto the injured side to help breathing.

Give rescue breathing if needed. If proper medical help doesn't turn up for a while, remove the seal for a few minutes every hour to avoid formation of a collapsed lung.

See flail chest below for more.

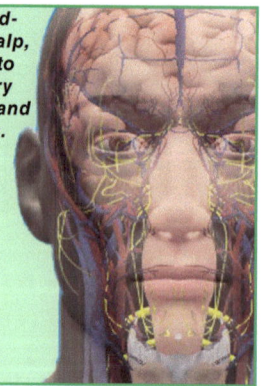

fig. 280 - If bleeding from the scalp, apply pressure to the temple artery or facial artery and apply bandages.

BLEEDING

For major **bleeding** seal the wound with your hand, applying firm pressure with the heel of your hand. If head wound (see fig. 280), apply padding over the wound and do not remove once soaked with blood, it might disturb clot formation and might restart bleeding.

If bleeding from the scalp, apply pressure to the temple artery or facial artery (fig. 280) and apply bandages. If bleeding on a limb, apply direct pressure to the wound, and if limb not broken, raise the limb enough to force blood to flow upwards and slow bleeding. Treat for shock.

SHOCK

In medical terms **shock** is caused by a reduction in oxygenated blood flow to vital organs as a response to severe physical trauma or blood loss.

Normal symptoms are pale and cold skin, dry mouth and feeling of thirst, nausea accompanied by vomiting, general weakness and sweating, quick shallow breathing and feeling dizzy, a weak and rapid pulse and general confusion and restlessness.

General treatment includes keeping injured person on his back, and do injury assessment as previously explained. If no injuries present, raise his legs 6-8 inches off the ground. Keep the patient warm but not hot. Watch out for vomiting that can be also provoked by sight of blood or injuries. So do not let him have a look at his wounds.

Loose any tight clothing and keep a calm and reassuring tone till qualified help arrives.

TRAUMA

Most of the injuries that you come across in a violent attack are the **trauma** type.

To understand trauma and its effect and mechanism it's important to learn a bit of the physics of such injury, that is the forces that produce injury and the types of injury that result. The law of conservation of energy (energy cannot be created or destroyed, but only changed in form) applies to all trauma accidents.

When two bodies collide, for example a person hitting the ground the kinetic energy (the energy of the falling person) does not just disappear, it must be absorbed.

The amount of energy absorbed by each body involved in the impact will be determined from the change of velocity and the masses involved.

If there is a big difference in mass between the two bodies involved, the smaller body (the person falling) will absorb the greater amount of energy.

Another physical law is Newton's first law of motion that says that a body will remain at rest or in motion at a constant velocity unless acted upon by an outside force.

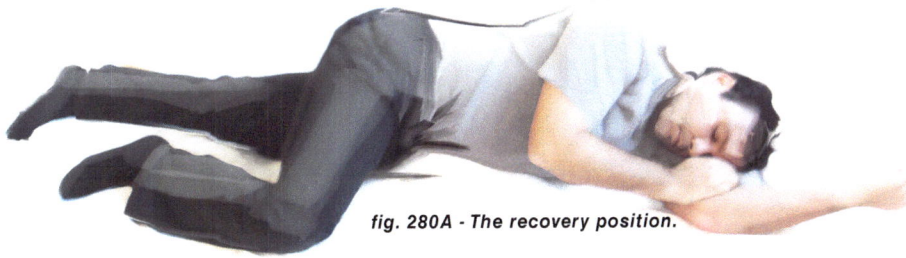

fig. 280A - The recovery position.

When a person hits the ground from height, there are two separate impacts each involving the transfer of kinetic energy.

The first impact is when the fall is abruptly stopped by the impact itself. The kinetic energy in this case is absorbed by the deformation of the person's body exterior structure. The second impact is when interior organs like the brain for instance, also hit against body structures, as the body decelerates, with the brain thrown forward and backwards in the scull, heart and lungs colliding violently with the chest walls. These laws are exemplified in blunt trauma, which occurs when the transfer of kinetic energy produces tissue damage without disrupting the skin.

We also further distinguish in penetrating injuries: these are injuries that involve a disruption of the skin, caused by knives or bullets.

The damage of a bullet, regardless of its velocity, has to do with two mechanisms: crushing the tissue in its path and stretching the surrounding tissue. As a bullet penetrates into tissue, it produces a permanent cavity of crushed tissue that maybe a cylinder of the same diameter of the bullet. At the same time, however, the kinetic energy of the moving bullet pushes tissue away from the bullet and forms a large temporary cavity that may be 30 times bigger in volume than the bullet itself. The higher the velocity of the bullet, the larger the cavity and the greater the stretch on surrounding tissues.

It's also worth remembering that most of the times bullets produce a small entrance wound, large damage inside and a larger exit wound, especially, for instance, when going through the thigh. Another factor influencing the seriousness of a gunshot wound, is the type of tissue that is being hit. Tissue of high elasticity like muscle for example, is better able to tolerate stretch (temporary cavitation) than tissue of low elasticity, like liver.

That's why if hit through the leg you can expect less damage than obviously if you are hit in the stomach.

Wound is any injury to the soft tissue, and they are normally divided into closed wounds, like a contusion or a bruise, and open wounds, when the skin is lacerated.

Treatment of extensive contusions is as follows:

1-ice should be applied to injured area, the cold constricts blood vessels, slowing the bleeding

2- compress the injured area, workbookly first then applying a splint

3- elevate the injured part above the heart to encourage drainage and decrease swelling

4- splint the injured extremities to prevent motion, therefore decrease bleeding.

Open wounds have potentially, as a consequence, serious blood loss.

They can also be vulnerable to infection and the treatment of open wounds should follow these general principles:

1- control bleeding by direct pressure, ideally using a sterile dressing but a clean cloth or a handkerchief will do if nothing else available, and should be kept till proper medical care arrives.

2- raising the injured part higher than the heart to slow down the bleeding.

3- applying pressure to the main arteries (see fig.281) you can apply pressure to the temporal artery (overlying the temporal bone of the skull) useful to control bleeding from the scalp.

Apply pressure to the brachial artery overlying the homerus to control bleeding from the forearm.

The femoral artery should compressed against the pelvis to control bleeding from the leg.

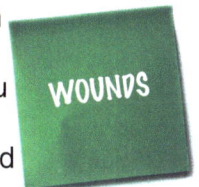

fig.281 - Blood circulation and pressure points.

Splinting is another way to control bleeding, to prevent movement of an extremity because motion promotes blood flow within the extremity.

After controlling bleeding, it's important to keep the wound as clean as possible, you could pour water over the area to clean it if necessary but do not pick out any foreign matter embedded in a wound.

Simply cover it with a dry, sterile dressing.

Open wounds are normally classified into abrasions, lacerations, puncture wounds and avulsions.

Abrasion is a superficial wound where part of the epidermis is lost after contact with a rough surface, **laceration** is a cut inflicted by a sharp instrument, like a knife or a razor blade, and controlling blood loss by direct manual pressure on the wound is the first priority.

Puncture wounds, is a stab from a pointed object such as a knife. Technically speaking a bullet wound is also a puncture wound

Generally these types of wounds do not cause significant external bleeding but they may cause extensive and even fatal internal bleeding, as well as further damage inside that cannot be detected at first sight.

In a puncture wound, if the pointed object remains embedded in the wound, **it's important not to try to remove the object, in other words, leave the knife in place, as efforts to do so may cause severe hemorrhage and further injury to underlying organs,** control bleeding by direct compression but not putting pressure on the object or the immediately surrounding tissue. Do not try to shorten the impaled object because any motion might damage surrounding tissues but instead stabilize the object in place with a bulky dressing and immobilize the extremity with a splint.

Avulsion occurs when a flap of skin has been torn loose, partially or completely.

If it's a large portion it's important to irrigate the part contaminated by dirt or debris and gently fold the skin flap back into place, holding it in place with dressing.

If a bigger part of the body is completely avulsed, as an amputation, it's important to try to preserve the amputated part to maximize the chances of successfully re implanting it.

Once you've stabilized the victim's injury, seal the amputated part in a plastic bag, if you could sterilize it with sterile saline it would be better, and then place it in a cool container like a can cooler.

But do not freeze or ever warm an amputated part, never place it in water, never place it directly on ice and bring it to the hospital in the shortest possible time.

To summarize: if for some immediate danger (incoming fast traffic for instance) you have to move the injured person and you are by yourself use the emergency drag (see fig. A) bearing in mind that you should never move the injured person from the side, always from the head.

Never lift from the head and feet, always keep the victim as horizontal and flat as possible, placing your hands gently in the armpits from behind.

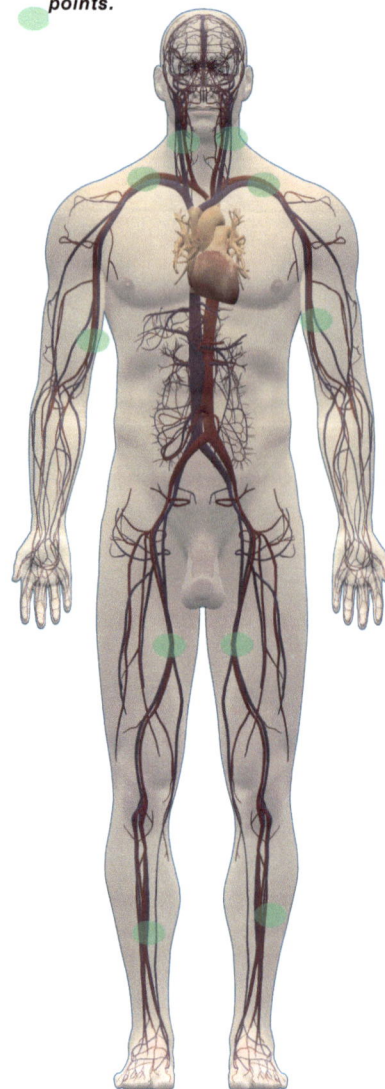

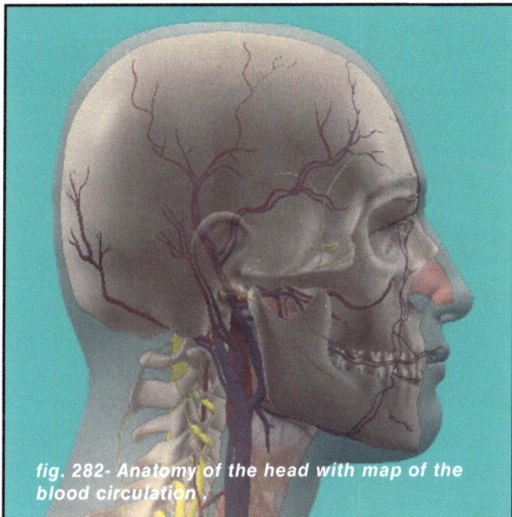
fig. 282- Anatomy of the head with map of the blood circulation.

INJURIES TO THE HEAD

Rest the person's head on your forearms, holding it tight so that it does no shift or turn. Two thirds of accidents involving motor vehicles or violent assault involvo **head injuries**. When head injuries are fatal, it is invariably because of associated injury to the brain.

The brain can be injured directly by a penetrating object, such as a bullet, but more commonly injury to the brain occurs indirectly as a result of external forces exerted to the skull. For instance, in a car accident, if an obstacle suddenly arrests the car's forward motion, the occupant continues to move forwards until his forward motion is arrested by the impact of his head with the windshield.

That impact causes a sudden deceleration of the skull, but the brain continues to move forward until its forward motion is arrested by impact with the inside of the skull. In fact, the brain is likely to crash into the skull twice - first in the original direction of motion, then, on rebound, against the opposite inner surface of the skull.

So, deceleration injuries to the brain may occur in either or both of two places: the point of initial impact (called "coup") or the side opposite ("contrecoup").

In either case, the response of the bruised brain will be similar to that of any other bruised tissue. It will start to swell. After several hours, an increase in cerebral water also starts to contribute to the swelling. Now we can appreciate the problem of having our brain inside a closed box.

When swelling occurs in an extremity, it is not ordinarily a critical problem, because the soft tissues have a lot of "give". But when swelling occurs within a rigid, closed box like the skull, there is no room in which the brain can expand. As intra-cranial pressure increases cerebral perfusion pressure inevitably falls, which means that blood flow to the brain decreases.

Clearly a decreasing cerebral blood flow is a potential catastrophe because the brain is dependant on a constant supply of blood to furnish the oxygen and glucose it needs to survive.

So the body attempts to resume cerebral perfusion pressure by raising the mean arterial pressure,that protective response will work only up to a certain point, if intra-cranial pressure continues to raise the resulting damage to brain parts will become irreversible, and death shortly follows.

HEAD INJURY ASSESSMENT

As for any other emergency, it starts with the ABC:

AIRWAY: If the patient is unconscious his airways are in jeopardy.

In opening the airway remember that any patient with significant head injury also has cervical spine injury until proved otherwise. If the forces that produced the head injuries are powerful enough to cause loss of consciousness, they were powerful enough to damage the cervical spine and the spinal cord within it

HEAD INJURY ASSESSMENT

 Act accordingly, and secure the airway without hyper extending the head or neck (jaw thrust or chin lift alone). In a head injury situation the airway might also be in jeopardy from vomiting, bleeding in the mouth or nose, or foreign objects such as broken teeth, hence it's necessary to make a quick inspection of the patient's mouth to remove obstructions.

BREATHING: Observe the chest during one or two respiratory cycles.

If there is any respiratory distress, expose the chest immediately for a more thorough examination because chest injuries may kill very quickly.

The most common cause for death on head injury is cerebral anoxia (lack of oxygen to the brain). If the patient's breathing is abnormally shallow or slow breathing, assist ventilation giving 20-25 breaths per minute.

CIRCULATION: Check for a pulse at the neck and the wrist (fig.275,285), and control major bleeding.

⚠️ **CAUTION** You can check the pupils and note their size whether they are equal and whether they constrict when a light is directed at them. Be aware that **the most important single sign in the evaluation of a head injured person is the changing state of consciousness.**

In addition to the ABC there are a few other supportive measures that should be taken while awaiting medical care for the head injured patient:

Do not allow the patient to become overheated, patients with head injury tend to develop a very high temperature that in turn may worsen the condition of the brain.

Do not cover the patient with blankets if the ambient temperature is 70 degrees Fahrenheit /21C or above. Cover wounds as needed. If there is an open fracture of the skull with brain tissue oozing out of the skull (it tends to resemble toothpaste), cover it lightly with sterile dressing, moistened with sterile saline. The same goes for leakage of blood from the ears, loose sterile dressings, and keep the area clean. Remember that objects impaled in the skull should be left where they are and protected from being jarred. Monitor the cardiac rhythm remembering that slow pulse (bradycardia) is a possible sign of increasing intra-cranial pressure.

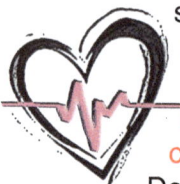

Do not give any medicines or liquids or foods. Immobilize the patient. It is worth noting that conscious head injured patients may not be entirely cooperative and may not wish to go to hospital.

However, every head injured patient who has had a period of unconsciousness must be evaluated in the hospital.

Do not attempt to stop the bleeding by direct pressure since the skull maybe broken.

Use padding only, applying pressure to the sides of the wound. 15% of head trauma cases involve neck injuries.

⚠️ **CAUTION** **Treat the injured as if a spinal injury is present.** Vomiting is very common following a head trauma.

fig.283 - Spinal cord with nerve distribution, side and back view.

CERVICAL NERVES — C 1- C8 — HEAD+NECK DIAPHRAGM ARMS-HANDS
THORACIC NERVES — T 1-T12 — CHEST MUSCLES ABDOMINAL MUSCLES
LUMBAR NERVES — L1- L5 — LEG MUSCLES
SACRAL NERVES — S1- S5 — BOWEL-BLADDER SEXUAL ORGANS

Symptoms of minor head trauma are dizziness, bruising and facial discoloration and headache.

In a major head trauma expect all of the above plus some or all of the following: slow pulse, breathing difficulties, severe localized headache, a generalized pain throughout the head, disorientation, staggering, drowsiness, unsteadiness when standing, bleeding or fluid drainage from mouth, ears or nose, dilated pupils, one pupil larger than the other, or failing to respond to changes in light levels, unconsciousness. Treatment for minor head trauma, if the injured person can stand with eyes closed and feet together without losing balance, consists in keeping the person at rest, or applying something cold.

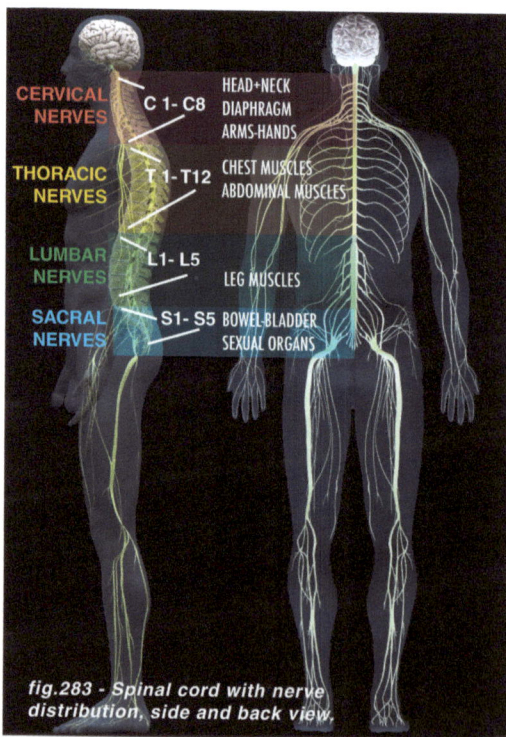

Don't forget that a minor head injury may evolve into a major one, doctors normally allow 24 hours after the injury to spot signs or symptoms as above. If they appear, treat as follows: keep airways clear, immobilize the person, especially neck and head, treat for shock, and do not allow them to eat or drink anything

INJURIES TO THE FACE

Injuries to the face may appear very dramatic but ordinarily are not life threatening in themselves. However, they should be taken seriously because they might be associated with airway obstruction, they may signal the presence of a closed head injury, as common as 55% of cases, and approximately 10% of all patients with facial fracture have cervical spine injury as well. Further more, facial injuries are extremely distressing to the person who sustains them, seriously worried about disfiguration.

SOFT TISSUE INJURIES TO THE FACE

Facial lacerations are treated as lacerations anywhere else, with direct pressure of control bleeding and sterile dressing.

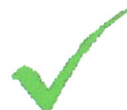

When a foreign object is impaled in the cheek the object SHOULD be removed because massive bleeding associated with cheek injuries may obstruct the airway.
This is probably the only instance in which an impaled object should be removed rather than stabilized. Carefully pull the object out from the same side as it entered, but if you experience difficulties removing it don't force it, just leave it.

Once the object has been removed, pack the inside of the cheek (between the teeth and the cheek) with sterile gauze, and apply contra-pressure with dressing on the outside of the wound. If bleeding is still profuse, position the patient so that blood will drain out of his mouth, rather than down his throat. A hematoma anywhere on the face can only be treated applying a cold pack, to minimize swelling and discomfort. Nosebleed (epistaxis) without fracture normally is controlled by pinching the nostrils together. It is normally self-limited unless associated with a fracture.

Remember that severe epistaxis is more frequently encountered among the elderly, and bleeding originating in the posterior part of the nose is only visible inspecting the back of the patient's throat, causing suffocation. In this case, turn the head or the whole body to the side to facilitate blood drainage.

MAXILLOFACIAL INJURIES

Maxillofacial fractures occur when the face absorbs the energy of a strong impact. The forces involved may be massive. It requires forces of up to 150 G for example to fracture the Maxilla, and forces of that magnitude can be expected to produce cerebral contusions and cervical spine injuries as well. Therefore, when you find a maxillofacial fracture, immobilize the spine and monitor neurological signs.

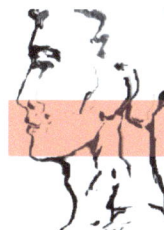

Clues to the presence of a maxillofacial fracture are usually ecchymosis, a black and blue mark on the face, or deep facial lacerations indicating that underlying bone may have been injured, as well as pain and palpation over a bone is also a sign.

The most common facial fracture is the broken nose, characterized by swelling, tenderness, and sometimes displacement from the normal position. Usually, there is crepitus, a crackling feeling on palpation, and epistaxis.

Next more common are fractures of the mandible.

There is at least a 50:50 chance that it is fractured in more than one place and will therefore be unstable for palpation.

There is likely to be ecchymosis and swelling over the fracture sight.

Teeth may be partially or completely avulsed. Maxillary fractures produce massive facial swelling, instability of the mid-facial bones, and malocclusion (abnormal bite).

There may be a black eye and the patient's face appears elongated.

Treatment to apply to all patients with significant maxillofacial injuries should be as follows: establish an AIRWAY, inspecting the mouth for obstructions, and if you find an intact missing tooth, even on the ground, pick it up by the crown, not the root, and place it in a container of cold fresh milk for storage, cushioning it with sterile gauze if possible.

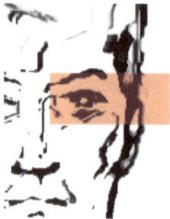

Notify medical personal you have recovered it, and preserving it so may increase the chance of re implantation. Apply cold packs to swollen parts to minimize swelling and alleviate pain. Always assume that there is cervical spine injury.

INJURIES TO THE EYE

Trauma to the eyes is very common and bears potential serious consequences.

The globe or eyeball is a spherical structure measuring about 1 inch in diameter housed within a bony cavity in the skull, called the eye socket or orbit.

There are two special fluids that help give the eye its shape and structure.

The aqueous humor fills the space between the cornea (crystal clear interior segment of the sclera or white of the eye, overlying the pupil and iris) and the lens.

Aqueous humor is produced behind the iris (pigmented tissue made up of muscles and blood vessels that can contract and expand to regulate the size of the pupil, that is the adjustable opening within the iris) and if lost through a penetrating injury to the eye it will gradually be replenished.

Filling the posterior chamber behind the lens (a transparent structure that can alter its thickness in order to focus light on the retina on the back of the eye) is the vitreous humor, a jellylike substance that maintains the shape of the globe. If the vitreous is lost, it cannot be replenished, and blindness will result. Treatment to eye injuries is complex: the eyes are delicate structures.

Generally, there isn't much you can do in the field and you could create serious damage trying to treat eye injuries, a simple contusion (black eye) can be treated gently applying cold pack to the injured part.

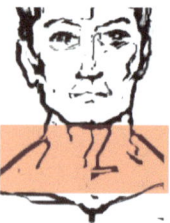

INJURIES TO THE NECK

The neck is a very vulnerable part of anatomy because it contains a critical portion of the airway (the larynx), major blood vessels to and from the head and the spinal cord, with its nerve supply to the whole body. Injuries to any of these structures can be disastrous, and any soft tissue injuries to the neck must be considered critical until proven otherwise. Blunt trauma to the neck may cause collapse of the larynx or the trachea, with consequent airway obstruction.

The most common finding during physical examination is hoarseness of the voice, or loss of voice altogether, and in some cases blood is coughed up.

Assisting breathing has to be done carefully to avoid cervical spine injury, so handle the patient carefully.

In case of penetrating injuries to the neck, if the trachea has been disrupted you will notice a frothy mixture of air and blood blowing through the penetrating wound. Such wounds must be sealed off. Penetrating injuries to the neck also carry a hazard of exsanguinating hemorrhage from the jugular veins, carotid arteries, or their branches.

One special danger associated with bleeding wounds of the neck, is the possibility of a fatal air embolism. If a major vein of the neck is disrupted, air can be sucked into the vein and from there be swept along with the blood flow into the heart, causing dysrhythmias and death.

When there is significant bleeding from the neck, therefore, the wound must sealed immediately, and hold pressure over the dressing by hand.

Do not bandage around the neck, it might interfere with blood flow on the other side of the neck and may also impair breathing.

Apply manual pressure only over the bleeding side. Position the patient on his left side, keeping the head down and feet elevated.

INJURIES TO THE SPINE

The majority of cases are a result of vehicle accidents and falls from great height.
Then as a consequence of falls, gunshot wounds and other penetrating injuries, and the rest from diving accidents, contact sports and other causes. It is important to remember that every victim from a multiple trauma has a spinal cord injury until proved otherwise.

The spinal cord connects the brain to all of the other organs in the body. If the cord is interrupted, all connections between the brain and muscle groups or organs below the level of cord damage are severed, the part of the body involved, becomes as useless as if it had been amputated. The higher the injury in the spinal cord, lets say about the 6th cervical vertebrae the more of the body will be paralyzed. (fig. 283) A bit higher, C4 or above, and the injury will paralyze the diaphragm as well making breathing virtually impossible. Any accident involving significant acceleration/deceleration forces, such as in a car accident, is likely to have snapped the victim's neck violently back and forth. Compression injuries, such as those that might be sustained in diving head first into a shallow pool or jumping from a height and landing on ones feet are also a likely source of spinal trauma. **In fact, any fall from a height should immediately taken as possible cause of serious spinal injury.**

Associated injuries, such as head trauma or facial trauma, must be assumed to have a cervical spine injury. and the same as crushing injuries, lightening injuries, which causes violent muscle contractions, and gunshot wounds especially to the head, neck, chest, back and abdomen.

Any patient found unconscious after trauma should be assumed to have a spinal cord injury. If the patient is conscious instruct not to move. It is important to apply some means of temporary stabilization to the cervical spine.

If there are a sufficient number of rescuers, the most sufficient and readily available means of temporary stabilization are a pair of hands or knees.

The object is to keep the head and neck in neutral position and prevent any flexion, extension, or movement to the side.

fig.283A - Spinal cord: nerves distribution seen from the back in relation to the vertebraes.

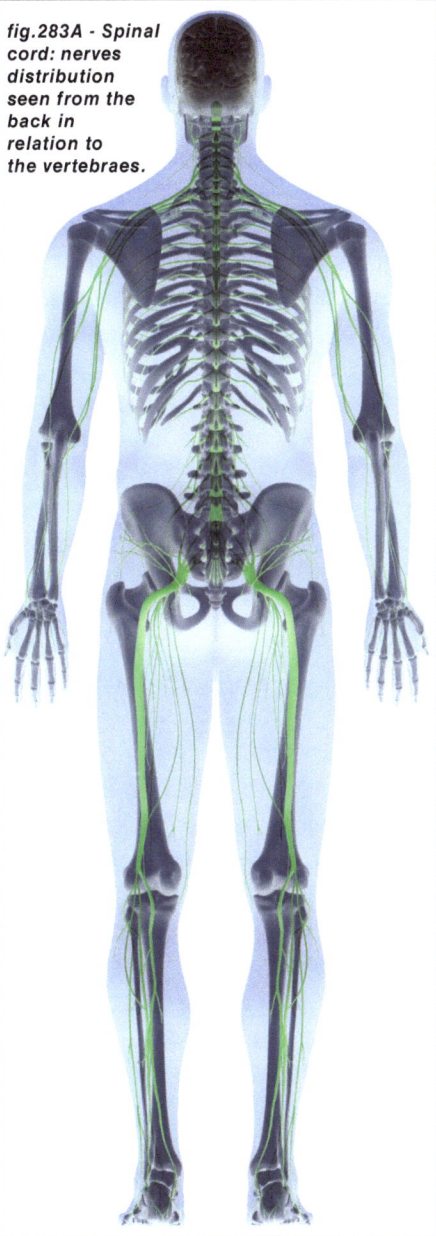

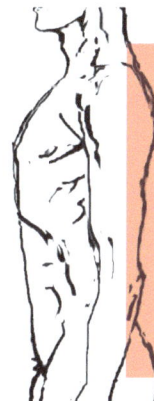

If the patient is unconscious the first priority is always to ensure an open airway. You can use a jaw thrust, chin lift, or jaw lift (fig. 277) without backward tilt of the head. Evaluate the patient's breathing since an injury involving the lower cervical or upper thoracic spinal cord may result in paralysis of the intercostal muscles.

Injury around C4 or higher will paralyze the diaphragm as well, causing severe impairment of recreation. You can assist breathing, making sure you keep the head and neck steady.

Circulation should be assessed meaning control of bleeding if any. Expose the patient by cutting away his clothes, to minimize motion of the spine. Do not try to change the victim's position in which he was found unless his airway is jeopardized. Victims of vehicular trauma have been known to walk away from the accident, only to become totally paralyzed hours later when an incautious nod of the head squeezed an unstable vertebral column against the spinal cord: even if a victim gets up and feels fine, you should convince him to go to hospital, or better, wait for an ambulance.

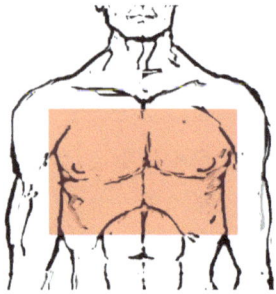

INJURIES TO THE CHEST

Injuries to the chest are the major cause of mortality in 25% of deaths due to trauma. In another 25% chest injuries contribute significantly to the fatal outcome. This shouldn't be surprising considering that the chest houses some of the most vital structures of the body: the heart, the lungs and the great vessels. Any significant injury to the chest can lead rapidly to hypoxia, circulatory insufficiency of both, and thereby threatens the whole organism. The thorax is a hollow cavity formed by the 12 pairs of ribs that join in the back with the thoracic spine and in the front with the sternum, to form a protective bony ring around the organs of the chest. The first four ribs are relatively protected by the shoulder girdle and are less likely to be fractured than rib 5 to 10. In fact, if ribs 1 and 2 were fractured, one has to assume that massive forces were involved.

The rib cage becomes stiffer with age, therefore, a blunt force applied to the chest of an older person is more likely to fracture ribs than the same force applied to the chest of a younger person. For that same reason, though, blunt trauma is more likely to injure the internal organs of a young person's chest, because the pliable rib cage of a young person is more easily compressed against the lungs and the heart.

The interior border of the thoracic cavity is formed by the diaphragm, which together with the intercostal muscles constitutes the main muscle of respiration.

The diaphragm is a domed muscle that arches up into the chest, therefore, some abdominal organs such as the liver and spleen are in fact located beneath the ribs and can be injured by trauma to the rib cage. For practical purposes remember that any injury below the level of the nipples is an abdominal injury as well as a chest injury.

Nearly the entire volume of the thoracic cavity is occupied by the lungs.

The heart lies just behind and slightly to the left of the sternum, so the heart is subject to injury when there is direct blow to the sternum or when deceleration forces cause the heart to collide against the sternum. The great vessels enter and exit the heart and they are the venea cavae and the aorta. Chest trauma may disrupt the trachea leading to airway problems that cannot be treated in the field. Your cause of action should be to clear the airway, and remember that noisy breathing means obstructed breathing.

An open pneumothorax is the result of a penetrating injury to the chest.

Small penetrating injuries such as entrance wounds from small caliber bullets, usually seal themselves off but larger injuries, such as shotgun wounds, may remain open.

In this case, air will move preferentially through the chest defect with each respiratory effort rather than into the trachea, creating a so-called sucking chest wound.

With the entrance of air into the pleural space on the involved side, the lung on that side collapses and cannot expand normally on inhalation. So the lung on the damaged side is soon depleted of its oxygen. Meanwhile, during exhalation, some air from the healthy lung is exhaled into the lung on the injured side. Then the same air is drawn back into the healthy lung with the next inhalation. Therefore, ventilation of the healthy lung is also impaired.

The symptoms and signs of open pneumothorax are respiratory distress, the open wound will be visible on the chest wall, and it will be possible to hear air being sucked into the wound on inhalation. Immediate treatment consists of applying a sterile or occlusive dressing such as petrolatum gauze or plastic wrap over the wound, covering it completely in a way that does not itself get sucked into the wound. If the patient is able to cooperate ask him to cough and then slap the dressing tight in place as he does so. Tape or secure the occlusive dressing on three sides only, leaving one side free to vent out any build-up of pressure within the chest.

The open end of the dressing must allow air to escape from the chest on exhalation, to avoid air accumulating within the thoracic cavity leading to tension pneumothorax.

TENSION PNEUMOTHORAX

Normally is the result of blunt chest trauma in which a damaged area of lung tissue does not seal itself off. Air enters the pleural space during inhalation but cannot escape during exhalation, so pressure builds up in the effected pleural cavity. As the pressure in the effected side of the chest increases the opposite lung is squeezed, thereby compromising it's ventilation as well.

Furthermore, the superior and inferior venae cavae become pink and compressed, hindering the return of blood to the right side of the heart.

As a result cardiac output falls and blood backs up in the systemic veins.

Tension pneumothorax presents itself with extreme dyspnea, restlessnesss and anxiety.

Breath sounds are diminished, and in addition the affected side of the chest may appear more expanded than the normal side and will move less with respiratory efforts. Treatment on the field can only be carried out by paramedics or doctors because if requires immediate decompression of the effected side of the chest using a through-the -needle catheter.

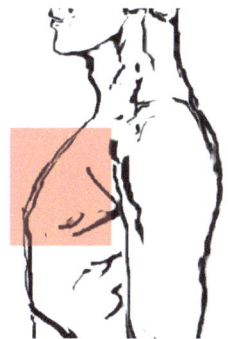

FLAIL CHEST

When several ribs, the sternum, or both are fractured in two or more places, an unstable or flail chest may result. The portion of the chest wall that is no longer in continuity with the rest of the thoracic cage, moves in a paradoxical fashion,expanding or bulging out during exhalation, and collapsing during inhalation.

Whenever the forces involved in an accident are sufficient to produce a flail chest, they are also sufficient to cause pneumothorax and serious injury to the underlying lung.

In addition, the collapse ot a segment of the rib cage during each inhalation leads to repeated contusion and further collapse of the lung beneath, with consequent impairment of oxygenation.

At the same time the severe pain characteristic of rib fractures prevents the victim from taking deep breaths. The consequence is hypoxemia and hypercarbia, so immediate treatment is aimed at correcting those, either administering 100% oxygen or assisting breathing.

The risk is to convert a simple pneumothorax into a tension pneumothorax with excessive positive pressure ventilation, so it's important to stabilize the flail segment by either applying constant firm manual pressure or by butressing the segment with sandbags or pillows.

INJURIES TO THE ABDOMEN

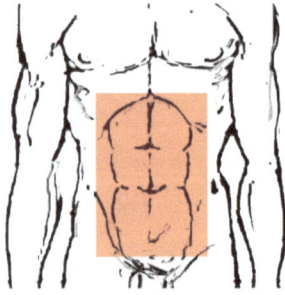

If the trauma is an open wound treat for bleeding as explained.

If organs are protruding do not attempt to place organs back into the abdominal cavity, and do not clean or touch the wound or the organs in any way. Keep the injured person on his back with his head turned to one side, unless spinal or neck injuries present. Watch for vomiting and do not let the person eat or drink anything whatsoever.

Significant abdominal injuries may sometimes be obvious as when the victim of a stabbing is found with half his intestines hanging out the stab wound.

CAUTION More often, however, the presence of potentially serious injury within the abdominal cavity may be very difficult to detect, even to people medically trained. We should also remember that part of the abdomen is in the chest, therefore, injuries to the chest might effect the abdomen.

Nearly all the organs of the abdomen are loosely suspended from the body walls by a delicate membrane called mesentery, which carries blood vessels and nerves to the abdominal organs.

The mesentery is easily torn, and because it is so vascular, can bleed profusely when lacerated. The abdominal cavity contains major portions of the digestive, lymphoid and genitourinary systems: abdominal injury is particularly likely to produce vomiting, which may jeopardize the airway, therefore, position the victim in the recovery position if possible to enable vomitus to drain out of the mouth rather than back down the throat. Impairment of breathing suggests associated chest or spinal injury. Sever compression injury to the abdomen may drive abdominal contents upwards and cause tears in the diaphragm.

A restless, anxious victim with cold clammy skin may very likely be bleeding into his abdomen. Don't forget that an injury to the chest anywhere below the nipple is also an injury to the abdomen. and that a distended, tender abdomen after injury means internal bleeding.

Penetrating injuries to the abdomen may result from knives, bullets and other blunt instruments.

Penetrating injuries might be much more serious than they appear from the outside: beneath the clean little bullet hole, for example may lie a disaster area of torn vessels, chewed up intestines and so forth.

Penetrating injuries most usually result in hemorrhage, from laceration of a major blood vessels or solid organ, and perforation of a hollow organ, usually a segment of the bowl. Treatment of a victim with penetrating trauma to the abdomen includes the following: attend first to the ABC (airways, breathing, circulation), cover open wounds with dry sterile dressings, if there is an impaled object in the abdomen, leave it there, stabilize the impaled object in place with bulky dressings and tape the dressing securely.

If viscera are protruding through a large open wound in the abdominal wall, do not attempt to replace the protruding organs into the abdomen.

Leave the viscera on the surface of the abdomen and cover them gently with sterile aluminum foil or with sterile dressings which have been soaked in sterile saline.

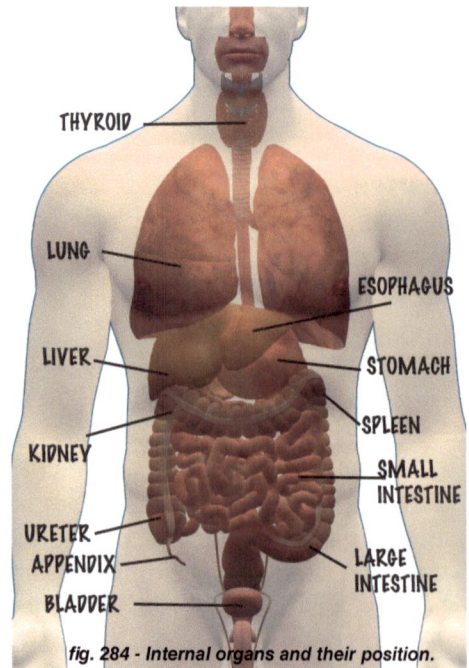

THYROID

LUNG

ESOPHAGUS

LIVER

STOMACH

SPLEEN

KIDNEY

SMALL INTESTINE

URETER

APPENDIX

LARGE INTESTINE

BLADDER

fig. 284 - Internal organs and their position.

Do not use dry dressings in direct contact with protruding viscera because they stick and are difficult to remove later.

Cover the foil or wet dressing with a clean towel or additional layers of universal dressings to minimize heat loss across the wound.

Give nothing by mouth.

Blunt abdominal trauma may have few outward signs.

Even bruises the usual indication of blunt impact may take several hours to develop. In a person who has sustained a blow to the abdomen mechanism of injury suggestive of blunt abdominal trauma include compression of the abdominal contents against the spine, direct blows (a kick in the belly), rapid deceleration (car accident).

Special attention for blunt abdominal trauma should be paid when a pedestrian is struck by a moving vehicle. The organs most commonly injured by blunt trauma to the abdomen (including the part of the abdomen that is within the chest) are the liver, spleen, pancreas, duodenum and mesentery of the small bowel.

The liver in the right upper quadrant of the abdomen, is easily torn by blunt injury, such as steering wheel trauma, and because of it's rich blood supply can bleed massively.

Similarly, severe hemorrhage may occur from rapture of the spleen. located in the left upper quadrant, also vulnerable to steering wheel trauma.

The spleen is the most commonly injured organ in blunt abdominal trauma, stashed up inside the ribs, the spleen in susceptible to rapture whenever there is a fracture of the left 9th and 10th ribs. With the majority of trauma to the abdomen be prepared for vomiting, and is really severe forces were involved expect also injuries to the spine.

Treatment of blunt abdominal trauma is principally aimed at anticipating shock and supporting the circulation. Attend first to the ABC, anticipate vomiting, immobilize the spine and don't forget that blunt abdominal injury might be more serious than it looks.

INJURIES TO THE GENITALS

genitourinary injuries may be produced by either blunt or penetrating trauma.

The kidneys, relatively well protected from injury by the ribs and heavy muscles of the back, therefore, any force powerful enough to damage the kidneys will usually produce other injuries as well, such as fractured ribs and vertebrae and damage to other abdominal organs. Any blow to the flank and to the lower rib cage in the back should arise suspicion of renal injuries.

The urinary bladder, located just behind the pubic bone is vulnerable to injury whenever there is a fracture of the pelvis.

Usually, people who have suffered genitourinary injuries will have suffered other more serious injuries, and treatment will usually be governed by the other injuries and overall condition.

Injuries to the external genitalia are rarely life threatening, even if often highly distressing to the victim. The kidneys are the most vulnerable part of the area and normally well protected by the ribs and the big muscles in the back.

Only when serious forces or blunt objects such as a knife or a bat and as well as heavy boots there could be injury to the kidneys.

The bladder, located in the pubic area, can suffer serious damage especially when a kick to the genitals has been received. Injuries to the external genitalia are rarely life threatening even if often seriously distressing for the person.

Treat as any other soft tissue injury anywhere else in the body.

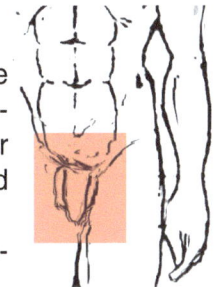

MUSCOSKELETAL INJURIES

MUSCOSKELATAL INJURIES.
We can distinguish these injuries into fractures, dislocations and sprains.

Fractures as a interruption in the continuity of a bone. They can be **closed**, when the skin is intact, or open if there is a wound and/or a bone is protruding.

Open fractures are more prone to infection and they obviously bleed. The main symptom of fracture is pain and well localized. Also the patient has probably heard something snapping or the sound of the bone breaking.

That is information that can be relied upon.

It will appear very tense to physical examination and the limb is in a unnatural position often looking shorter than the other; swelling is present and also an ecchymosis is quite apparent.

Often it can be determined by the way the patient is holding his limb such as the wrist or the shoulder, almost to protect it.

A fractured bone is often tender to palpation and crepitus (crackling sound) is present. Fractures are normally low priority injuries unless they are bleeding or cause respiratory problems, although they can produce shock.

A **dislocation** is when a bone is displaced from his natural position. The principal symptom is of increased pressure on the joint together with loss of motion.

The joins mostly affected normally are shoulder, elbow, fingers, hips and ankles. Dislocations in these locations might produce a compromise in the nerve and blood supply to the extremity, therefore always check distal pulse and if loss of sensation is detected the patient should be transported to hospital as soon as possible.

Sprains are injuries involving a ligament that is thorn, often because of sudden twisting or extended past its normal range of movement. Knees and ankles are most commonly affected and in these locations pain and swelling as well as discoloration, because of blood circulation difficulty, is often present. In practice though is not that easy to differentiate among these types of injuries. For this very reason is always best to treat severe strains or dislocation as if were fractures.

To sum it up the assessment to carry out in case of an injured joint is proper blood circulation (check if discoloration of the skin is present) and assess nerve supply checking the sensory reactions.

On the field the first action in case of most musculoskeletal injuries is immobilization normally referred as splinting. Splinting and relief from pain ease the patient's stress preventing shock, avoiding further damage to muscles and nerves as the patient would suffer going into shock or becoming agitated, thus preventing a close fracture from becoming an open fracture.

To perform proper splinting of extremities cutting clothing may be necessary, expose the wounds before splinting to air and check proper sensation in motor function and make a note of it.

But unless you really know what you are doing is better not to straighten a damaged joint especially when involving the shoulder or elbow, better to restrain them in the position in which you find them and also in the case of exposed fractures do not push the bone back underneath the skin, just cover it with sterile dressing.

fig.285 - How to check distal pulse on the foot.

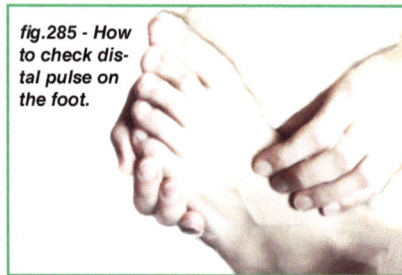

And on the wrist.

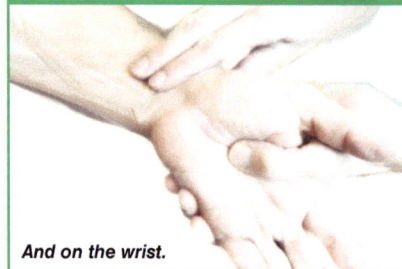

fig.286 - How to control hyperventilation using a paper bag.

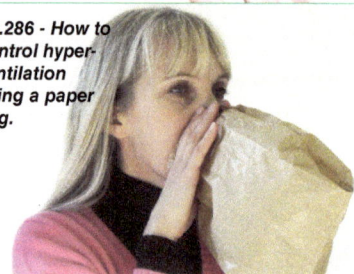

A sling is useful for immobilizing injuries of the shoulder and elbow.

A dislocation of the knee is often the result of basic hyperextension's injury, it is easy to spot because the knee will be heavily bruised and swollen. Quite often a heavy percussion results into the popliteal artery compromising circulation of the foot.

Knee fractures are often a result of a blow and can be extremely painful, like most fractures keep cool and immobilize, organize transport or rescue as quickly as possible.

Snake Bites normally can be quite painful, but not necessarily all snakes are poisonous or not necessarily all poisonous snakes are deadly.

In case you are bitten remain calm, becoming agitated will increase blood circulation and carry the venom more quickly. Control your breathing, if you are hiperventilating cup your hands in front of your mouth or breath into a bag for few seconds (fig.286) to bring the level of carbon dioxide back to normal. Make some notes on the snake appearance as quickly as possible, if snakes still present take a picture of it with your phone, it will help medical personnel later on to give you the correct antivenom. Do not try to kill the snake, but if you or one of your companions did bring the snake with you for identification. If you can examine the bitten area do so and check if the bite looks poisonous or not (fig. 248 and 249 page 163) In any case ask for help. Rinse the area with water, do not cover or cut around the wound and **DO NOT SUCK out the poison with your mouth**.

If you have a sucking device apply it as soon as possible, it can remove more than half of the injected poison if applied promptly. Do not apply any tourniquet or bandage and remove jewellery and rings. Swelling in the bitten area will happen within 5-10 minutes, together within increasing localized pain. Within 30 minutes to one and half hour you might experience dizziness, nausea, pounding headache as well as vomiting and an increased heart rate and breathing rate. If close enough to a medical centre or help it is safe to walk for up to two hours at normal pace, but keeping most of the movement or your weight off the stricken part. The majority of bites are NOT lethal and the survival rate is quite high, even the most poisonous snakes do not inject all the venom in their sack all the time they bite and an adult of good fitness level can survive easily. Bites from other animals must be treated according to severity, if superficial rinse part under running water and disinfect and treat as per abrasion. If more severe see earlier advice and seek qualified medical help.

SNAKE BITES

CAUTION

CPR QUICK REFERENCE

fig.286A - Keeping your arms straight give 80-100 chest compressions per minute, 2 inches deep.
Every 15 compressions give 2 full breaths, making sure that the chest raises.

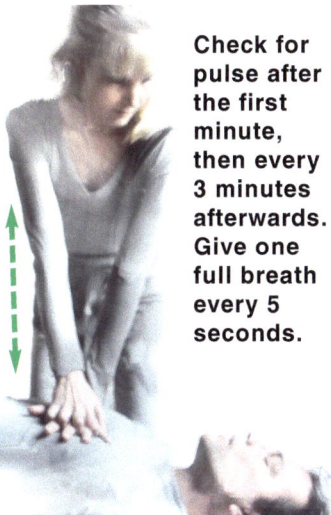

Check for pulse after the first minute, then every 3 minutes afterwards. Give one full breath every 5 seconds.

Start with 4 slow, full breaths, lasting 1 1/2 seconds. Continue rescue breathing, one full breath every 5 seconds. Monitor the chest.

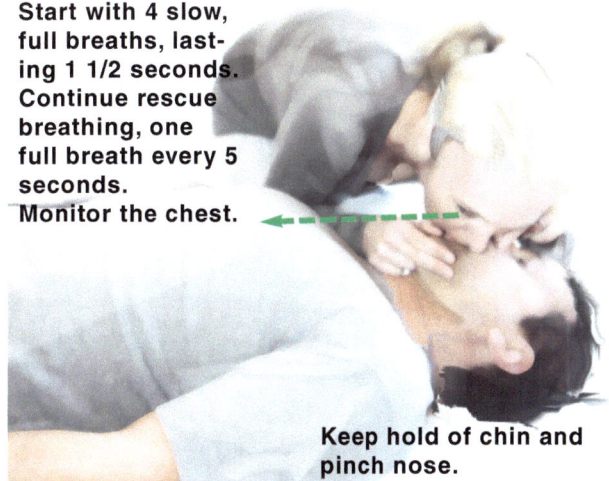

Keep hold of chin and pinch nose.

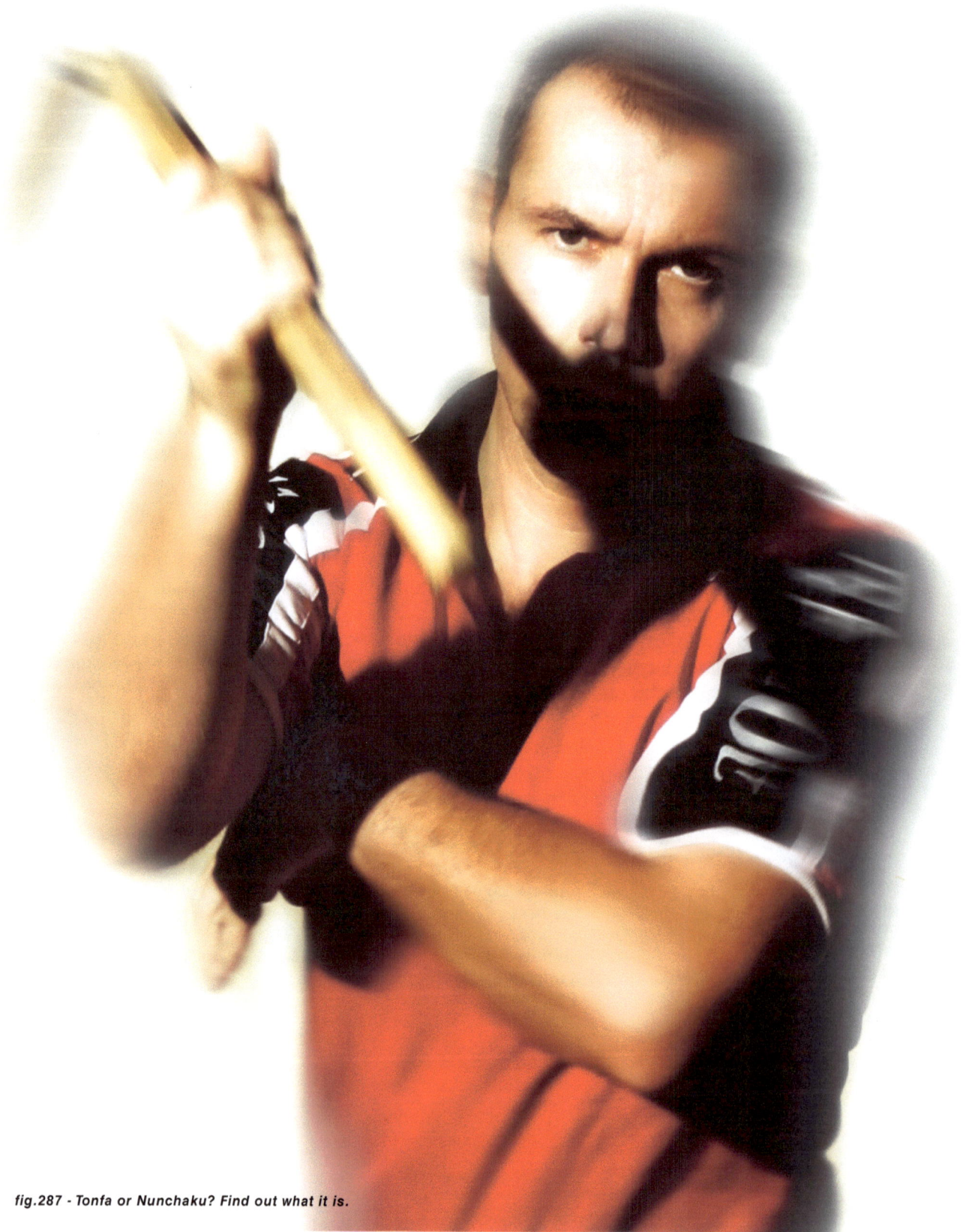
fig.287 - Tonfa or Nunchaku? Find out what it is.

419 (internet scam) named after section 419 of the Nigerian penal code, a section that deals with the prohibition of this kind of fraud and it is also known as the Spanish Prisoner Of War Scam dating from the 16th century, a confidence trick dating back to 1588. In its original form, the confidence trickster (con man) tells his victim (the mark) that he is in correspondence with a wealthy person of high estate who has been imprisoned in Spain (originally by King Philip II) under a false identity. The alleged prisoner cannot reveal his identity without serious repercussions, and is relying on the confidence trickster to raise money to secure his release. The trickster offers to let the mark supply some of the money, with a promise that he will be rewarded generously when the prisoner returns both financially and by being married to the prisoner's beautiful daughter. However, once the mark has turned over his money, he learns that further problems have arisen, requiring yet more money, until the mark is cleaned out and has no money left to send. In 419 advance fee fraud, a valuable item might need to be ransomed from a security company, bank, warehouse, customs agent, or a lost baggage facility before the authorities or thieves recognize its value.

In the Nigerian variation, a self proclaimed relative of a deposed African dictator or a relative of wealthy minister or businessman offers to transfer millions of illegally acquired dollars into the bank account of the victim in return for small initial payments to cover bribes and other expenses.

ACUPUNCTURE part of Chinese medicine using needles inserted into body points (meridians).

AD-WARE Unwanted programs that, once installed, bombard users with unwanted adverts. Often those pushing the ad-ware programs get paid for every machine they manage to recruit. Some ad-ware poses as fake computer security software. It can be very hard to remove.

AIKIDO (Way of Spiritual Harmony) created by MORIHEI UESHIBA who developed it in the early 1930s in Japan, borrowing from JUJUTSU and comprehending throws, joint locks and weapon work. It's based on the principle that you apply your technique the moment you make contact, with techniques against an armed opponent. The practitioner is called AIKIDOKA.

ARNIS DE MANO (hand's harness) martial arts from Philippines using canes, kicks, arm locks and throws. Linked to ESCRIMA.

ATEMI Strikes aimed at vital points of the body. Used in JUJITSU and KARATE but prohibited in JUDO.

BACK DOOR Hidden software or hardware mechanism used to circumvent security controls. Synonymous with trap door.

BALISONG Philippine term for BUTTERFLY KNIFE. Mostly used in ESKRIMA and KALI.

BANDESH Combat form originating from India designed to render the aggressor inoffensive without killing him.

BANDO Burmese martial art introduced in the West by Mung Gyi in 1962. The techniques are named after 12 animals: wild boar, bull, cobra, red deer, eagle, monkey, bird, panther, piton, scorpion, tiger and viper.

BANSHAI Martial art originating from Burma that employs weapons such as stick, sword and spear.

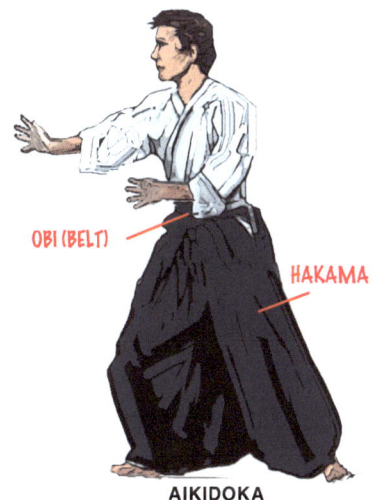

OBI (BELT)

HAKAMA

AIKIDOKA

BARATERO or ARTE DE MANEJAR LA NAVAJA EL CHUCHILLO Y LA TIJERA DE LOS GITANOS published in Madrid in 1849; is the first known workbook on knives handling in combat. The art of knife handling was very popular in Spain and in Italy and then became popular in the colonies as well as Argentina, Uruguay, Puerto Rico, Mexico. In ESCRIMA practitioners use a particular knife called BALI SONG and the Americans, once they took over from the Spanish, called it KLIK KLIK because of the sound it makes when it opens, or BUTTERFLY KNIFE.

BERSILAT Malaysian Martial art derivative of PENTJAK-SILAT. Practiced in Giava and Sumatra.

BINOT Ancient martial art from India without weapons, 3000 years old.

BLACK BELT The first meaningful degree in martial arts grades. In Japanese it is called "SHODAN".

BLACKHAT A hacker that uses his skills for explicitly criminal or malicious ends, writing destructive viruses or jamming websites offline. Now it is likely to refer to those that steal credit card numbers and banking data with VIRUSES or through PHISHING.

BO Stick about six feet long used in combat in many Japanese martial arts from Okinawa.

BODHIDARMA Indian guru who introduced Buddhist Zen concept to China, and then taking in the Shaolin temple the basics of the famous Kung-Fu.

BOK HOK PAI Chinese method of Kung-Fu based on the moves of the white crane.

BOK MEI PAI Kung-Fu style based mostly on speed of execution, it means "white eye-browed man" from its creator Bok Mei. Legend says that he was expelled from the Shaolin temple after killing one of his own pupils in a fight.

BOKH (strength) or Mongolian wrestling is celebrated during Nadam Festival. It originated 2,000 years ago as military training, the match has no time or weight limit and the loser is the one who touches the ground with any part above his knee.

BOKKEN Solid sword made out of wood used for training in Kendo and other martial arts.

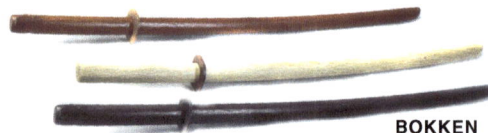

BOKKEN

BOT The name given to an individual computer in a larger botnet mostly a PC running Windows. The name is an abbreviation of "robot" to imply that it is under someone else's control.

BOTNET A large number of hijacked computers under the remote control of a single person via net-based command and control system. The machines are often recruited via a virus that travels via e-mail but increasingly DRIVE BY DOWNLOADS and WORMS are also used to find and recruit victims. The biggest botnets can have tens of thousands of hijacked computers that can be hired by criminals for few cents for each machine.

BOTNET HERDER One of the names for the controller or operator of a BOTNET.

BOXER REBELLION European term given to the internal war in China of 1900 because many of the rebels belonged to the secret society I HO CHUAN practicing Kung-Fuand Chinese boxe.

BOXING combat sport with two fighters of similar weight exchanging blows with their fists during one or three-minute rounds. The knockout or KO is obtained when the opponent is sent to the ground and is counted by the referee to 10, or if he is deemed too injured to continue (called technical knockout) or by the referee's decision the side ring judges' scores. There are many different styles of boxing around the world, THAI BOXING, BURMESE BOXE, FRENCH BOXE etc.

BUDO (Martial Arts) all martial arts practiced today have come down to us from ancient BUJUTSU (military techniques). Originally BUDO was strongly connected to the BUSHIDO, the ethical and philosophical life of the SAMURAI. The BUDO techniques comprehended not just hand combat techniques developed in case the SAMURAI would be separated from his weapons, but included the secrets of the bow, the sword, the javelin and horse riding. The BUJUTSU became more than just a practical way to neutralise the enemy, more a way of life. Martial arts became an art during the Edo-period, the first part of the 17th century when BUSHI (warriors) had plenty of time in their hands because of a long period of peace. BUJUTSU grew more theoretical borrowing from Zen Philosophy, Confucianism and Taoism. The age of the SAMURAI died with the advent of the Meiji period in 1868, when firearms became the weapon of choice. BUJUTSU found new fame with the modern wars, first against China (1894/95), Russia (1904/05) and the two World Wars. Especially KENDO and JUDO grew in popularity, together with the rise of nationalism, the glorification of physical strength, courage and honour. After Japan's defeat in World War II the allies tried to prohibit the practice of martial arts, but the spirit of BUDO resisted till today. In 1964 JUDO became an Olympic sport bringing new life to this sport around the world. SUMO, the most ancient of wrestling still remains strong with all its pomp and rituals.

BULLET-PROOF HOSTING A company that guarantees that its servers will not be shut down even when the request to do so comes from law enforcement agencies. These hosting companies are often located off-shore or in nations where computer crime laws are lax or non-existent and where extradition requests will not be honoured.

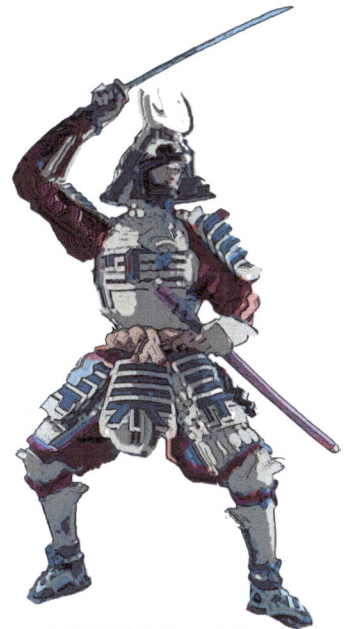

SAMURAI followed the BUSHIDO code.

BUSHI In Japanese the expert warrior of martial arts who follows the honour code BUSHIDO.

BUTTERFLY KNIFE Short Chinese knife used in some Kung-Fu styles (wing chun and hung gar). The true name is 'both jum do'. The BALISONG is also called BUTTERFLY KNIFE, but has a different shape and the blade flick opens with a movement of the wrist.

CALECON Swiss wrestling which took its name from the short trousers the wrestlers wear. Matches last 6 minutes and are based on a grip on the opponent's trousers (one hand must always grip) and it is won throwing the opponent to the ground onto his shoulders, arms and back of the head.

CAPOEIRA fighting style originally from Angola, which found huge popularity in Brazil. Performed to music, it's a martial art disguising its highly technical kicks and punches as dance moves. It was disguised when the Spanish domination made it illegal as a combat form.

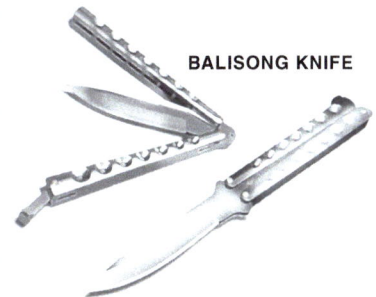

BALISONG KNIFE

CARDER Someone who steals or trades exclusively in stolen credit card numbers and their associated information.

CASH-OUT An euphemism that means to steal money from a bank account or credit card to which someone has gained illegal access. Hackers who grab credit card data often do not possess the skills or contacts to launder the money they can steal this way.

CAT STANCE Used in some Karate and Kung-Fu styles. The weight of the body is all on the one leg making the practitioner look like a cat ready to jump.

CATCH or CATCH-AS-CATCH-CAN USA originated but derived from Indian wrestling or from a type of wrestling from Lancashire (UK). The winner throws the opponent to the ground on his shoulders holding him there till the referee whistles, or making him surrender with a painful hold.

It became famous when Primo Carnera, the Italian boxing champion, started practicing it after losing his world title.

CENTRAL LINE Fundamental theory of WING CHUN KUNG FU: it's the line that crosses the body in the middle where all the vital energy concentrates and must be protected at all cost.

CH'AN or CHAN Chinese word for Zen (meditation). In India is called Dhyana.

CH'AN or CHAN Chinese word for Zen (meditation). In India is called Dhyana.

CH'IN-NA It is a Chinese martial art which uses seizing and immobilising, a type of fighting technique that demands sophisticated anatomy studies.

CHANG SAN-FENG Mithical thaoist philosopher who would have founded TAI CHI CHUAN.

CHANG-HON YU Taekwondo School created by Choi Hong Hi (which means small blue house).

CHI SAO Exercises in Wing Chun Kung-Fu in order to develop coordination in the arms.

CHI The inner energy that can be activated with breathing exercises known as Chi Kung, or Gung, to achieve good health and physical form. It is the base of the practice of TAI - CHI and Hsing-i.

CHIEN or CHEN The most ancient form of Tai Chi Chuan encompassing 108 positions, original of the Chinese village of Chien.

CHOY LI FUT Southern style Chinese boxe, descending from the system of the Shaolin temple and created in 1836 by Chan Heung.

CHRONIC As opposed to acute, a chronic condition is prolonged, or slow to heal.

CHUAN FA Chinese term that means "way of the fist". It is the modern correct way of describing what is normally designated as KUNG FU.

CHUDAN In Japanese martial arts it is the median part of the body or thorax, In Karate it is one of the three main points considered the main target of the body.

CHUNIN The intermediate man. One of the three degrees of the Ninjutsu.

CIRCULATORY SYSTEM The system providing blood to the body. It includes the heart, arteries, arterioles, capillaries, veins, blood, plasma, and lymphatic vessels and fluid.

COMPRESSION Act of pressing or squeezing together, important in pressure point action.

COOKIES are pieces of information generated by a Web server and stored in the user's computer, ready for future access. Cookies are embedded in the HTML information flowing back and forth between the user's computer and the servers. Cookies were implemented to allow user-side customisation of Web information. For example, cookies are used to personalise web search engines, to allow users to participate in WWW-wide contests (but only once!), and to store shopping lists of items a user has selected while browsing through a virtual shopping mall.

CRANE One of the five animals of Shaolin style in Kung-Fu as well as a well known Kung-Fu stance.

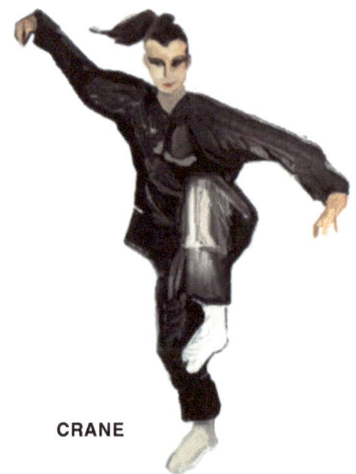

CRANE

CROSS-SITE SCRIPTING This is a sophisticated phishing attack that exploits weaknesses in the legitimate websites of financial institutions in order to trick people into handing over confidential details. A successful use of Cross-site scripting will make it look like all the transactions are being done on the website of the real bank or financial institution.

DAISENSEI Great master, title only given it to high level masters.

DAISHO The Japanese long and short sabres carried together by Samurai in the era Tokugawa.

DAITI RYU Style of Aiki Jutsu from which Aikido was developed from.

DAITO Japanese sword more than 60 cm long, used mostly by Samurai.

DAN Japanese term in order to indicate who has a black belt.

DDoS Stands for Distributed Denial of Service. This is an attack in which thousands of separate computers, usually part of a botnet, bombard a target with bogus data to knock it off the net. DDoS attacks have been used by extortionists who threaten to knock a site offline unless a hefty ransom is paid.

DEAD-DROP A hijacked PC or server used to store personal data stolen by key loggers, spy-ware

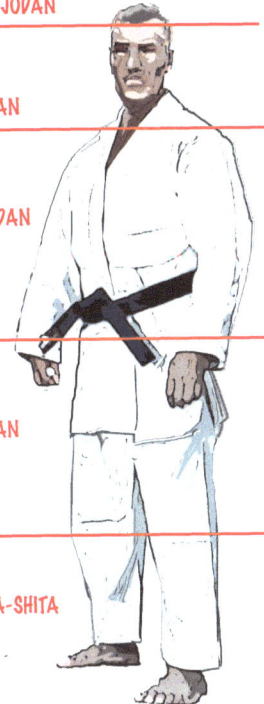

DAI-JODAN

JODAN

CHUDAN

GEDAN

HIZA-SHITA

or viruses. Criminal hackers prefer to keep their distance from this data as its possession is incriminating. Dead drops are often found and shut down in few days of the associated phishing e-mails being sent out.

DEHYDRATION Depletion of body fluids, to the point of illness.

DIM MAK The legendary deadly single strike to the famous meridians known in acupuncture on which a blow performed by a great master could provoke death hours or even days later.

DISLOCATION Displacement of bones at a joint.

DISPLACEMENT is to move a limb (eg shoulder) out of its normal position.

DIT DA JOW Ointment made of plant extracts and other secret substances preventing lesions during training in martial arts.

DO Japanese word for way or path, the end component of words like Kendo, Judo and Aikido.

DOJO This is a training hall in which one practices Japanese martial arts.

DOSHIN-SO Founder of Japanese religious schism and SHORINJI KEMPO.

DRAGON One of five styles of Shaolin KUNG FU, symbolizes the spirit.

DRIVE-BY DOWNLOAD Malicious programs that automatically install when a potential victim visits a booby-trapped website. The majority exploit vulnerabilities in main internet browser. Sometimes it is obvious that a drive-by download has occurred as they can replace bookmarks and start pages or install unwanted toolbars.Increasingly cyber criminals are using them to install key loggers that steal login and password information.

DRUNKEN MONKEY Style of KUNG FU based on the behaviour of a drunken monkey.The style is to wave around the opponent to provoke a wrong movement that will create an opportunity for a strike.

EDEMA A condition where fluid accumulates in spaces between cells, swelling tissues.

ELBOW STRIKES Technique found in many martial arts, especially MUAY THAI Thailandese.

ESCRIMA martial arts from Philippines mixing staff and hand combat. It was originally disguised as stage plays, linked to ARNIS DE MANO (from the Spanish word for fencing).

EXPLOIT Vulnerability in software that malicious hackers use to compromise a computer or network. Exploit code is the snippet of programming that does the work of penetrating via this loophole.

FIREWALL Program or feature built into hardware that sits between a computer and the internet to filter incoming and outbound traffic stopping net-borne attacks such as worms reaching your PC.

FIVE ANCESTORS refers to the five survivors of the pillage of the Shaolin temple, who allegedly funded the triads.

FIVE ANIMALS These are the animal movements of crane, dragon, leopard, tiger and snake which inspired the Shaolin KUNG FU system.

FLOS DUELLATORUM Ancient Italian study (1409) by Fiori Dei Liberi, a famous fencing master who wrote a lot on how to defend yourself if you lose your sword in a fight. It is interesting to see that some of the techniques in the original drawings show a FIGURE FOUR LOCK.

FOCUS PADS also called target pad, are flat or curved, hand-held pads that are about 12 inches in diameter. They are made of dense foam covered in leather or vinyl. They are used in boxing and martial arts training to improve speed and accuracy, as well as learning how to quickly adapt to a target change of direction. The pads are held at different ranges and angles.

FORMS These are a series of choreographic movements that unite different techniques from many martial arts. Also known as KATA in Japanese martial arts.

FRACTURE Any break in rigid body tissue, including bones, cartilage and teeth.

FOCUS PADS

FU JOW PAI Kung-Fu style meaning "tiger claw" developed in the Shaolin temple.

FULL CONTACT is a form of Karate in which all strikes are performed with full force against an adequately padded opponent.

GEDAN Body's area from the belt down in Japanese martial arts (see also CHUDAN).

GENIN Lowest degree in the NINJA hierarchy, operating in the field executing assassinations.

GI Uniform worn in Japanese martial arts. In Karate it is called Karate-gi, in Judo, Judo-gi.

GICHIN FUNAKOSHI Founder of Shotokan who introduced Karate in 1922 in Okinawa.

GLIMA original combat style from Iceland similar to the Swiss CALECON. The winner is the one that makes the opponent touch the ground with any part of the body. In 1908 London Olympic Games there was a famous exhibition of this wrestling style.

GOJU KAI A branch of Goju Ryu Karate founded by Gogen Yamaguchi, called "the cat", he was a student with the great master Miyagi.

GOJU RYU One of the more important styles of Karate from the style Naha Te from Okinawa.

GULAT A type of combat created in Giava derived from SUMO.

GUNG FU Cantonese pronunciation for KUNG FU.

GURU Term of Indian origin to indicate the master in some martial arts. In Japanese it is SENSEI.

GYOJI The referee in SUMO wrestling.

HACHIDAN This is the Eighth degree dan black belt. In the martial artsit indicates one of the highest grades. Sensei Bruno Carmeni is one of the few westerners to have achieved that in Judo.

HADAN Term of Taekwondo to indicate the zone under the belt. In Japanese GEDAN.

HAKAMA It means skirt-pantaloon. It covers legs and feet and it is used in AIKIDO, KENDO and other Japanese martial arts. It is useful in order to hide from the opponent the leg movements, adding an element of surprise to most attacks.

HAN Disciple of Bhudda and name of the first techniques taught by Bodhidharma to Shaolin monks

HAPKIDO (Way of coordinated power) martial art from Korea mixing punching, kicking, blocks and throws. Very popular in the US police forces, similar to Aikido.

HARIMAU The style of the tiger in the PENTJAK-SILAT.

HEIAN The name of the five basic kata in Karate. In some schools are called PINAN kata.

HEMATOMA Internal bleeding produced by a broken blood vessel causing a dome under the skin.

HO JUTSU The art of the SAMURAI firing weapons.

HOJO-JUTSU The Japanese art of binding or rope tying. A somewhat complicated method used by the samurai in order to tie up prisoners.

HONEYPOT An individual computer or a network of machines set up to look like a poorly protected system but which records every attempt to compromise it. Often the first hints of a new rash of malicious programs come from the evidence collected by honeypots. Now cyber criminals are tuning their malware to spot when it has compromised a honeypot and to leave without taking over.

HOP GAR Style of Kung-Fu fashionable in the age of the Ching dynasty in China; it was used from Manchui emperors and their guards. There were two styles, white crane and low horn. This is also known as "blade Kung-Fu".

HORSE STANCE Popular starting position in many martial arts, in particular in the Chinese Hung Gar and the Japanese Karate (called KIBA DACHI).

HSING I A Chinese martial art created from the great warrior Yueh Fei, based on the five elements in nature and sometimes it indicates a type of boxe.

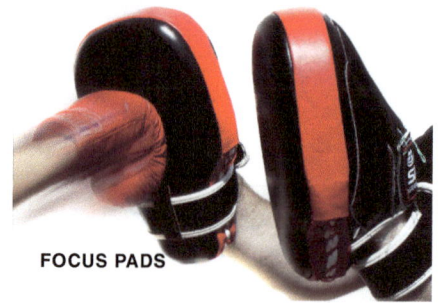

HSING-I CHUAN (mind's form) martial art from China using techniques borrowed from the movement of the bear, eagle, falcon, cock, dragon, horse, swallow, monkey, tiger, turtle and snake. It relies heavily on fancy footwork.

HUNG GAR From the name of its creator called HUNG (GAR meaning family) popular style of KUNG FU based on the movement of the tiger and privileges low stances, like the "sei ping ma" horse stance, and powerful hand techniques, such as the bridge hand and the tiger claw.

HWARANG DO A martial art from Korea mixing ancient techniques proper of the Samurai. It is still practiced in some part of the United States.

HYPERXTENSION When the angle between bones of a joint is greater than normal, common in KICKBOXING when kicking.

HYUNG kicking, punching, and blocking combinations in TAEKWONDO. Equivalent to KATA.

AI JUTSU A martial art from which derived the IAI DO, the art to extract and put away the sword in the fastest way during battle.

IAI DO (Way of Simultaneous Actions) Martial arts from Japan, similar to KENDO, where the emphasis is on extracting your sword and simultaneously killing your enemy with one move. Its techniques cover striking from any position, including lying down.

IGA Remote Japanese mountainous zone where the NINJA lived.

INFLAMMATION A reaction to injury that may include redness, heat and swelling.

IP ADDRESS The numerical identifier that every machine attached to the internet needs, to ensure that the data it requests returns to the right place. IP stands for Internet Protocol.

IRC An abbreviation for Internet Relay Chat - one of the net's hugely popular text chat systems. this technology is also used by botnet herders to keep tabs on and control their flock of machines.

JEET KUN DO Style of Kung-Fu invented and developed by Bruce Lee

JODAN In Japanese martial arts the high part of the body over the shoulders. See also CHUDAN.

JODO (Way of the Staff) Martial art from Japan using a staff about 1 metre long. Like the IAIDO it's also related to Kendo.

JONIN A high ranking NINJA of great experience and skill.

JUDO (The Gentle Way) Martial art from Japan developed by Jigoro Kano from JUJUTSU. It relies on throwing, sweeping, strangling and similar techniques, often using the laws of physics and the attacker's momentum against him. If practiced properly it does not need a lot of strength. Kano summarized this principle as "SEYRYOKU ZEN YO" (efficient use of energy). Contrary to JUJUTSU, JUDO places more emphasis on RANDORI (free style fighting) than KATA (fixed exercises) making training more dynamic.

JUDOKA Who practices Judo.

JUJUTSU (The Gentle Skill) Martial art from Japan using throws, locks, sweeps as well as striking techniques and weapon handling. It borrowed techniques from Chinese martial arts as well as fighting techniques developed by the people of Okinawa, where generally martial arts were developed. Around 1870 an edict from the Emperor forbid all Samurais to carry weapons, and this increased the popularity of martial arts favouring empty-handed techniques.

JUKEN DO The way of the bayonet: martial art fought with a bayonet mounted rifle, similar to the combat style developed with spears or sticks.

JUTSO or JITSU In Japanese ability or art.

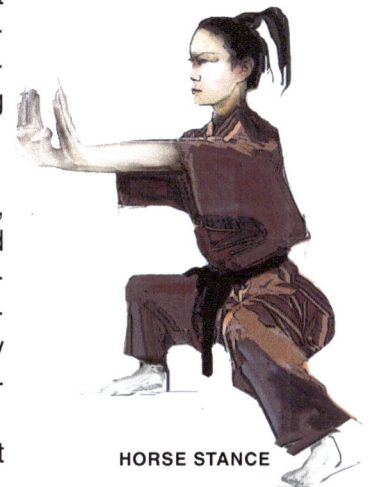

HORSE STANCE

JUTTE or JITTE Thin iron stick with grip and a side hook used to block strikes. It was used by soldiers with police duties (called a Doshin) in Japan during the Edo period.

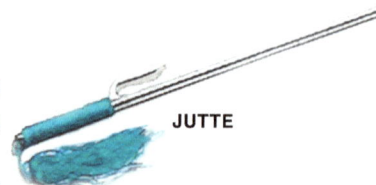

KALARAPYIT and many similar way of spelling it is a very ancient martial art from India that encompasses various empty hand strikes as well as weapon work.

KALI martial art from the Philippines similar to ARNIS DE MANO, made up of twelve disciplines.

KAMA Ancient Okinawa agricultural instrument similar to a sickle.

KARAKUSAK see KIRKPINAR

KARATE (Art of the empty hand) a martial art from Japan relying on punching, kicking and blocking. It is one of the most popular martial arts worldwide. Funakoshi Gichin made Karate popular at the beginning of 1900, modernizing it and making it available to the public, creating his own style called Shotokan (Shoto was his nickname and Kan means institution or school). Among the styles developed over the years by other people, presently more than fifty in Japan alone, are GOJURYU, WADORYU and SHUKOKKAI.

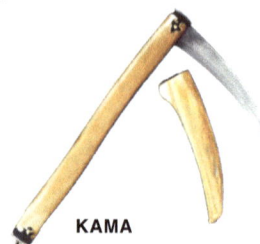

KARATEKA Karate practitioner.

KATA is a series of movements in which the Martial Artist defends himself from an imaginary enemy.

KATANA The Japanese sword.

KEMPO or KENPO is the Japanese translation of the Chinese term "quanfa". Under this name there are several different martial arts, mostly resembling KARATE and THAI BOXING.

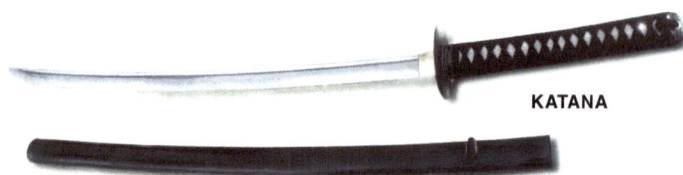

KENDO (Way of the Sword) martial art originating from Japan where opponents using a SHINAI, a sword made out of bamboo, fight each other, protected by the DOGU a body armour including the MEN, the traditional face mask with grills.

KENJUTSU martial art that originated KENDO, originally developed by BUSHI and made popular by Samurais. It became KENDO thanks to SAKAKIBARA KENKICHI.

KENPO originally from China, developed by the military for self-defence using thrusts and blows with fist or open hand (chopper). The body is kept relaxed and fluid.

KEY LOGGER Program or hardware installed on a computer that records every keystroke that a user makes, for stealing login and password details. However, the data that is stolen often has to be heavily processed to make it intelligible and to extract names and numbers.

KI It means energy, living power, spirit, the vital energy.

KIAI The loud outcry that accompanies an attack in Japanese martial arts in order to increase the energy and confuse the opponent.

KICKBOXING Probably invented by Japanese BOXING promoter Osamu Noguchi for a variant of MUAI THAI and KARATE he created in 1950. There are several styles today and it does combine punches and kicks, often quite spectacularly, with sweeps. Knee and elbow strikes are not allowed in competition, but are practiced in training.

KIHON (fundamentals) Normally refers to the basic techniques that are the foundation of most Japanese martial arts.

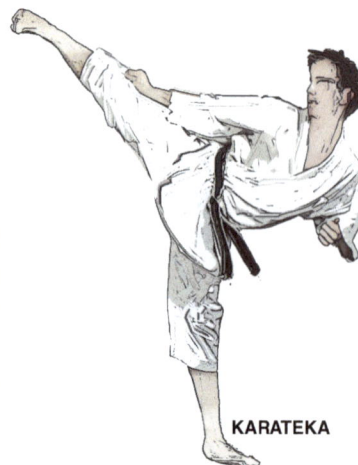

JUTTE

KAMA

KATANA

KARATEKA

KIRKPINAR (Forty Springs) originally from Turkey, it was originally a celebration during funeral rites, and since 1360 it takes place in the city of Edirne, the wrestlers have their body smeared with oil and wear strong trousers called Kispet made out of buffalo skin. It's based on strength more than agility and it's very tough. There is also a version without oil called KARAKUSAK.

KOBUDO (old martial way) martial art form originating from Okinawa organizing all the weapons handling systems.

KUBOTAN Close-quarter self-defence tool that fits onto your palm. It can be used as a pressure point and pain compliance instrument. It comes with a flat or point tip, normally made of aluminium and a ring to be used as a keying everyday. It is illegal in the UK and many other countries. Always check your local laws before purchasing any self-defence tool.

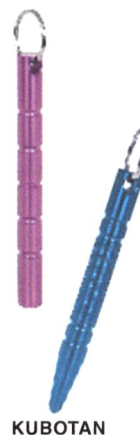

KUBOTAN

KRABI KABBONG Thailand combat art using two short and extremely sharp swords.

KRAV MAGA (contact fight) developed by grandmaster Imi Sde-Or (Lichtenfeld) for the Israel Defence Force, combining several techniques focusing on simplicity and speed. Quite effective against armed attacks, it does require a good level of general fitness.

KUMITE A Japanese term indicating generic sparring in Japanese martial arts.

KUNG-FU (Human Effort) martial art from China combining a range of styles, including weapons and developed by the Shaolin monks in the Shaolin-Temple in North-China. It was Bodhidharma, a Buddhist teacher from India, who approximately. in the 5th century arrived in the temple and turned the monks' discipline into a proper fighting style. Kung-Fu can be divided in 5 main styles, all based on movements borrowed from different animals. The HUNG GAR (adapted from the Tiger style of Shaolins) is the most adapt foe hand combat, with its low stance and powerful leg work combined with long reaching hand strikes. KUNG FU was made famous by Bruce Lee whose master Yip Man who was teaching Win-Chun (Bright Spring).

KUP One of the eight degrees of the Taekwondo, comparable to the Kyu in Japanese martial Arts.

KUSARIGAMA Weapon in the shape of a small shear joined to a long chain with a weight to the other extremity. Used mostly by NINJAs.

KYOKOSHINKAI (the way of the last truth) founded by Korean Masatatsu Oyama who used to fight bulls with bare hands and achieved the record of the highest number of broken roof tiles with a single blow.

KYUDO (Way of the Bow) originated in Japan, originally known as KYUJUTSU applied both in battle and hunting. The bow is very long, more than 2 metres and so is the arrow, and great emphasis is put into the spiritual training.

LATHI or LATHE Indian technique of combat with a stick.

LIGAMENT A tough cord of tissue that connects bone to bone or cartilage to bone. Torn ligaments are a common injury when kicking.

LUMBAR The lower back region.

MAKIWARA A tapered wood beam embedded in the ground and rising to about chest height with straw, rope, or leather wrapped around the top of the board. It is used by Karate practitioners to toughen hands and feet through repetitively striking the board. There is also another type solid to the wall.

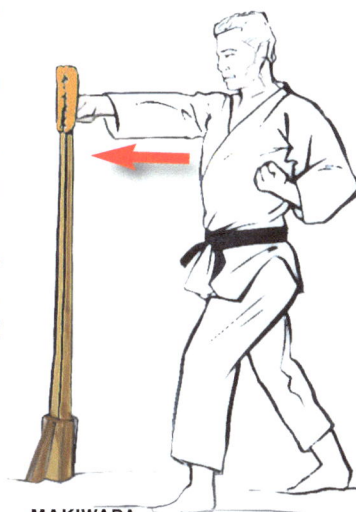

MAKIWARA

MAL-WARE Portmanteau term for all malicious software or any unwanted program which makes its way on to a computer. The word is derived from Mal(icious soft)ware.

MAN-IN-THE-MIDDLE A sophisticated attack in which a criminal hacker intercepts traffic sent between a victim's computer and the website of the organisation, usually a financial institution,that they are using. Used to lend credibility to attacks or simply steal information on online accounts.

MANRIKIGUSARI (=strength of thousand men) A metal chain approximately 3 feet in length with both ends terminating in a heavy metal tip or handle, used by the SAMURAI. The techniques encompass some fancy moves, darting out the tips in a thrust or swinging it in different directions. It can be quite lethal.

MEN The face guard in KENDO.

MOO DUK KWAN Korean term for Academy of martial arts.

MOON JOONG Wooden mannequin of human form for training in Kung-Fu.

MUAY THAI Correct name for THAI BOXE.

NAGINATA (halberd) originally from Japan, it was a martial art practiced mostly by women for self-defence and by children of the SAMURAI to learn the fundamentals of weapon work. It employs a long halberd made of wood, normally oak, with a curved bamboo-blade on one end. The total length is over 2m long. The blade can be used to cut, slice sideways and to deflect blows. The butt-end lends itself to thrusts, strikes and parrying.

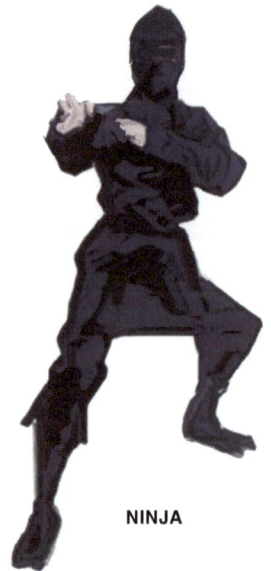

NINJA

NINJA A secret society in Japan that trained adepts and practitioners in the art of assassination and espionage (see NINJUTSU).

NINJUTSU (the Art of Invisibility) originated in Japan where Ninjas formed a special social class of their own in some areas. These mythical figures were in reality expert assassins, skilled in different weapons like the famous SHURIKEN (blade hidden in hand, normally star-shaped) as well as experts in poisons and drugs. Their skills reached such perfection that people started believing they could be invisible and capable of walkng on ceilings. The term NINJUTSU is also used to describe the arts and techniques of the ninja; originally NINJAS were called SHINOBI (=invisible, stealthy).

NUNCHAKU Is shown in fig.287. For more see RYUKYU KOBUJUTSU.

PA KUA Style of Kung-Fu based on circular motions with blows performed open palm. It is also known as "boxe with the palm in eight directions".

PACKET SNIFFING This is the practice of examining the individual packages of data received by a computer to find out more about what the machine is being used for. Often login names and passwords are sent in plain text within data packets and can easily be extracted.

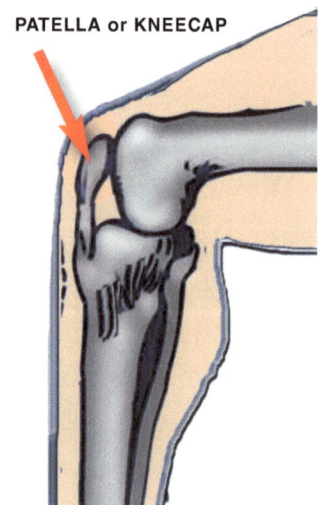

PATELLA or KNEECAP

PAKUA (the Eight Hexagrams) originated in China and mostly consisting in a sudden change of direction while performing palm-strikes and evasion techniques, resembling Kung-Fu.

PATELLA (of the knee) knee cap or kneepan, is a bone articulating with the femur and covering the knee joint. It is responsible for the extension of the knee, being attached to the tendon of the quadriceps femoral muscle and the vastus intermedialis muscle. Quite prone to breaking when falling frontally.

PENCHAK-SILAT (Lightening Combat) originating from Indonesia and Malaysia, combining striking techniques, weapons and groundwork. Heavily ritualistic it often resembles a choreographed dance with sweeps and elbow strikes.

PHARMING Similar in nature to e-mail phishing, pharming seeks to obtain personal or private (usually financial related) information through domain spoofing. Rather than being spammed with malicious and mischievous e-mail requests for you to visit spoof Web sites which appear legitimate, pharming 'poisons' a DNS server by infusing false information into the DNS server, resulting in a user's request being redirected elsewhere. Your browser however will show you are at the correct web site, which makes pharming a bit more serious and more difficult to detect.

Phishing attempts to scam people one at a time with an e-mail while pharming allows the scammers to target large groups of people at one time through domain spoofing.

PHISHING attacks using email or malicious web sites to solicit personal, often financial, information. Attackers may send an email seemingly from a reputable credit card company or financial institution which requests account information, often suggesting that there is a problem. When users respond with the requested information they are tricked into handing over confidential details.

PRAYING MANTIS Kung-Fu Style from China, invented by Wang Lang observing two mantis fighting each other over food. Also called "The Gates of Praying Mantis" (Tang Lang Men).

PORT The virtual door that net-capable programs open to identify where the data they request from the net should be directed once it reaches a computer. Web browsing traffic typically passes through port 80, e-mail through port 25.

RANDORI multiple-person attacks in martial arts training.

ROKUSHAKU BO Long stick (6 feet) used in Martial Arts originated from Okinawa (Roku = the number six, shaku = foot measure, bo = stick)

RONIN see SAMURAI

ROOTS This is a slang term for networks that have been hacked into by criminal hackers. It derives from the type of (root), access that system administrators typically use on a network or computer. The login details to get root access are often sold to spammers and phishing gangs who then use these networks to send out millions of e-mail messages.

RUPTURE Tearing apart of a tissue.

RYU In Japanese it indicates school or style.

RYUKYU KOBUJUTSU (the Art of Weapons) originated in the island of Okinawa/Japan and is a system combining farmers' tools like the handle of a millstone to grind rice called

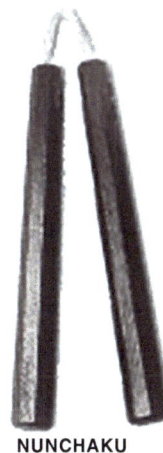

NUNCHAKU

TONFA and the NUNCHAKU, originally a tool to beat rice and corn or an instrument carried by the village night watch, made of two blocks of wood joined by cord. Hitting the wood together would alert villagers about fires and other dangers. The TONFA has become in our days the weapon of choice of many police forces and it consists of a heavy wooden staff, about half a metre long with a handle fixed at 90º three quarters up. The NUNCHAKU (as pictured in photo 287) consists of two wooden sticks, octagonal or cylindrical about 30cm long, linked by a rope or a chain. Other weapons are the SAI, a forked dagger, the KAMA, a sickle with a long handle, the EKKU, a wooden oar, the TIMBE and ROSHIN, a small shield and a short spear, the TAKKO, resembling a knuckle duster and the BO, a long staff.

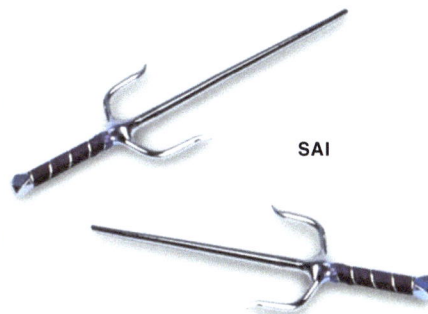

SAI

SAI Short iron fork with two curved prongs (called yoku) extruding from the handle and a straight longer one in the middle that, contrary to what most people believe, is not a blade.

SAMBO (SAMozashchita Bez Oruzhiya) = "defence without weapons", Russian Special Forces combat system born in 1923, merging Judo and Karate and wrestling styles. Emphasis is given to strangling and lethal strikes. There is an even more lethal secret style simply called the SYSTEM.

SAMURAI Japanese warrior, in the Bushi era; the samurai without a lord to serve was called RONIN.

SANCHIN Exercise of 20 respiration movements used in the Okinawa KARATE.

SAVATE or BOX FRANCAISE developed in France by Michel Casseux in the early 1800s in Paris; it resembles a combination of boxing and Karate.

SCRIPT KIDDIE An unskilled hacker who steals code, techniques and attack methods from others. Many viruses and worms on the web today are simply patched together from other bits of code that malicious hackers share.

SENSEI In Japanese it means master or instructor.

SHAKEN Chinese name for SHURIKEN.

SHAOLIN Place of birth of Kung-Fu in the Songshan mountains of North China.

SHIAI It is a Japanese term for "contest", used mostly in Kendo.

SHINAI Blade made up of four stripes of bamboo replacing a steel blade in Kendo.

SHINOBI Ancient name for NINJA; it means invisible, stealthy.

SHORINJI KENPO (Boxing of the SHAOLIN) born quite recently in Japan and resembling a mix of JUJUTSU, KARATE and AIKIDO. It is regarded and registered as a religion but obviously it is in its physical aspects a martial art.

SHOTOKAN Karate style, amongst the most diffused in the world and founded by Gichin Funakoshi.

SHUAI CHIAO One of the first combat methods of ancient China, 1300 years old; it is still an official sport in China.

SHURIKEN (hand hidden sword) Japanese concealed weapon also known as death stars, made out of metal they were used as an additional weapon to the KATANA. Legend makes it the Ninjas favourite weapon. They can have many shapes, from a simple small spear (a long nail), cross shaped or as an elaborate star. They have become collector's items, and are illegal in many countries.

SIFU Chinese instructor of Kung-Fu (means father) corresponding to the Japanese SENSEI.

SIKARAN Martial art from the island of Luzon in the Philippines with prevailing use of legs strikes.

SIL LIM TAO First module in WING CHUN, about elbows position and protection of the body's centre.

SIL LUM Cantonese name of Shaolin temple.

SIU TIN LUNG also known as Tziu Huo Long, meaning Celestial Fire Dragon, is a rare style of Kung-Fu original of the Emei Mount (centre-south of China). Created originally in the XV century, it is characterised by fluid and circular movements focusing on contact sensitivity. Currently it is practiced only in Italy and Peru.

SO JUTSU The Japanese art of handling the spear in combat.

SOFT TISSUES All tissues in the body except bone.

SPIM Spam that is sent over Instant Messaging. Like spam, spam can contain worms, viruses and other malicious code.

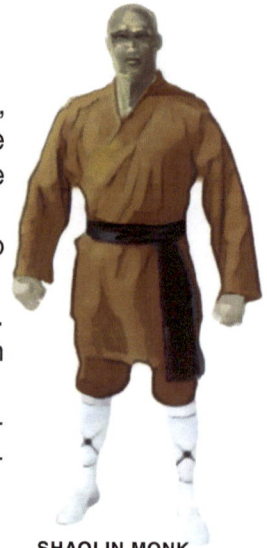

SHAOLIN MONK

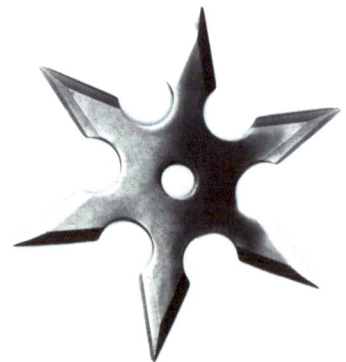

SHURIKEN, star shaped.

SPLINT Any rigid material meant to immobilise a damaged part of the body.

SPOOFING An unauthorised use of legitimate identification and authentication data, however obtained, to mimic a subject different from the attacker. Impersonating, masquerading, piggybacking, and mimicking are forms of spoofing.

SPRAIN Any injury where fibres of a ligament are stretched or torn.

SPYWARE Any software using someone's Internet connection in the background without their knowledge or explicit permission. Spy-ware applications are typically bundled as a hidden component of freeware or shareware programs that can be downloaded from the Internet; however, it should be noted that the majority of shareware and freeware applications do not come with spy-ware. Once installed, the spy-ware monitors user activity on the Internet and transmits that information in the background to someone else. Spy-ware can also gather information about e-mail addresses and even passwords and credit card numbers.

STEEL PALM This is a lethal technique in Kung-Fu in order to kill with a single blow.
The hand and the forearm are trained for years in order to become hard like steel.

STRAIN Any injury where a muscle or tendon is stretched or torn.

STUN GUN also known as TASERS (brand name) is a mechanical device that gives an electroshock incapacitating the receiver. They are used by Police as a less lethal weapon. It is a controversial weapon because it is allegedly used as a torture device in some countries.

SUMO It is an ancient Japanese wrestling art. Two opponents wearing only loincloths have only their bare hands to knock or push their opponent over. Being large and heavy is a distinct advantage but a smaller wrestler's perfect technique can win against an opponent double the size. Even if the wrestlers are often huge they are extremely agile and have lightning reflexes. SUMO wrestlers reach star status if winning, and they are highly respected in Japan.

SUN TZU or TSU is the Author of the Art of the War on which he based the NINJUTSU.

SWEEP Technique designed to make the opponent lose his balance, normally using your foot. Sweeps are very useful against bigger opponents using their momentum.

TAEKWONDO originating from Korea, it was developed by general CHOI HONG HI, a keen practicant of the ancient Korean art TAE KYON. He mixed KARATE and TAE KYON and in the late 50s created the TAEK-WONDO, a martial art that relies heavily on high kicks and very tough training in repeatedly hitting targets really hard.

TAI CHI CHUAN ("Supreme art of combat") Ancient Chinese martial art based on the Taoist concept of YING YANG, the eternal alliance of opposites. Born as self-defence system has transformed over the centuries in a refined form of exercise for health and welfare even though some schools continue to teach and exercise as real defence system. The practice of Tai Chi Chuan consists mainly of a series of circular movements reminiscent of a silent dance, but in fact mimic the fight with an imaginary opponent.

TAI CHI CHUAN practitioner

There are different styles of Tai Chi Chuan, the most popular are Yang and Chen.
The first is the most practiced, Chen requires much more complex and difficult exercise. In addition to the concept of Yin and Yang, the expression that describes this technique is the concept of "Form", a system of linked movements that are performed in a slow, uniform and seamless way.

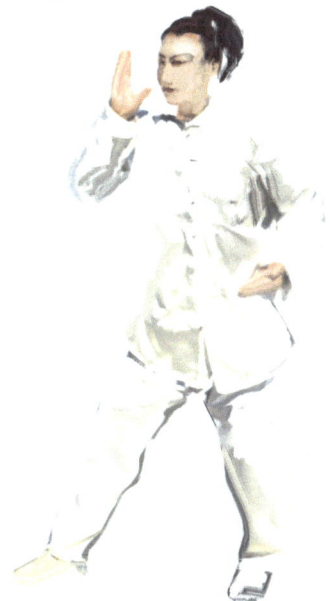

These movements can be performed with bare hands or with the support of weapons. There is also a set of exercises that are performed in pairs and are called TUI SHOUS. The study of Tai Chi Chuan should start with the sequence of movements called "slow form``". Gradually you learn to relax the mind, moving the body in a relaxed and controlled way, regulating your breathing. The careful and constant practice of these techniques due to their softness, the roundness and the slowness, with which they are executed, makes the body more supple and harmonious, improves posture and has a beneficial effect on the nervous system and blood circulation.

TAI WHO CHUAN One of the three styles of Kung-Fu based on the extreme fluidity of extremely slowly executed movements.

TAMASHIWARI A Japanese technique using the body to hit different material such as wood or bricks. This is done to test the power of the strike. Highly successful in the West but not so popular in Asia.

The author performing TAMASHIWARI with bricks.

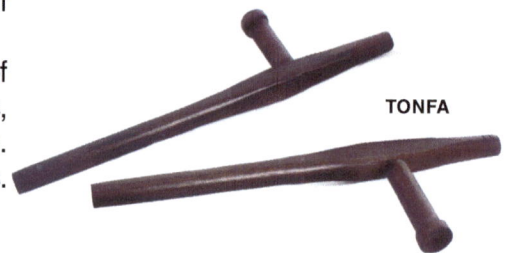

TANG SOO DO Korean martial art has techniques similar to Japanese shotokan Karate; created in 1949 by Hang Kee.

TCP Abbreviation for Transmission Control Protocol, indicating the series of specifications which define the format of data packets sent across the internet.

TENDON The cord of fibrous tissue connecting a muscle with another part (e.g. bone).

THAI BOXING combat sport originally from Thailand combining kicks, punches and elbow strikes. In the '30s the violence of THAI BOXING matches reached such an extreme (1 in 3 matches ended with the death of one of the contestants) that new regulations were introduced forbidding certain strikes like an elbow strike to the temple and to use regular gloves instead of the ones in use, made of hardened jute fabric with pieces of glass glued onto it.

THAING This is a term which groups different Martial arts of Burma, such as Bando (hand to hand) Banshay (using swords, staff and spears) Lethwei (similar to Boxing) Naban (wrestling).

TONFA

TOBOK Protective gear worn by TAEKWONDO practitioners.

TONFA see RYUKYU KOBUJUTSU

TRAUMA Any wound or injury to living tissue.

TROJAN This is a malicious or harmful code contained inside apparently harmless programs or data. The code is disguised as something pleasant to the recipient. The Trojan can get control and do its chosen form of damage, such as ruining the file allocation table on your hard disk. Many of the attachments on virus-bearing e-mail messages carry Trojans.

TUI SHOUS see TAI CHI CHUAN.

URUMI An Indian sword with four blades that can open suddenly.

VERTEBRAE The bony segments of the spinal column.

VIRUS A malicious program - usually one that requires action to successfully infect a victim. For instance - the malicious programs inside e-mail attachments usually only strike if the recipient opens them. Increasingly the word is used as a portmanteau term for all malicious programs - those that users must set off or those that find their own way around the net.

WADO RYU Derivative style from Shotokan Karate developed by Grand Master Hironori Ohtsuka.

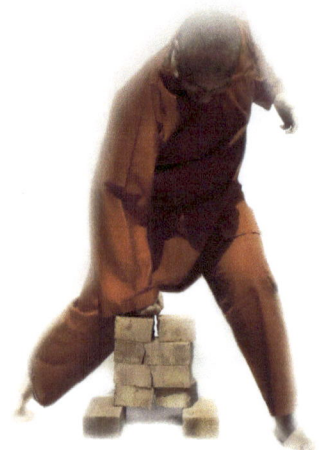

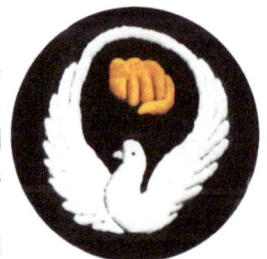

WADO RYU symbol

WHITE BELT In many Japanese martial arts it indicates the beginner.

WHITEHAT A hacker that uses his or her skills for positive ends and often to thwart malicious hackers. Many Whitehat security professionals spend their time looking for and closing the bugs in code that Blackhats are keen to exploit. See also BLACKHAT.

WING CHUN It means "beautiful spring". It is a Martial art from China created after a woman named Yim Wing Chun; considered it to be very effective, it has influenced Bruce Lee's JET-KUN-DO.

WORM Independent program that replicates from machine to machine across network connections often clogging networks and information systems as it spreads. It distinguishes itself from a virus that requires user action to compromise a machine. Worms can infect and take over computers without any help, just because the machine is not made secure.

YING YANG symbol.

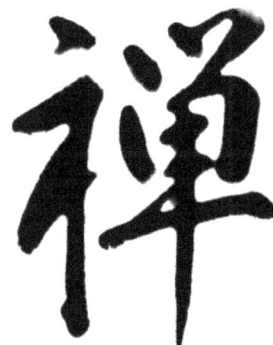

WU SHU Generally "military art", now the name for a highly acrobatic Chinese martial art.

YANG STYLE A style created by Yang Lu-ch'an, hired by the Chinese Imperial family to teach TAI CHI CHUAN to the elite Imperial Guards in 1850; it contains the 13 original positions of TAI CHI.

YARI Japanese spear with a straight blade that replaced the NAGINATA in battle.

YING YANG is a circular symbol divided in half each looking like a interlocking water drop., called Ying and Yang. Ying is white with a black dot and has the point of the tear pointing upwards. Yang is black with a white dot and the tear point aimed down. This juxtaposition symbolizes two sides of everything, the light and the dark, happiness and sadness, good and evil and so on. The Ying represents good/light/day, in other words all the positive energy and Yang is a symbol of all the negative energy. Ying, in a ying-yang symbol, is always on the left side.

They interlock meaning that one needs the other to exist.

YOKO ARUKI A way of walking practiced mostly by NINJA, keeping the body parallel to the plane of travel, crossing the legs and swinging the arms, designed to walk through tight spaces in the dark.

YOKOZUNA Highest rank achieved in Sumo wrestling.

ZANSHIN The state of calm and awareness of mind in Japanese martial arts, achieving control of self and total readiness.

ZEN (meditation) A school of Buddhism originally from China, specifically the Shaolin Temple, by the monk BODYDHARMA who developed a form of meditation to achieve enlightenment.

It enjoyed widespread diffusion, reaching Japan eventually.

ZERO DAY A Zero day vulnerability is one on which the code to exploit it appears on the first day that a loophole is announced. As most of the damage done by exploiting bugs occurs in the first few days after they become public, software firms usually move quickly to patch zero day vulnerabilities.

ZHURKANE This is a Persian term indicating a very ancient form of hand combat going back to the kingdom of Darius. Very similar to some type of wrestling it relies on strength and physical condition.

ZOMBIE Another name for a hijacked computer that is a member of a botnet.

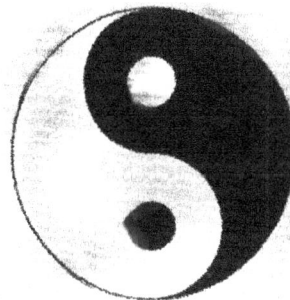

ZEN written in KANJI

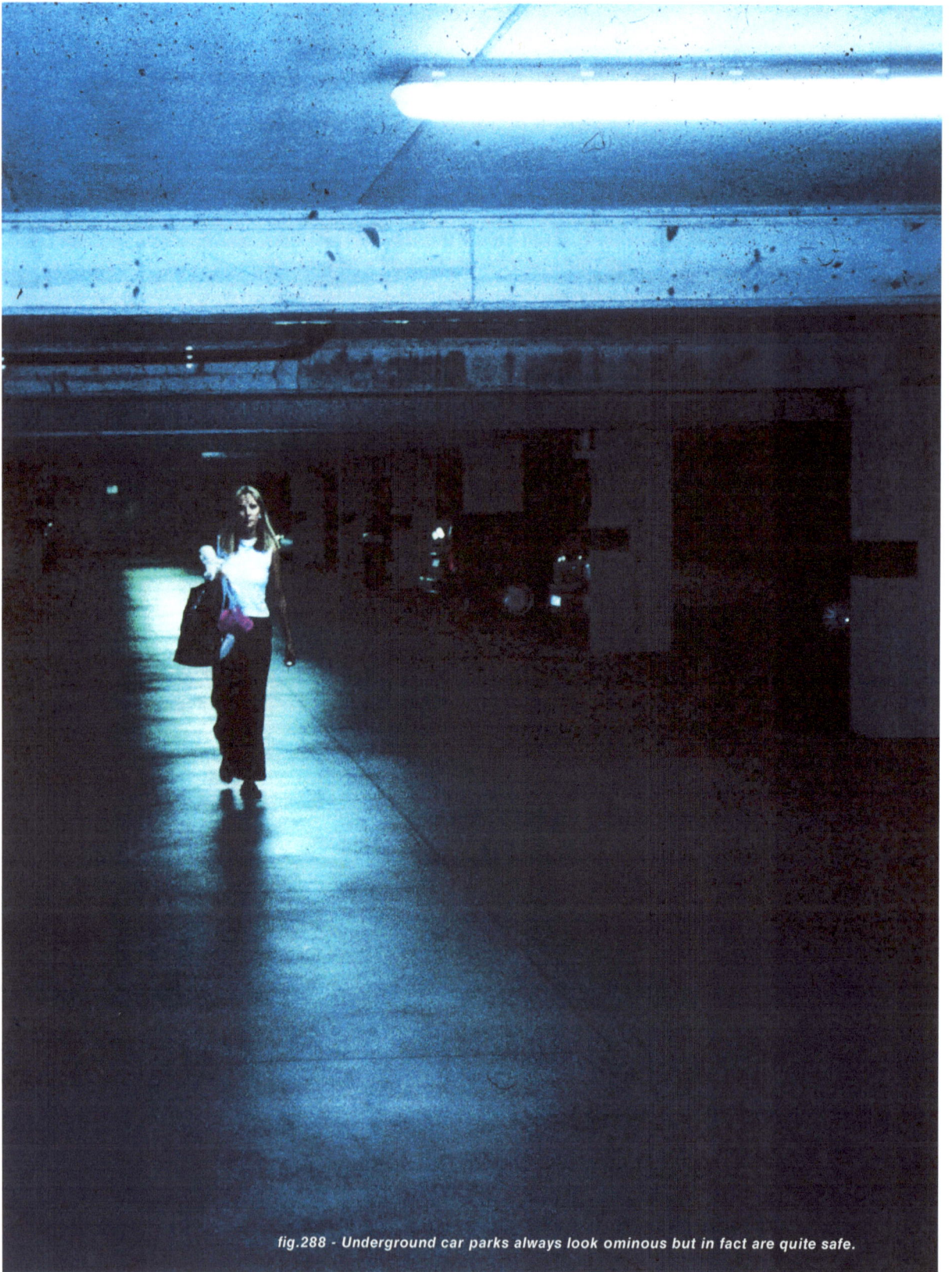

fig.288 - Underground car parks always look ominous but in fact are quite safe.

scenarios

What follows are simplified scenarios, a quick reference to what we discussed throughout the book. It is more important that you build a natural attitude to defend yourself more than trying to remember the scenario by rote and what to do.

Nevertheless it is easier to jog your memory going through particular situations that can occur and the course of action that can be taken when and "if" needed.

Obviously we are not implying that for instance taking a taxi is dangerous, or using an underground car park can get you into trouble, quite the opposite but normally during the practical courses that we hold these are the questions that a lot of attendees want answers to, both in an INDOOR and OUTDOOR situation. Obviously you can use techiques from one similar scenario and apply to another similar one. For instance if you are woken up by an intruder within your bedroom the same action applies if that happens in a hotel room.

AT HOME DAYTIME If you live/work on the ground/basement/first floor keep main doors and windows locked at all time. If you have to keep some windows open install grills or at least chain locks that allow you to leave the window partially open but does not allow easy entry.

If you hear someone breaking/entering while you are in, grab a phone and lock yourself in the nearest room. Call emergency services talking very loudly, making yourself heard. If this is not possible, grab whatever is within reach that can help in fending off an attacker, kitchen knife, baseball bat, and hairspray. Shout very loudly that you are armed and you have called the Police and he should leave. Remember that half of all home attacks happened after someone "conned" his way in with an excuse, such as that they have a delivery for you or informing you of a neighbour's, accident, utility reading, impersonating law enforcement or authority, etc. If you are meeting someone you don't know for whatever reason (prospective buyer, work colleague) make sure that they have the impression that someone should be home any moment.

You can even call your own number pre-dialling it on your mobile and pretending that someone has been delayed but is coming soon.

NIGHT TIME Make sure that all windows and doors are locked, including balconies or any other windows or doors even if they are on the top floor. Burglars can climb up a drainpipe/tree/nearby building and access your roof/balcony. Make certain to fit chain locks even to windows.

Keep a mobile/ phone next to your bed. If you are woken by an intruder make some noise and dial the emergency services. If it is possible to, lock yourself in the bedroom. If the telephone is out of reach or not in the room with you pretend you are calling the Police. If you are attacked and pinned onto the bed or on the floor see GROUNDWORK (page 82). If you are within a room see OBJECTS (page 132) . Remember if you are fighting to defend yourself within a room that you can maximise your strikes or pushes using the walls or furniture as leverage. (fig.63)

BUS or **COACH/TRAIN/TRAM/UNDERGROUND METRO** If the bus is really empty do not sit on the upper deck or at the back by yourself, but find a seat next to the driver. If you are not sure stand next to the driver if possible. Do not sit next to the windows, but near a corridor. Someone can easily sit next to you holding a knife and block your escape route. Choose seats that allow you to have as much visibility as possible should someone sit next to you. Choose to sit next to someone who you think might help you if needed. If you are threatened move

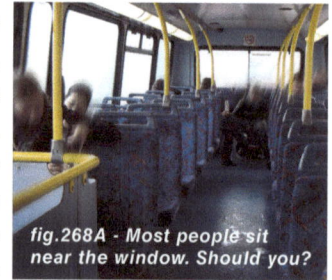
fig.268A - Most people sit near the window. Should you?

away towards the driver or start pressing the alarm/ring repeatedly. Always choose a coach/carriage containing as many people as possible. Most public transport vehicles have safety hammers/axes/extinguishers; use them if you fear for your own life. If necessary, push the attacker away using a seat/window/side of bus to push from. Do not intervene to tell someone off who is smoking or putting his feet on the seat. Let the authorities deal with that. It was all over the news about a woman who told off someone for smoking on a train platform and she was pushed onto the rail, barely surviving the fall on the high voltage line. Be wary as you walk down a deserted train corridor, especially at night, someone might just drag you into his compartment, in that case resist being dragged into it, pin yourself against a door frame, divider, grab the handle, but do not be dragged inside at any cost.

BOAT or **SHIP** If you are on board a large vessel such as a cruise ship, follow the same advice as per Hotel situation. Do not walk around by yourself especially at night on a big ship, especially on the lower decks or parts of the ship reserved for personnel. You need to familiarise yourself with the locations of escape routes. It is useful to try to locate alarms and fire extinguishers. If you are on a small vessel make sure

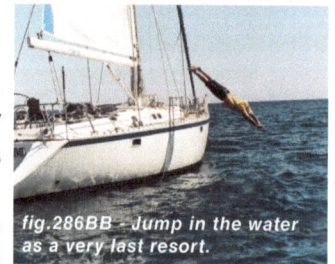
fig.286BB - Jump in the water as a very last resort.

that you know what you can use in case someone decides to have a go for you, on a boat there are plenty of tools that can turn into useful defensive weapons. Always locate where the fire extinguisher is, when mooring make the access to the boat more difficult. If attacked always try to go on to upper levels, bang repeatedly against the wall (they resonate loudly) scream and grab anything that can be used as weapon. Jump in the water as a very last resort if everything else fails. If mooring in the harbour with your own boat make access to the boat more difficult during the night. There are alarms and other devices on the market that can help to secure a boat from unwanted visitors.

HOTEL or **HOSTEL ROOM** If you can choose a room choose one in the middle of the corridor, not at the end of it, so that if something happens you can bang on either wall and people will hear you. If you cannot lock yourself in using the door key (do not trust electronic keys, someone can easily duplicate them) jam a chair against the door knob. The same goes if you are staying in a bungalow or similar accommodation, don't choose the most remote location unless you have someone able bodied with you. If someone enters while you are asleep see HOME – night time described previously. If you need to shout something, shout "FIRE" not "help". (See STRONG page 24).

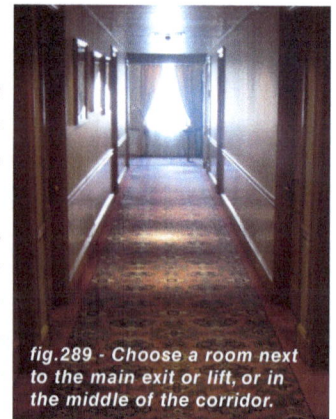
fig.289 - Choose a room next to the main exit or lift, or in the middle of the corridor.

As a norm try not to carry your key with the room number in view, or avoid asking for your key at reception loudly. Do not open the door unless absolutely sure of who is calling.

If you are walking down the corridor late at night and come across rowdy people or in any case someone who makes you feel uneasy, it is better to go back to a common area or reception and ask a member of staff to escort you to your room or just wait for a while before going back.

If you are attacked while in the corridor do shout, there are people behind the doors.

If necessary press the fire alarm or use the fire extinguisher, there are plenty of extinguishers about in any hotel. If you are attacked within a room trash everything within reach and make as much noise as possible, people will complain and someone from the hotel staff will come and check. If a phone is within reach take the receiver off and dial zero. Locate fire extinguishers and fire alarms. Don't forget that unfortunately a woman by herself at the hotel bar is sometimes mistaken for a prostitute since often hotels bars are fertile ground for them to pick up customers.

TAXI or HIRED DRIVER

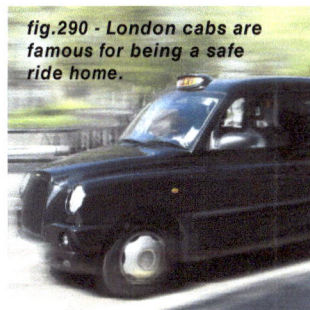

fig.290 - London cabs are famous for being a safe ride home.

If possible always choose a reputable authorised taxi service. Do not take a taxi that stops asking to take you anywhere even if it looks legitimate enough. Make sure someone knows that you travelling by taxi and with which company especially if coming back from a party at night. Sit BEHIND the driver, it makes it more difficult for him to threaten you or try to reach for you. Familiarise yourself with how the door opens. Hold your mobile phone in your hand. Remove expensive jewellery before entering the taxi (away from view).

Make sure that if you are talking on the phone you do not reveal any personal details, including your mobile number (you can always text it to the person asking on the phone. Do not assume the driver cannot listen to you or that he does not speak/understand your language even if he doesn't seem to. Do not give him your exact address; just close enough, even one or two door numbers different. Make sure he has disappeared from view before going to your door. Pretend you are looking for keys or go to neighbour's door. If a driver takes an unfamiliar route or you are sensing something odd ask him to go back urgently because you have forgotten your purse/wallet. If he ignores you get out of the car at the first opportunity to do so safely. If this is not possible attract the attention of passers by/other cars, lower window and call for help. Call emergency services after you have noted WHERE you are, name of street etc.

UNDERPASS / ALLEY / SECLUDED STREET

If you are confronted or feeling uncomfortable as you go through an underpass/alley or staircase try to go back to where you have just come from. Do not feel embarrassed or stupid about it, the threat might be real. Avoid walking close to the bushes or the wall, stay away from secluded entries/doorways and be aware of hidden spots, Walk in the middle or near the pavement edge. See if there are any objects that you can grab in case you need to defend yourself, a fire extinguisher for instance or loose pipes. If you are attacked use the walls to your advantage, push

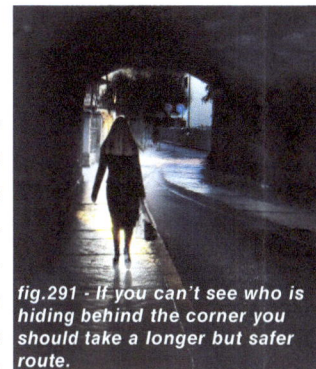

fig.291 - If you can't see who is hiding behind the corner you should take a longer but safer route.

away from them or back against it and push away your attacker. If you can turn him (push/pull action) against the stairs going down push him as hard and suddenly as you can to make him fall. If you are able to wait until someone else passes by who seems trust worthy and follow him/her.

Always walk facing the traffic flow, if someone harasses you it's easier to run in the opposite direction than the one you are facing already. Always run towards heavier traffic or a more built up area. Do not engage in conversation with anyone who stops in a car. If you decide to help keep your distance. Never accept a lift from a stranger.

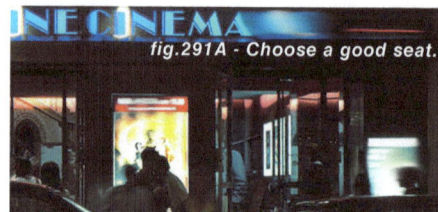
fig.291A - Choose a good seat.

CINEMA/THEATRE or VENUE If you find yourself threaten or molested in this type of venue try and move towards the MAIN exit as soon as possible. Do not sit in a corner alone or near a column, always try and sit close to a group of people, family or near a main aisle. Do not let children go to the toilet by themselves. If the attacker has you cornered shout "FIRE!" or attract the attention of staff or nearby people. Remember all public venues have fire extinguishers and fire alarms, use them if necessary. Locate all emergency exits and escape routes if possible on initial entry to the building.

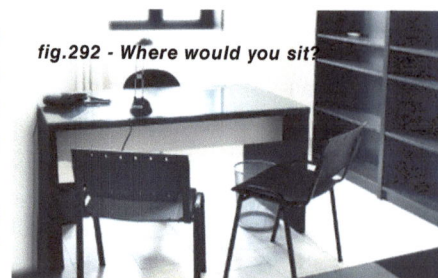
fig.292 - Where would you sit?

JOB INTERVIEW or MODEL/ACTOR AUDITION If you are asked to go to an interview make sure that at least two friends or family members know the exact address where you are going and at what time you will be there and who you will be meeting with.

Do not go to private homes, reputable companies will not do that, if unavoidable suggest a cafe or other venue where other people are/will be present. Do not go to interviews past 6 pm, unless you can go accompanied by someone. Sit three quarters facing the exit route and familiarise yourself with the exit route on the way in. If you feel uncomfortable about any aspect or tone of the person you are meeting make an excuse that you need to exit a moment to put money in the parking metre or because you have forgotten your mobile downstairs/outside. make sure you say clearly that you will be back in few minutes. Pretend your phone is ringing (even if it doesn't it could have been on silent/vibrate mode) and you need to leave the room for a moment and then leave. If you are attacked while in the office with an interviewer use what is on the desk, pencils, scissors, staplers etc, or within the room such as a plant, chair, vase or any heavy object. Never accept a dinner invite after a job interview or a lift back home, it gives the wrong signal and a true professional would never do that in any case.

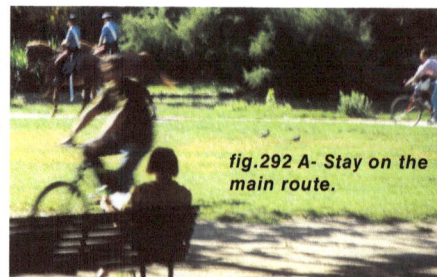
fig.292 A- Stay on the main route.

PARK or GREEN SPACE If walking alone or with your dog or jogging alone in a park make sure you do so near main routes/walkway, do not go in undergrowth or places away or hidden from main activity. Familiarise yourself with map/surroundings, know where you are at all times.

Do not be convinced to follow anyone even in an emergency, call for help from your mobile phone. Avoid regular patterns and using the same route at the same time everyday. Do not take a park or green space as a short-cut no matter how short if deserted or in the dark. It is always the perfect spot for an ambush. Avoid stopping in isolated or screened section of the park to do some stretching or exercises, keep near the main path and near groups of people.

Do not have music in your earphones at too high a volume, just low enough to hear what is happening around you. Take with you an insect repellent spray, the strong type, it can be very useful to spray onto someone's face if you are attacked, it works even on dogs if aimed at the nose/eyes. Beware of animals such as dogs/swans etc, if jogging slow down and walk until past them. If you are attacked remember to use soil/sand/branches to fight back, run into lake/pond or climb up tree. If you have been followed and have lost your bearings aim for a wide open space, downhill, there are more chances of meeting someone. If necessary, use a large feature such as a tree, fountain, bench as an obstacle to put in between you and your attacker.

BEACH or RIVER/LAKE

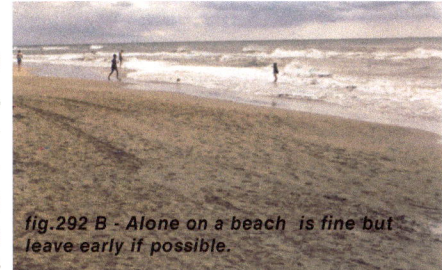

fig.292 B - Alone on a beach is fine but leave early if possible.

Do not lie on a deserted beach alone, always go with friends or where people are present. Beware of going to facilities by yourself or without other people knowing. Do not rest/fall asleep in a secluded area. Familiarise yourself with your surroundings and check possible exit routes or where you can go for safety. Remember if you are attacked or if you realise that you are about to be that going into the water can be a good solution, especially if you are a good swimmer. Do not go on the beach by yourself after dark. If in a wild country remember that rivers at night attract large animals to drink and most predators in warm countries hunt at night near rivers. Sharks and other sea animals feed towards dusk or at night time. Always check local customs so you do not end up offending locals or worse breaking local laws. Some countries carry heavy fines or punishment for sunbathing alone or "being indecent". Make sure you are not the last one to leave a beach or other secluded space, especially in the late afternoon.

CAR PARK or UNDERGROUND GARAGE

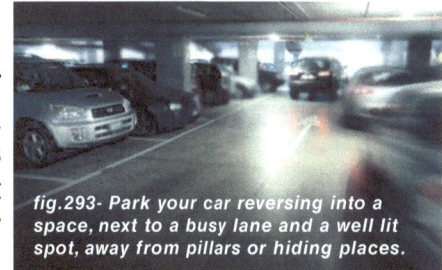

fig.293- Park your car reversing into a space, next to a busy lane and a well lit spot, away from pillars or hiding places.

Always park your car with the front facing towards exit (see fig. 293) and near a main route, not in a secluded/hidden spot such as near walls or heavy foliage If you are parked closer to the main entry/exit better. Reverse into a parking slot. Be aware as you exit/entry car, that is vulnerable moment. Check where alarms/fire extinguishers/fire axes are located. Make a note of the exact spot/row number/level on your mobile phone so that you don't walk around needlessly trying to find your car. If you sense danger going back to your car or you see a person around your car do not confront him or carry on towards your car and seek help as you go back. As you walk towards your car be aware of people sitting in cars parked close to yours or loitering nearby sometimes pretending to give leaflets away. Avoid parking next to vans or very big cars with blackout windows. If you are attacked do not let the person drag you into a car or van, fight with all your might. Make sure that when you return to your car you have your car keys ready in your hand. If the attacker wants your car key throw it at them and let them have it. Make sure if it's an underground car park that your mobile phone has a signal, if not (very possible) try to go back to your car with some other people. If you don't feel comfortable do not chance it, take a taxi home or ask the car park personnel for help. If you are attacked as you are loading your shopping or groceries (the most common moment of attacks on women) use what is at hand, a bottle for instance from your shopping. See also CARJACKING.

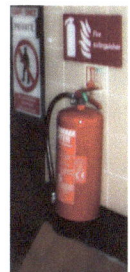

218

CARJACKING Lock yourself inside the car the very moment you get in, before doing anything else, even before putting the key in the ignition. If it happens while you are getting into your car, it is best to let them take the car, as long as they're not trying to take you or your child with it.

You should never let the carjacker take both you and the car but if you find yourself in the car with the carjacker (now a kid-

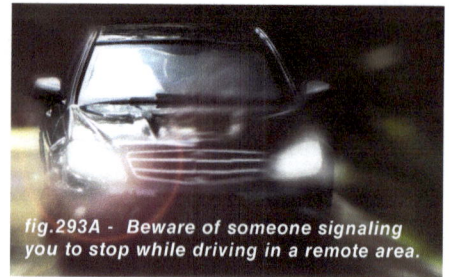
fig.293A - Beware of someone signaling you to stop while driving in a remote area.

napper), try to make the car crash by grabbing the steering wheel, or attacking the kidnapper's eyes. If you are the one who's driving and you know the area go to the nearest Police station or stop the car next to a Policeman or Police car.

In any case act as early as possible and do it in an urban area, if you wait too long and allow him to drive you outside town you have less chances of survival.

Remember that more often than not compliance does not mean making it safely, more often it is the opposite. If you are put in the trunk, use your mobile phone to call for help, or kick out a tail light and wave your hand through the opening.

Carjacking is more common in some countries than others, especially in cities where the car is a very important means to get around, and the majorities of carjackers use a weapon to make you comply. Do not resist, just get out of the car and run.

Carjacking occurs most of the time while the victim is entering or exiting their vehicle while parked, sometimes right on home doorsteps, often within five miles from home. Carjackers target people on their own and want car keys readily available, car door unlocked and a quick getaway.

Most targeted people are men, young and single/divorced, since they tend to have flashy cars or in any case go to places more exposed to this type of crime.

As a rule never pick up hitch-hikers, never mind how harmless they seem.

Carjacking target locations are parking lots, gas stations or any place where you might either drive through slowly (fast food) or you might stop quickly to get something and back to your car, such an ATM or convenience store. Shopping centres are also at risk, be aware of your surroundings when loading groceries/shopping in car. As you approach the car look around, under and inside it and start your car and drive away immediately. Traffic lights intersections/crossroads are also high risk. A carjacker will jump off his vehicle, drag you out at gun point out of your car and drive away. Normally this happens at deserted junctions to avoid other drivers reporting it to the police in real time, that's why you should always drive with your car doors locked and windows shut. Another technique is to crash into the back of your vehicle and as you get out to assess damage the car-jacker will take your vehicle while the accomplice drives away. If you are bumped by a car from behind, with young males on board, be alert. Be wary if someone points out that you have a flat tyre and he can help to sort it out.

If you are forced to drive, crash your car near a busy intersection to attract attention.

To avoid been attacked while asking for help if the car breaks down join a rescue service (such as AA or RAC in UK). Have some loose coins in your car in case you need to make a phone call and your mobile runs flat. ALWAYS Keep a spare phone charger in the car. Keep a large torch (Maglite is best for that) in your vehicle and a fire extinguisher. Both can be very useful in many ways. If you are attacked as you are sitting hold onto the steering wheel and kick him off fighting like a wild cat, start the car and drive off. If you are dragged by your clothes come out of the car in an explosive way, head butting your attacker. Remember that this type of crime is opportunistic; therefore you must avoid giving an opportunity to a criminal.

RAILWAY STATION or SHOPPING CENTRE/MALL Any sit-
uation where a large setting offers a lot of hiding places or op-
portunities for crime should have your full attention.

A busy harbour/railway/buses/subway station normally has a
lot of people carrying valuables with them, such as money for
their trip/holiday. Also people going through these environments have a lot on their mind or in any case their attention

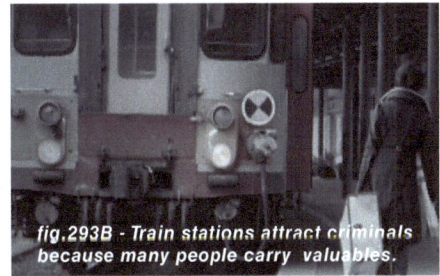
fig.293B - Train stations attract criminals
because many people carry valuables.

is constantly challenged, looking up at the board to see what platform or what delay and so on,
in any case they will have suitcases/shopping or their hands full or in any case are multitasking.
If you are queuing to get your tickets or are retrieving your pre-booked ticket at a vending machine
be aware of your baggage, put a leg in the strap if you need to have it on the floor and keep it in
front of you, NOT BEHIND. Be aware of people bumping onto you or offering help with your lug-
gage.As you go up the escalator make sure you have the person behind you at a reasonable distance. If it is not possible because it is too crowded keep your bags in sight and make sure nothing
on you is easily accessible to a pick pocketer. If you are travelling with a rucksack on your back
make sure you have it in front of you while queuing and if you are waiting for something/someone
lean against a wall. Remember that public facilities such as toilets are often targeted by criminals.

NIGHTCLUB or DISCOTHEQUE/BAR Stick to well known rep-
utable venues. Avoid places with a dubious reputation or
which are known for fights breaking out all the time.

If you are not sure ask the locals or do a search on the internet adding "trouble" or "disturbances" next to the venue's
name.

If while having a drink you have the feeling that you are not
welcome there or people are trying to set you up just leave.
Pretend you are making a phone call and need some quiet

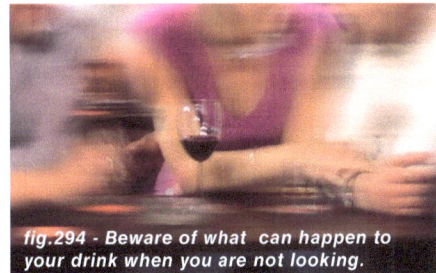
fig.294 - Beware of what can happen to
your drink when you are not looking.

spot then leave immediately. You can always ask the doormen (or bouncers) to let you leave via
another exit so people won't realise you have left and will not follow you.

If you are desperate just use the emergency exit and if the alarm goes off as you open the door
so be it. In the event that a fight breaks out do not intervene, just leave, the beefy security guys
who will turn up won't make any difference and they will see you just as one of the troublemakers
and no matter what excuse you come up with they will just remove you from the venue in no time
and not very gracefully.

Always stay within the club, it is safer to be where there is a crowd, the moment you go into a secluded space or even the car park by yourself you can become a target.

Always go with someone, even for just a quick cigarette. If you meet someone that you like make
sure that the people with you meet him as well.

Think twice about leaving with someone you have just met, the sweetest person can turn out to
be different once alone with you. If you really want to leave with the stranger, make sure that whoever came with you knows that you are leaving or knows where you are going. If you decide to
leave early and the others prefer to stay make sure that you have someone picking you up that
you can trust or a reputable taxi company.

ATM MACHINE/CASH WITHDRAWAL If you need to withdraw lots of cash, even just few hundreds is considered "lots" you have to be on your guard even if you make the transaction inside the bank. Some criminals might decide to follow you afterwards and rob you at the first opportunity.
Most ATM crime is committed between 7pm and 4 am by young males alone. ATM robbers usually position themselves

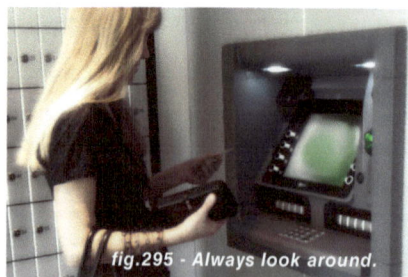
fig.295 - Always look around.

nearby (50 feet) waiting for a victim to approach and withdraw cash. Half of the ATM robberies occur after the cash withdrawal. Many ATM robbery victims are women and were alone when robbed. Most claim that they never saw the robber coming. Most ATM robbers use a gun or claim to have a concealed weapon when confronting the victim and demanding their cash.

WALKING/SHOPPING If you are walking on the footpath, carry your handbag on the opposite side of the road, to avoid bag snatchers grabbing your bag while riding a scooter. Wear your bags strap across your body if possible, making it more difficult to grab. If you are cycling keep the bag on your body, not on the front or rear basket. If carrying a rucksack wear it on the front, more difficult to cut the pockets open. Remember that if you are pushing a pram you are more likely to be subjected to a bag snatch, criminals know you wouldn't go after them and leave the pram there. Do not keep money and values in your bag, better to keep them on your person, or at least split it. If someone grabs your bag and is riding a scooter let the bag go. It's not worth the danger of getting hurt: if you are dragged with it you might sustain serious head injuries, or even die. If you are quick enough you can apply a takedown to a bag snatcher on foot, see TAKEDOWNS page 52 . If you walk in a deserted street or late at night stay away from side of buildings or parts that offer a hiding place, as you turn around a corner stay "wide" so you can quickly spot trouble instead of walking right into it. Remember if there is a bar or any other activity nearby or as you walk past, in case you need to go back and ask for help. If you need press any or even all doorbells on an entry phone or throw something onto the windows to attract attention.

LIFT ELEVATOR OR STAIRCASES If you take a lift, especially during unsociable hours, make sure that you never have your back to the doors, while you wait for it and when travelling in it. Stay more than an arm length from the doors, to avoid someone dragging you inside. If you find yourself in an lift and you feel uncomfortable about the other people or someone in particular get off at the first chance even if it is not your

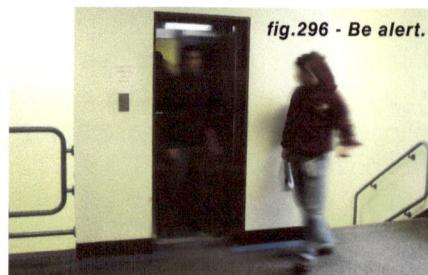
fig.296 - Be alert.

floor., in any case exit with the person before the last one. Keep close to the buttons and make sure you know which one is the alarm button. If the lift is the one to your home and you are with people you don't know, exit at the floor before yours, so they do not know which floor you live on. Many attacks in lifts happen as the doors are about to open or close, therefore stay more alert when that happens, especially as you enter. If possible avoid at all cost being trapped in the cabin, if it is too late, fight pushing away from the walls and use elbows/eyegauging/headbutting.
As you go up or down staircases try to see what is around the corner before you turn and avoid using your mobile phone , instead keep an eye on what is around you, especially side doors or hidden spots.

DRIVING OR ROADRAGE If you find yourself subject to abuse by another motorist (or motorcyclist/cyclist) it is best to stay in the car (never get out of the car or lower your window) lock yourself inside, raise hands and apologise. If you are able to do so, drive away. If you are chased, drive to a busy road, not to an out of town or deserted road. Stop at a police station. You can call the emergency services and provide the vehicle

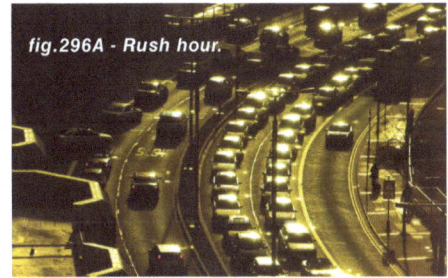
fig.296A - Rush hour.

registration number, or you can pretend you are doing so. Make sure that the other person understands what you are doing. If the window is open say in a very loud voice, "police, hello a driver is etc...registration number" often that should work. Do not engage in conversation; do not gesture except to clearly apologise and a big smile. If the other person hits your vehicle DO NOT STOP, stay within the traffic flow, other people might report what is happening. Stay calm, it's only damage to a car, but if you stop and get out you might be seriously hurt or even killed.

DOG OR ANIMAL ATTACK If you come across a dog being walked on a leash keep a safe distance between yourself and the dog, keep children well away, dogs and other animals generally attack the smallest. Stay away from barking, snarling, sleeping, eating, or nursing dogs.
If a dog approaches you do not stare into its eyes, turn sideways and slowly move away.
You can't outrun a dog, and showing your back to the dog might provoke an attack.
Speak in a calm and soft tone "Good dog, it's OK" keep repeating calmly; do not wave your hands.
Put an obstacle such as a tree, car, fountain or bench between you and the dog.
If you are attacked, put something between you and the dog's mouth, coat, purse, large stick.
If you fall to the ground get up as soon as possible. If the dog has grabbed your arm in his mouth push towards the back of his throat, do not pull away. Be aware of unleashed dogs in the street or in the wild, stay away or walk together with other people. Climb on a parked car roof if necessary. The majority of wild animals such as BEARS, MOUNTAIN LIONS, and COYOTES etc will shy away if you make yourself big, spread coat/mantel to appear so.
Do not enter caves unless sure it is empty. Never turn your back on an animal. Playing dead, rolling into a ball has worked with some bears some times but there is no guarantee, it does not work with other animals. In SNAKE infested country walk making noises and carrying a long stick, inspect before sitting on rocks, grass.
Carry poison extractor and antivenom. Move back slowly if you startle a snake, keep your hands close to your body and offer a long stick for the snake to bite if the snake moves towards you. In SHARK infested waters stay away from fish/turtle farms or fishing boats, do not swim at night or dusk. While surfing do not go off on your own.
If you are attacked do not play dead, hit the shark's head with all your strength, aiming for the eyes/gills/snout. Scream underwater, I am sure you will feel up to that if confronted.

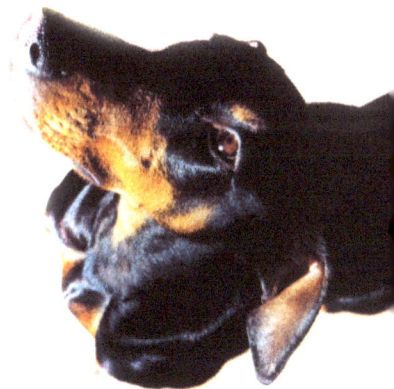
Bfig.296B - Good doggy.

ALWAYS STRETCH BEFORE TRAINING

ALL EXERCISES ARE FOR MEN OR WOMEN IRRESPECTIVELY.

THIS COLOUR INDICATES THE AREA YOU ARE SUPPOSED TO "FEEL" STRETCHING THE MOST.

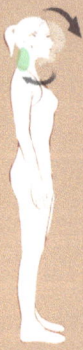

HEAD UP+DOWN, DO NOT ROLL WITH CIRCULAR MOVES.

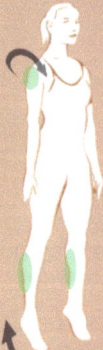

LIFT YOUR HEELS, ROTATE SHOULDERS (BOTH WAYS).

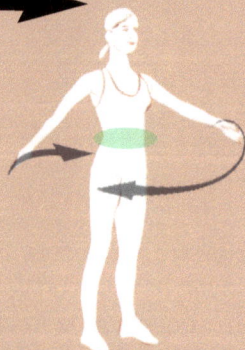

SWING YOUR ARMS, ROTATING ON THE SPOT.

EXTEND YOUR BACK, LOOK UP. LOWER/RAISE ARMS

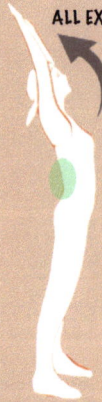

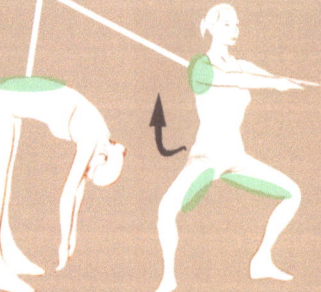

BEND DOWN, TRY TO TOUCH YOUR TOES.

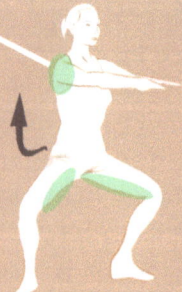

SQUAT, LEG WIDE, HANDS FORWARD.

START WITH YOUR NECK, END WITH YOUR LEGS.

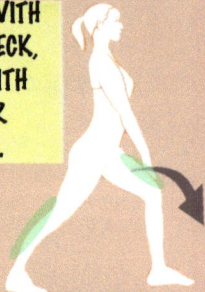

LOUNGE FORWARD, KEEPING YOUR BACK STRAIGHT.

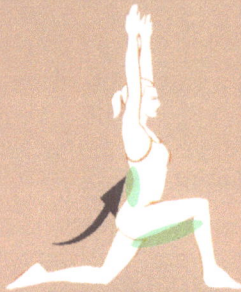

SAME AS BEFORE (LEFT) BUT WITH KNEE ON THE GROUND.

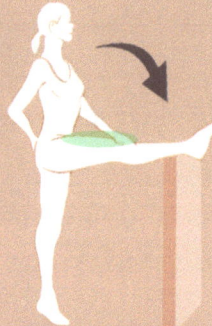

REST ONE LEG ONTO SOMETHING, AT A RIGHT ANGLE, SLOWLY BEND ONTO IT.

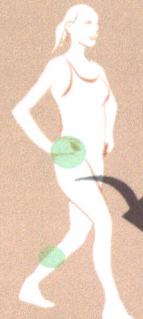

LOUNGE FORWARD ADDING A LITTLE TWIST TO YOUR HIPS.

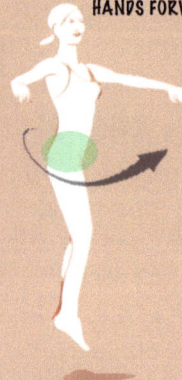

JUMP ON THE SPOT AND TWIST, BEND KNEES AS YOU LAND. KEEP YOUR SHOULDERS FACING FORWARD.

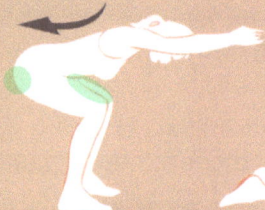

SQUAT AND STRETCH ARMS FORWARD.

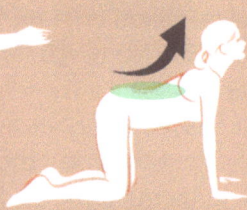

ON ALL FOURS, BEND UPWARDS

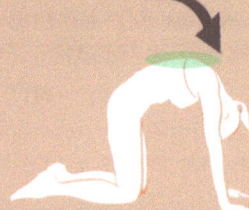

ON ALL FOURS, ARCH YOUR SPINE.

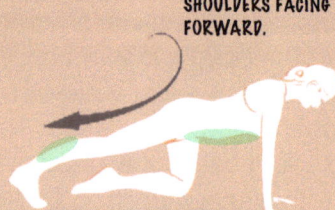

ON ALL FOURS, EXTEND ONE LEG AND THEN THE OTHER.

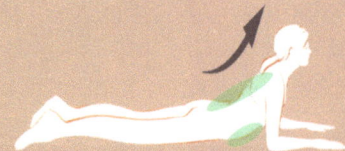

LAY DOWN, PUSH UP FROM ELBOWS, KEEPING HIPS ON FLOOR

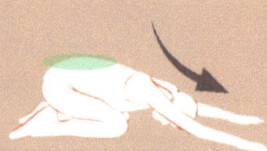

SINK DEEP INTO POSITION, REACH FORWARDS WITH ARMS.

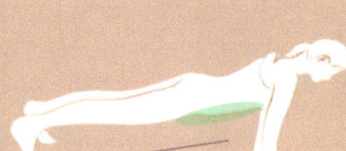

MANTAIN STRAIGHT LINE, TIGHTEN ABS.

HEAD RESTING ON ARM, DRAW FOOT TO BUTTOCK.

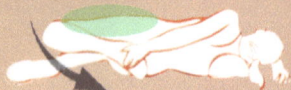

HEAD FACING OPPOSITE DIRECTION TO KNEES, STRETCH BOTH SIDES.

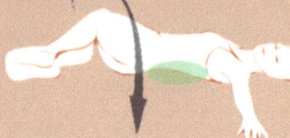

FEET TOGETHER HOLD CALVES AND BEND FORWARD.

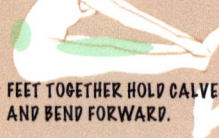

SAME AS BEFORE, LEGS WIDE. LEAN ONTO EACH LEG, THEN INTO THE MIDDLE.

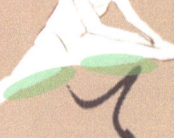

223

A muscle with good elasticity is a faster muscle, allowing you to deliver faster strikes in less reaction time and it is less prone to injury. Everyone should always stretch before training, beginning with some warm-up, rotating your joints to lubricate them with synovial fluid performing slow circular movements, clockwise and anti-clockwise.

Follow this order: fingers, knuckles, wrists, elbows, shoulders, neck, waist, hips, legs, knees, ankles, toes. Once completed do some light aerobic work for at least five minutes, eg. jumping or skipping. This raises your core body temperature and to increase blood flow in the muscles to improve muscle performance and flexibility and to reduce the likelihood of injuries.

Now you are ready for some static stretching. Start from the biggest muscles and work your way down: your back, pectorals, legs etc. (see fig.298) After that you can do some dynamic stretching, ideally consistent with the activity you are doing later on (punching, kicking etc).

Once you have finished training stretch again to cool down, this will help eliminating the lactic acid accumulated in your muscles and can reduce cramping and soreness in fatigued muscles as well as making you feel better afterwards. Perform all exercises slowly, holding each position for at least 20 seconds. Always stretch both sides equally (both shoulders, both hips etc). The general rule is to increase the intensity of the exercises gradually, breathe slowly and regularly during the stretch and never hold your breath during a lengthening exercise, an important factor because proper oxygenation attenuates the tension. Do not swing or move up and down, the aim of stretching is to increase muscular flexibility. The environment temperature should not be less than 18° C (64° Fahrenheit), as cold temperature hardens muscles structure and inhibits innervations. Stretching stimulates the production or retention of lubricants between the connective tissue fibres, preventing the formation of adhesions. It is possible to improve the capacity of muscles and connective tissues to stretch, regardless of age, a few minutes every day and an active life surely helps, because reduced use of the connective tissue produces a significant resistance and limits flexibility.

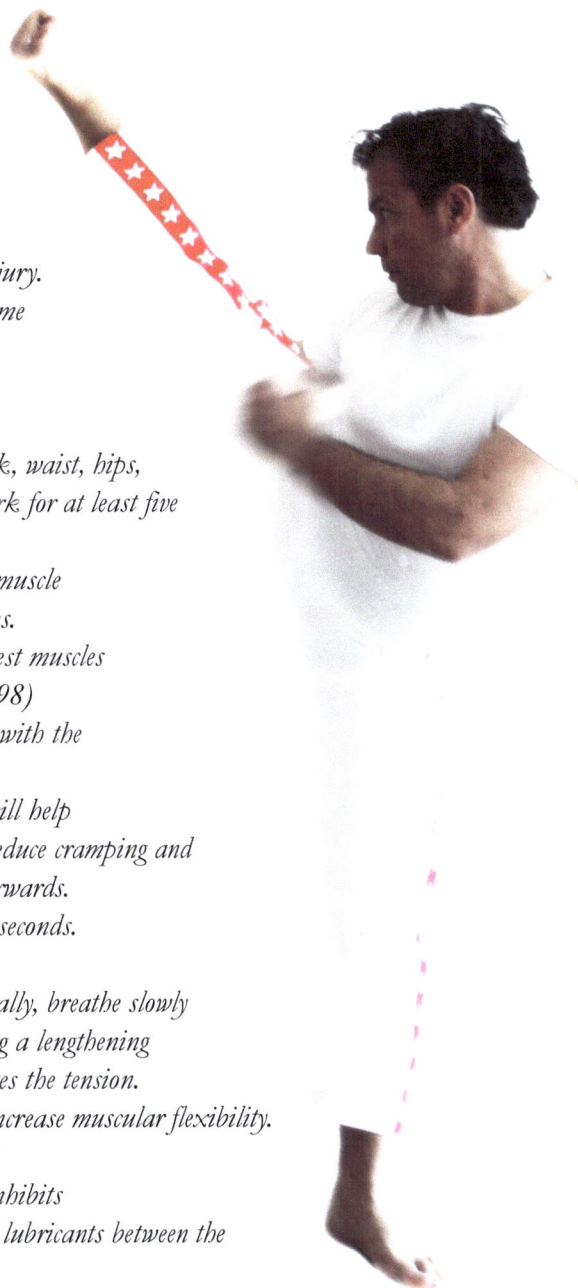

fig. 297- Strive to achieve a good stretch form.

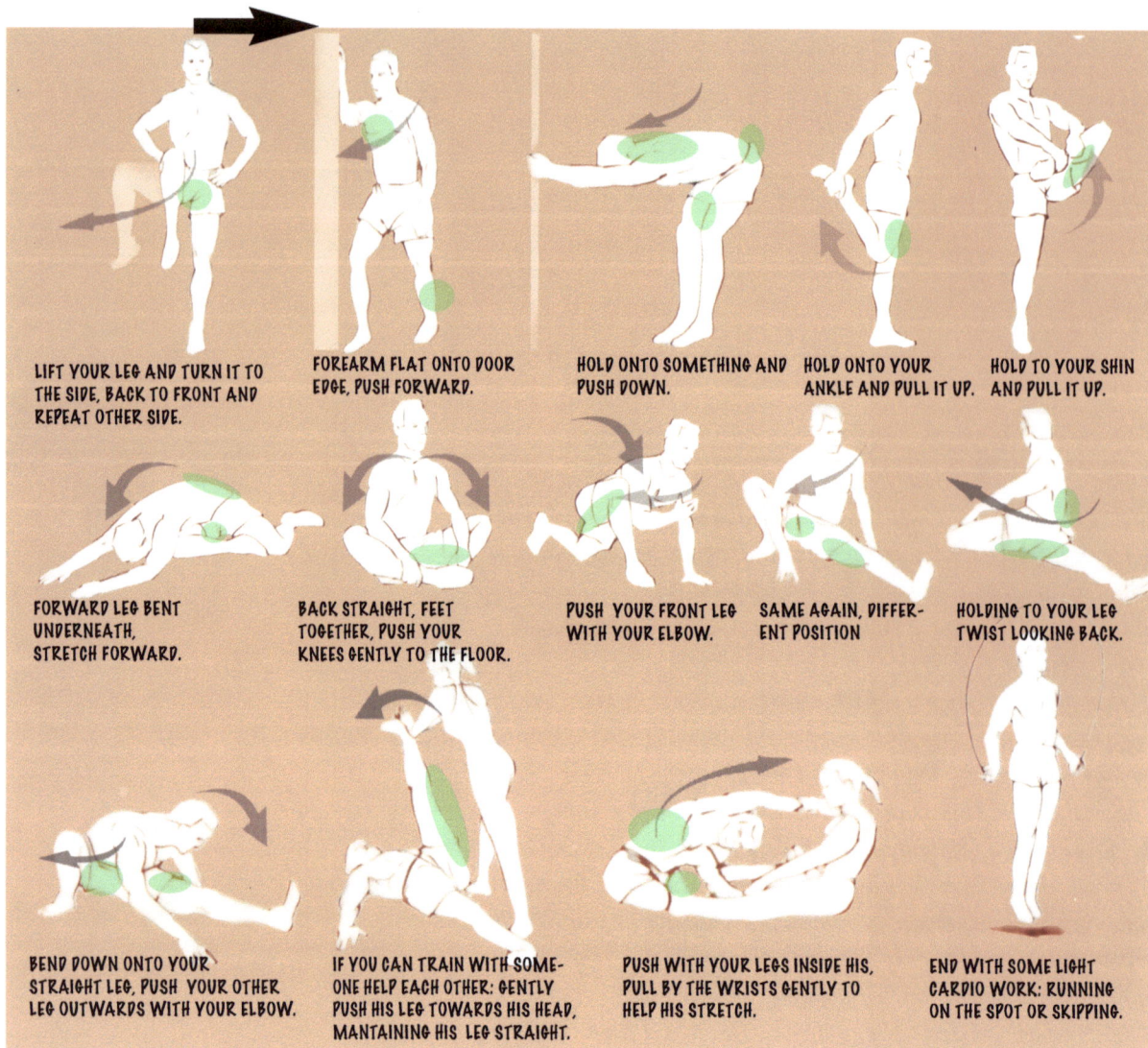

LIFT YOUR LEG AND TURN IT TO THE SIDE, BACK TO FRONT AND REPEAT OTHER SIDE.

FOREARM FLAT ONTO DOOR EDGE, PUSH FORWARD.

HOLD ONTO SOMETHING AND PUSH DOWN.

HOLD ONTO YOUR ANKLE AND PULL IT UP.

HOLD TO YOUR SHIN AND PULL IT UP.

FORWARD LEG BENT UNDERNEATH, STRETCH FORWARD.

BACK STRAIGHT, FEET TOGETHER, PUSH YOUR KNEES GENTLY TO THE FLOOR.

PUSH YOUR FRONT LEG WITH YOUR ELBOW.

SAME AGAIN, DIFFERENT POSITION

HOLDING TO YOUR LEG TWIST LOOKING BACK.

BEND DOWN ONTO YOUR STRAIGHT LEG, PUSH YOUR OTHER LEG OUTWARDS WITH YOUR ELBOW.

IF YOU CAN TRAIN WITH SOMEONE HELP EACH OTHER: GENTLY PUSH HIS LEG TOWARDS HIS HEAD, MANTAINING HIS LEG STRAIGHT.

PUSH WITH YOUR LEGS INSIDE HIS, PULL BY THE WRISTS GENTLY TO HELP HIS STRETCH.

END WITH SOME LIGHT CARDIO WORK: RUNNING ON THE SPOT OR SKIPPING.

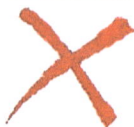

Do not bounce, instead relax and increase the stretch slowly.
Do not stretch any muscle to painful levels.
Do not force the stretch, stay within the muscles maximum stretch capability.
Do not hold your breath while performing a stretch.

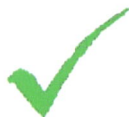

Always warm up before stretching, some light aerobic work will do.
Move slowly and maintain tension of the stretch throughout.
Concentrate on the muscles that you are stretching.
Keep your breathing slow and regular.

In fig.298 you can see the locations of the muscles and tendons, and it would be a good idea if you familiarise yourself with the position within your body of all the major muscles. Knowing what and where you are stretching will improve your stretching capability as well as avoiding stretching muscles the wrong way.

As you can see all muscles are interconnected and every movement we do involves several muscles at the same time.

A simple smile can involve the majority of the 36 muscles responsible for facial expression in humans amongst the 43 muscles that are present in the face, most of which are controlled by the seventh cranial nerve.

Lack of activity and aging causes elastin (a protein in connective tissues that is elastic and allows tissues to resume their original shape after stretching) to begin to fray, it becomes less elastic and collagen becomes stiffer and denser. Aging has effects on connective tissue as much as lack of activity does, with the addition of progressive dehydration, a greater loss of calcium and the replacement of muscle fibres with collagen fat fibres. This is why greater intake of water contributes to greater mobility, therefore keep drinking plenty of water every day, the average adult is 65 percent water. Health organisations suggest at least eight glasses, each containing eight ounces (168 ml), of water per day, a total of 64 fluid ounces, or 1.89 litres), and if you exercise regularly more than that. Most of the 600 plus voluntary skeletal muscles of the human body are connected to the bones via tendons crossing joints. Understanding these relations help to perform and achieve better stretch and gain more flexibility.

KNOWING HOW MUSCLES ARE CONNECTED HELPS IMPROVE FLEXIBILITY.

MUSCLES AND TENDON LOCATION

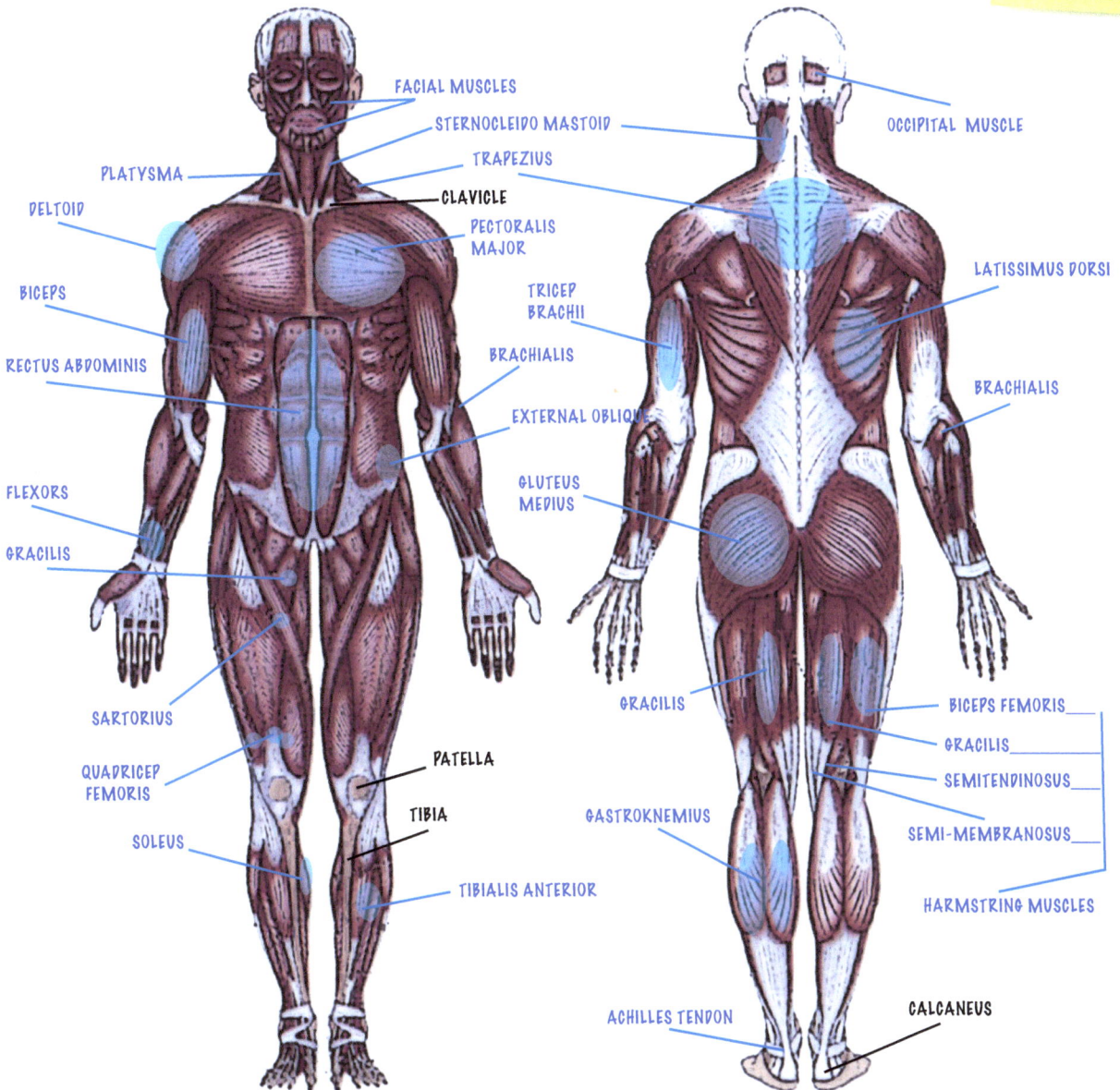

FACIAL MUSCLES
STERNOCLEIDO MASTOID
OCCIPITAL MUSCLE
TRAPEZIUS
PLATYSMA
CLAVICLE
DELTOID
PECTORALIS MAJOR
LATISSIMUS DORSI
BICEPS
TRICEP BRACHII
BRACHIALIS
RECTUS ABDOMINIS
BRACHIALIS
EXTERNAL OBLIQUE
FLEXORS
GLUTEUS MEDIUS
GRACILIS
SARTORIUS
GRACILIS
BICEPS FEMORIS___
QUADRICEP FEMORIS
PATELLA
GRACILIS_____
SEMITENDINOSUS___
TIBIA
SEMI-MEMBRANOSUS___
SOLEUS
GASTROKNEMIUS
TIBIALIS ANTERIOR
HARMSTRING MUSCLES
ACHILLES TENDON
CALCANEUS

LITTLE WEIGHT AND LOTS OF REPETITIONS

THIS COLOUR INDICATES THE AREA YOU ARE SUPPOSED TO "FEEL" AS YOU WORK OUT. ALL EXERCISES ARE FOR MEN OR WOMEN IRRESPECTIVELY.

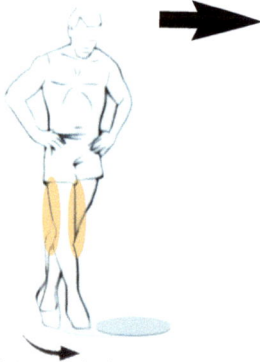

PUSH A 10 KG PLATE WITH THE INTERNAL PART OF YOUR FOOT, ACROSS THE FRONT (ADDUCTORS).
IF YOU PUSH WITH THE EXTERNAL PART OF YOUR FOOT THE OUTER ABDUCTOR WORKS.

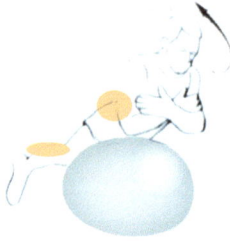

LEGS STRAIGHT. LEAN PRONE ON THE SWISS BALL, ARMS CROSSED ON CHEST, NOW LIFT YOUR CHEST OFF THE BALL.

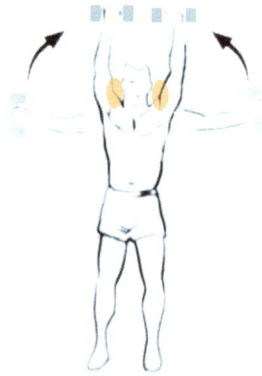

KEEPING THE DUMBELLS ALWAYS IN LINE LOWER THEM, THEN ROTATE HALF WAY DOWN.

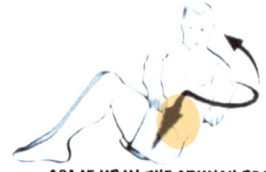

COME UP IN THE CRUNCH POSITION AND TWIST YOUR TORSO AS YOU COME UP, ARMS STRETCHED OUT AHEAD.

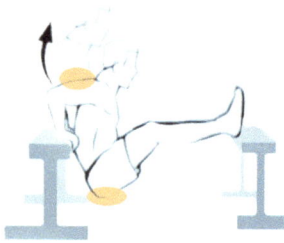

FEET ON A BENCH AND PALMS ON ANOTHER BENCH OPPOSITE, SLOWLY BEND YOUR ARMS LOWERING YOUR TORSO, KEEP YOUR LEGS AS STRAIGHT AS POSSIBLE.

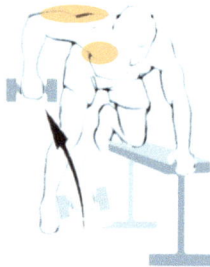

KNEE ON BENCH, HOLD ON TO BENCH WITH SAME SIDE HAND AND RAISE DUMBELL FROM FLOOR TO SHOULDER HEIGHT.

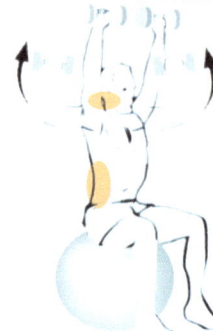

SITTING ON THE SWISS BALL PUSH DUMBELLS UP IN LINE WITH YOUR SHOULDERS.

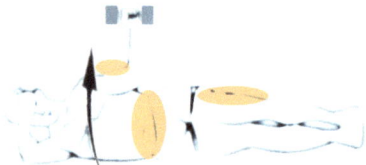

ROTATE YOUR FOREARM HOLDING THE DUMBELL UNTIL YOUR ARM IS PARALLEL TO THE FLOOR. HOLD FOR A FEW SECONDS AND GO BACK.

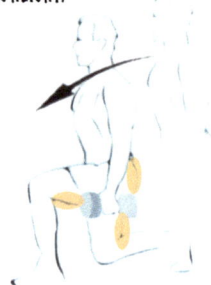

STAND WITH LEGS ONE IN FRONT OF THE OTHER, BEND KNEES KEEPING TORSO STRAIGHT.

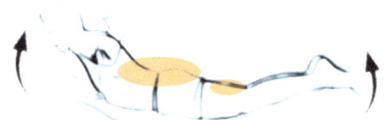

FACE DOWN, LEGS STRAIGHT AND ARMS OUTSTRETCHED LIFT TORSO AND LEGS SIMULTANEOUSLY.

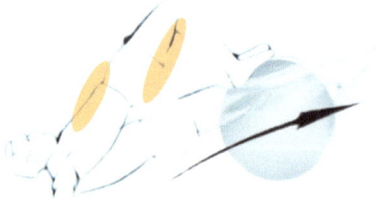

WITH YOUR BODY IN LINE WITH THE SWISS BALL PULL THE BALL TOWARDS YOU BENDING KNEES AND EXTENDING HIPS. GO BACK SLOWLY TO ORIGINAL POSITION

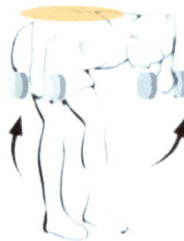

LEGS SLIGHTLY BENT, TORSO AT 90°, LIFT DUMBELLS TO SHOULDER HEIGHT.

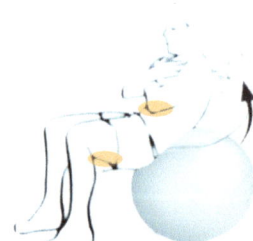

LIE BACK ON THE SWISS BALL, KNEES AT 90°, CRUNCH UP SLOWLY HOLDING YOUR HIPS STILL.

Strength

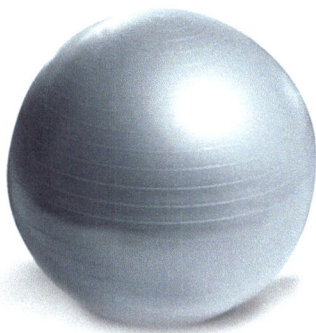

**fig.299 - Exercise, stability or Swiss ball.
Choose the right size for you.**

*Keeping fit is fundamental, even though it is important not to become obsessive.
Lets say that it is better to exercise 20 minutes everyday than once a week for a
couple of hours. One day of the week should be kept as a rest day from intense
exercise. To increase strength without losing speed follow the exercise table on the
left, equally suitable for both sexes, bearing in mind that you should try and do
as many repetitions as you can with little weight, instead of trying to lift a lot.
Ideally it would be better avoiding using weights whatsoever; a big muscle is very
rarely a fast one. Therefore try and follow this very simple training programme,
you should feel free to mix and match as you please; avoiding training the same
group of muscles for too long.
If you work the legs then follow up with some abs, if you work out your torso then
add some legwork.*

*Always start with a warm up, do some stretching and at least twenty minutes of these simple exercises.
They are thought out to increase strength where you need it the most and to help increase the speed of execution, without building mass.*

*Strong legs kick better, toned arms
strike faster.*

*Remember that you should rest at least
45 seconds between each set.*

*Rest is as important as physical work
and your muscles need that time to absorb the work done.*

*A typical strength building training ses-
sion should be like this:*

*Number of exercises per session: 3
Number of sets per exercise: 6
Number of repetitions per exercise: 5
Rest interval between sets: maximum 3
minutes. How can you easily find out
how fit you really are?
It very much varies with age, sex and
genetic predisposition.*

BODY MASS INDEX (BMI)

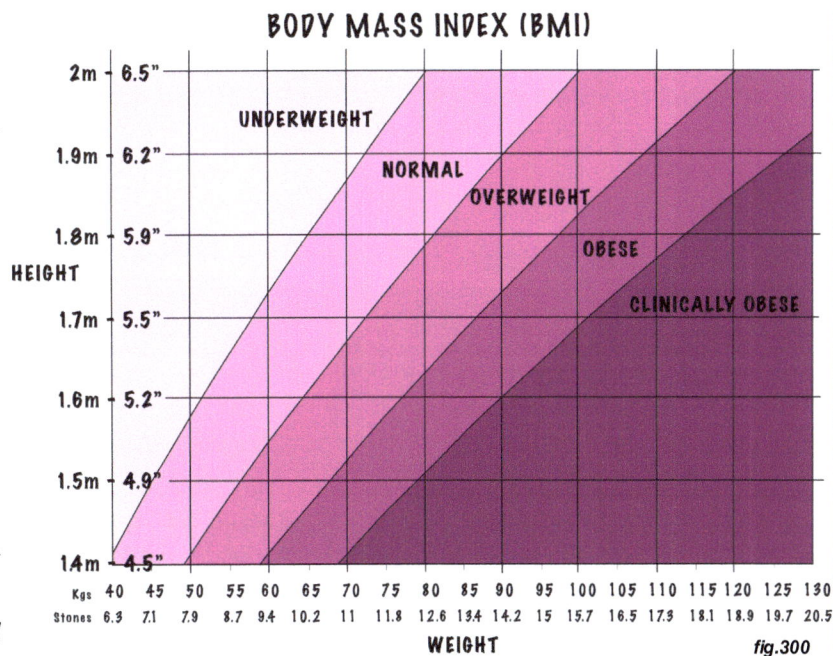

HEIGHT		UNDERWEIGHT	NORMAL	OVERWEIGHT	OBESE	CLINICALLY OBESE
2m	6.5"					
1.9m	6.2"					
1.8m	5.9"					
1.7m	5.5"					
1.6m	5.2"					
1.5m	4.9"					
1.4m	4.5"					

Kgs	40	45	50	55	60	65	70	75	80	85	90	95	100	105	110	115	120	125	130
Stones	6.3	7.1	7.9	8.7	9.4	10.2	11	11.8	12.6	13.4	14.2	15	15.7	16.5	17.3	18.1	18.9	19.7	20.5

WEIGHT

fig.300

This chart is only an approximation and should not be taken as an accurate measurement.

228

Assuming you are not terribly overweight (see BMI chart fig. 300) and in good health, you can try the following simple home tests, in the following order, to see how fit you are compared to the average fit person.

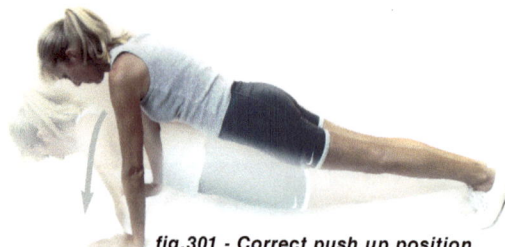

fig.301 - Correct push up position.

PUSH UP TEST

Men put hands and toes on the floor, women do the same or in "bent knee" (fig. 302) position. Do as many push ups as you can counting them and when you stop because you cannot do anymore check with the values below:

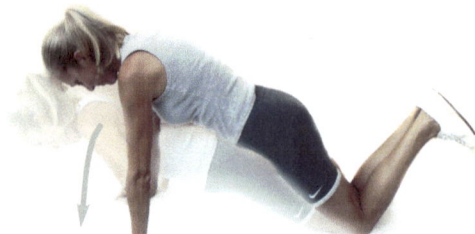

fig.302 - Alternative push up position for women.

Age	17-19	20-29	30-39	40-49	50-59	60-65
Men average	19-34	17-29	13-24	11-20	9-17	6-16
Women average	11-20	12-22	10-21	8-17	7-14	5-12

SIT UP TEST

How many sit-ups can you do in 1 minute? Find out how good your core stability is.

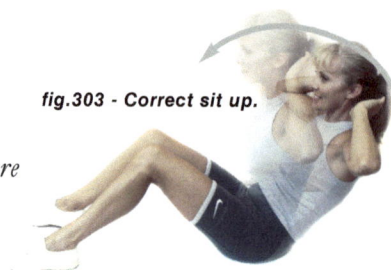

fig.303 - Correct sit up.

Age	18-25	26-35	36-45	46-55	56-65	65+
Men average	35-38	31-34	27-29	22-24	17-20	15-18
Women average	29-32	25-28	19-22	14-17	10-12	11-13

SQUAT TEST

Position yourself in front of a exercise bench or chair keeping your feet apart in line with your shoulders, keeping your hands on your hips. Squat down caressing the chair with your buttocks before standing back up. What is the maximum you can perform?

Age	18-25	26-35	36-45	46-55	56-65	65+
Men average	35-38	31-34	27-29	22-24	17-20	15-18
Women average	29-32	25-28	19-22	14-17	10-12	11-13

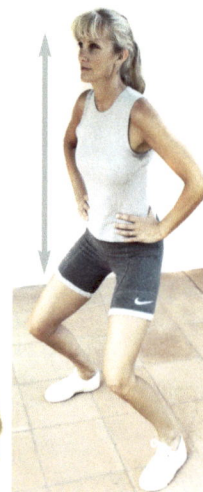

fig.304 - Proper squat.

STEP TEST

For this all you need is a 12" high step or sturdy wooden box of the same height and a stopwatch. Now step on and off for three minutes, up one foot and the other follows and repeat (down with one foot and the other follows). Keep a steady regular pace, it helps if you say loud "up...up...down...down..." Once the three minutes are up, measure your heart rate taking your pulse for one minute. You can now compare your heart rate with th table below, the lower the rate the fitter you are, more accurately your cardiovascular endurance).

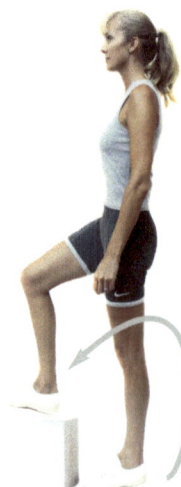

fig.305 - This is how you should do steps.

The lower your heart rate is after you completed the exercise, the fitter you are (the values that follow are pulses per minute).

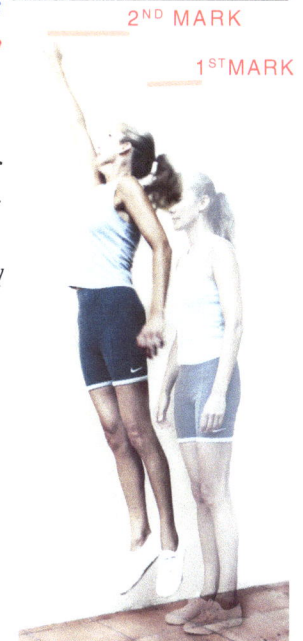

Age	18-25	26-35	36-45	46-55	56-65	65+
Men average	100-105	100-107	104-112	106-116	104-112	104-113
Women average	109-117	112-119	111-118	116-120	113-118	116-122

VERTICAL JUMP TEST

Position yourself next to a wall, making sure that the ceiling is high enough and the floor is not slippery or uneven. Reach with one hand (staying as close to the wall as you can) as high as you can. This is your starting measurement, the standing reach height, now make a note or mark that height (you can use masking tape). Move a little away from the wall and jump as high as possible and try to touch the wall as high as you can. Mark that. The difference between your first standing reach and the second you achieved with your jump is the result. You can try as many times as you wish and in whatever way you prefer, the aim is to jump as high as possible and measure your legs explosive power.

Men average	(inches)	(cm)	Women average	(inches)	(cm)
	16 - 20	41-50		12 - 16	31-40

2ND MARK

1ST MARK

fig.307 - How to execute the jump for the test.

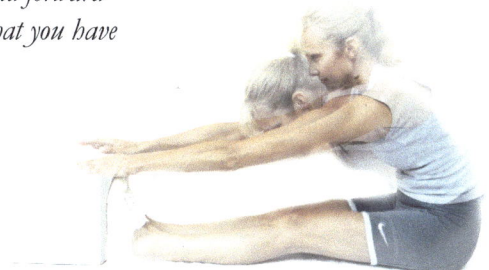

FLEXIBILITY TEST

Leave this test until last so that you are warmed up to perform the required stretch. Positioning yourself as in fig.308 measure how far you can go as you bend forward one hand on top of the other, do it slowly. Measure the farthest reach that you have managed with the tips of your fingers and that you managed to hold for at least three seconds. Keep your knees flat to the ground.
If you haven't managed to reach or pass your feet, take in any case a measurement of how far you are away from your toes.
You can also perform this test standing on a step at least 20 cm high, feet together, and as you bend forward measure how far you can reach of the step. This is a "negative" measurement and it is the one you should improve upon. Practicing the exercises in the STRETCHING TABLE at page 223 and 225 you will be able to improve your flexibility.

fig.308 - How to execute the flexibility test.

Men average	(inches)	(cm)	Women average	(inches)	(cm)
	0 to +2	0 to+5		0 to +2	1to +10

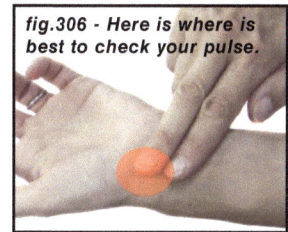

All these tests are just a simple and practical way to find out with good approximation your fitness level, by no means can it substitute a proper examination and accurate tests carried out in a dedicated facility by qualified professionals.

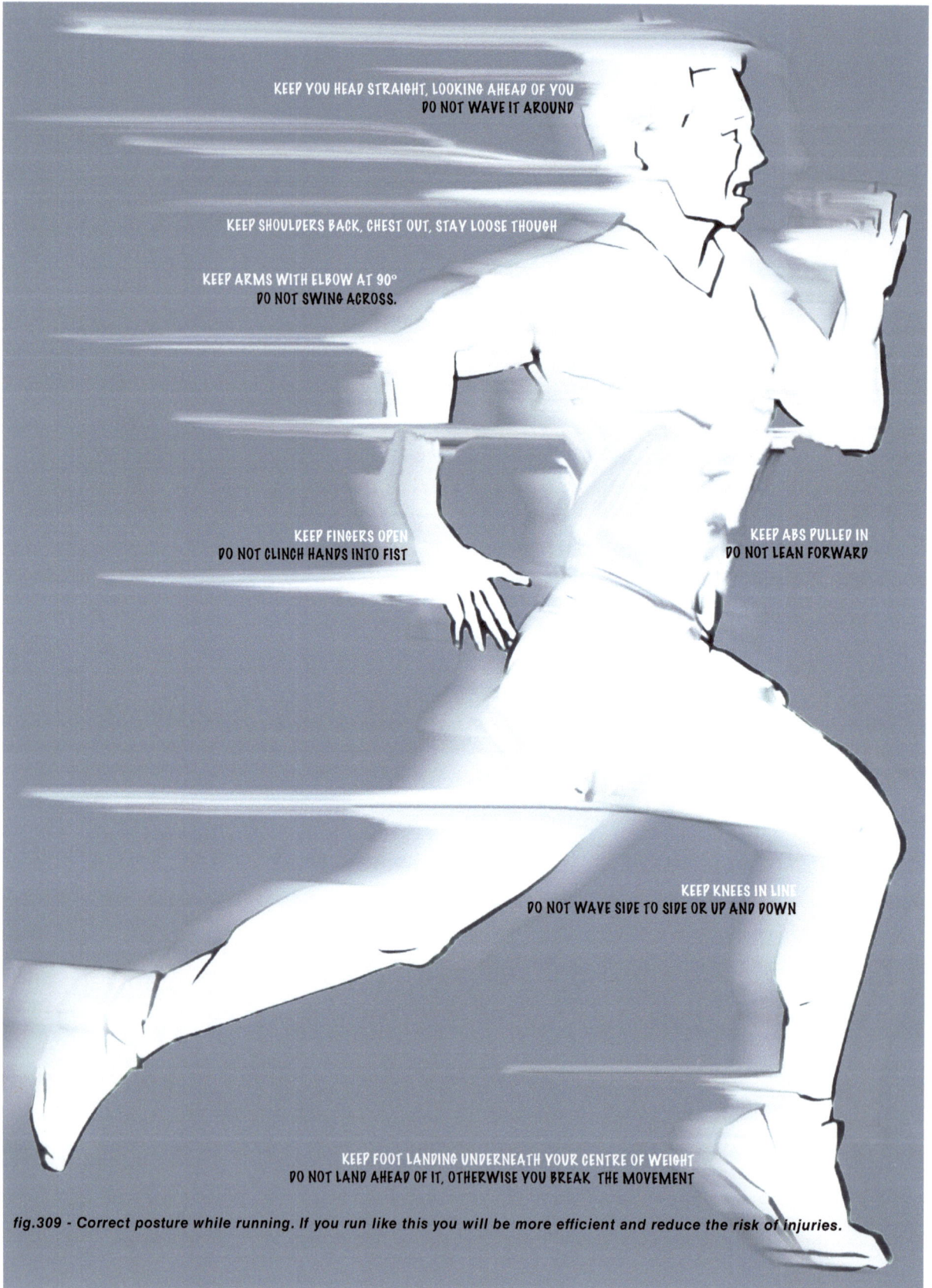

KEEP YOU HEAD STRAIGHT, LOOKING AHEAD OF YOU
DO NOT WAVE IT AROUND

KEEP SHOULDERS BACK, CHEST OUT, STAY LOOSE THOUGH

KEEP ARMS WITH ELBOW AT 90°
DO NOT SWING ACROSS.

KEEP FINGERS OPEN
DO NOT CLINCH HANDS INTO FIST

KEEP ABS PULLED IN
DO NOT LEAN FORWARD

KEEP KNEES IN LINE
DO NOT WAVE SIDE TO SIDE OR UP AND DOWN

KEEP FOOT LANDING UNDERNEATH YOUR CENTRE OF WEIGHT
DO NOT LAND AHEAD OF IT, OTHERWISE YOU BREAK THE MOVEMENT

fig.309 - Correct posture while running. If you run like this you will be more efficient and reduce the risk of injuries.

Speed

You better believe me when I say I am probably the worst runner you may ever run across.
But I always made an effort to run and learn how to run well because running is very important to keep your condition as well as absolutely necessary in case you need to escape an attack or chase someone.
Let's see what makes a good running posture. As you can see on fig.309 it is important to keep your back straight and to achieve that you must look ahead and keep your chin up, do not move your head side to side or up/down. Keep your shoulders back, pushing your chest out without stiffening up, stay loose. Your elbows should be at a 90° angle with your arms that should not swing across. Fingers should be kept open, don't run with clinched fists.

Keep your knees as much as you can in a straight line, not waving them sideways or up and down.

All this advice is coming from people who make a living out of running or athletics, but what about if, it doesn't matter what, you find all this very difficult?

Probably you are running with the wrong shoes for your type of foot, so let's make sure you have the right shoe for the right foot.

The fact that you are wearing your "normal" shoe size does not mean you are wearing the right shoes for your foot.

The main thing that anyone should always remember is never buy a shoe by size only, but by fit, and it is best to follow "the rule of thumb": when trying on a shoe you should be able to measure half to full thumb width from the end of your big toe to the end of your chosen shoe.

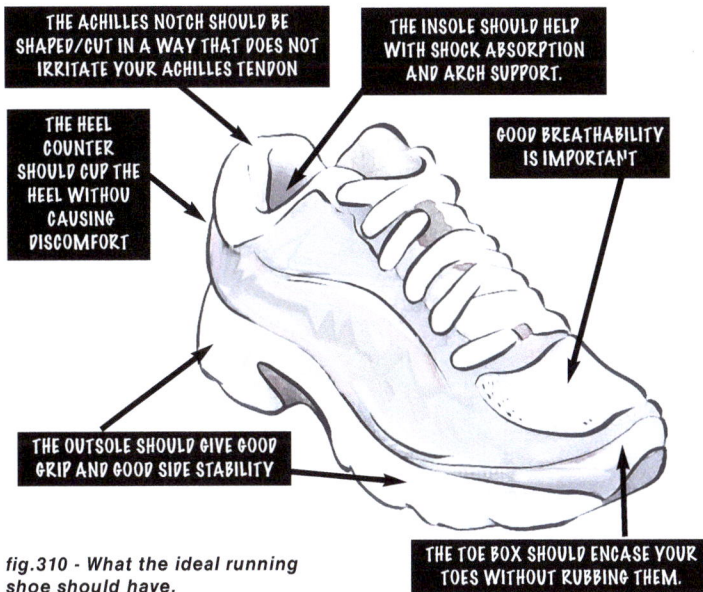

THE ACHILLES NOTCH SHOULD BE SHAPED/CUT IN A WAY THAT DOES NOT IRRITATE YOUR ACHILLES TENDON

THE INSOLE SHOULD HELP WITH SHOCK ABSORPTION AND ARCH SUPPORT.

THE HEEL COUNTER SHOULD CUP THE HEEL WITHOU CAUSING DISCOMFORT

GOOD BREATHABILITY IS IMPORTANT

THE OUTSOLE SHOULD GIVE GOOD GRIP AND GOOD SIDE STABILITY

THE TOE BOX SHOULD ENCASE YOUR TOES WITHOUT RUBBING THEM.

fig.310 - **What the ideal running shoe should have.**

Running on grass is more difficult because it slows you down (grass offers more resistance than tarmac or concrete) but is better for your joints, especially your knees, since it cushions the impact of the foot on the ground. Avoid running on wet grass, it's very slippery, and you should wear running shoes with a good grip. Be aware of possible holes or natural asperities of the terrain that could make you trip over or strain an ankle. Overall you should always choose grass to run on to any other type of commonly available surface.

Having said that you should also be able to pinch material between your toes, and you should also be able to arch the foot slightly within the shoe without feeling too much constriction. Colour, stripes or a cool logo should not be your first priority, really.

In the past there was just standard sizes for all, because all sizes matched the "Brannock" that is a foot measuring device looking more like an Inquisition torture device. Nowadays though because shoes are produced without using that standardised measuring tool you will easily find that a size 10 varies even considerably across brands.

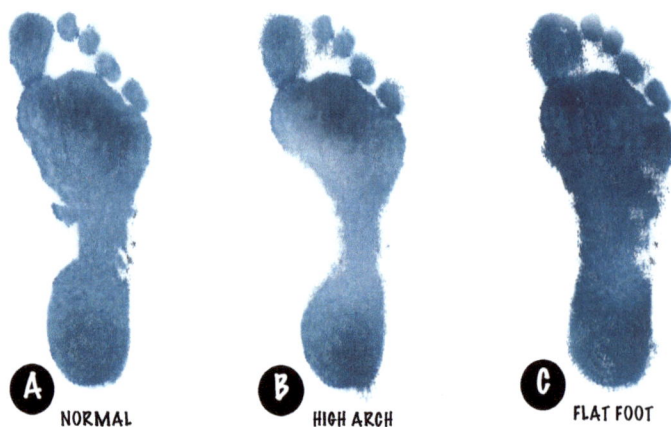

fig.311 - How to check your pronation.

A NORMAL **B** HIGH ARCH **C** FLAT FOOT

Another consideration in choosing a running shoe (but any shoe really) is how much your foot might swell as you run or walk, as well as on what type of terrain you will end up practicing the most, be it tarmac, grass, sand or dirt.

You should know approximately how much your foot expands, taking into account also that in hot weather it might expand more, and if running uphill a lot (or a combination of uphill-downhill) it will swell in a different way. Because the foot naturally dissipates the shock of the impact on landing with an inward roll motion called "pronation", it is clear that anything affecting this action, either the foot's natural shape or the wrong type of shoe forcing the foot to pronate the wrong way, is a cause of problems. A correct pronation allows the foot to roll onto the ball of the foot avoiding burdening the heel with all the impact of the weight landing on it at speed that is quite brutal.

Feet are arched differently from person to person (fig.311): a foot arched normally like **A** has normal pronation, meaning that it impacts the ground in a stable and uniform manner, dissipating the weight and energy equally along the foot surface. Someone like **B** will have an overly arched foot, with a tendency to underpronate; therefore they need a shoe with very little cushioning to encourage a more natural landing of the foot.

And lastly, someone with a flat foot like **C** clearly overpronates, needing a shape of the inner sole and a shoe build to correct and stimulate more arching of the foot while walking and especially running.

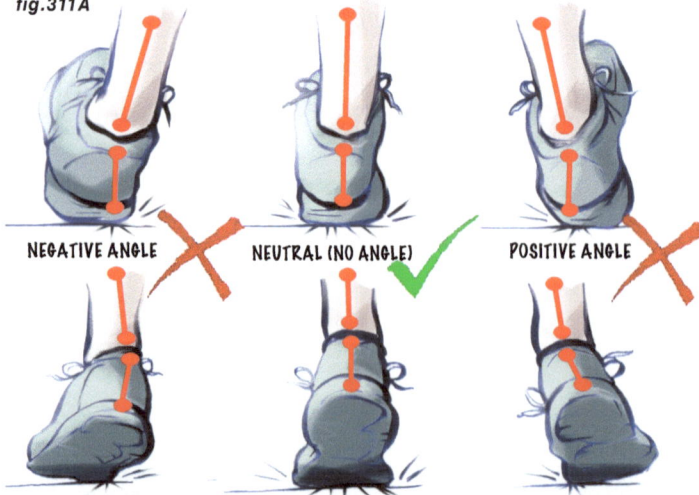

FOOT LANDING ON THE GROUND (NOTE IMPACT AREA)

fig.311A

NEGATIVE ANGLE NEUTRAL (NO ANGLE) POSITIVE ANGLE

FOOT LEAVING THE GROUND

You can check quite easily what type of foot you have by wetting your foot and walking onto a terracotta or porous floor, or on a newspaper laying on the floor. Another way to find out if you're a pronator or supinator is to look at your shoes: a pronator's outer soles wear down along the inside of the ball of the foot tending to have flat feet, the supinator's outer soles wear down along the outer edge because their feet tend to have high arches. To sum it up: pronation is the inward (medial) roll of the foot and in particular the heel and arch which occurs naturally at the heel strike as a cushioning mechanism, while overpronation is when the feet roll inwards too much. (fig.311A)

Underpronation, also known as supination, is the opposite of pronation where the feet don't roll inward enough.
Wearing the wrong type of shoe will lead to painful shins and joints, or even injury.
Good running shoes are designed to control these problems, make sure you choose the one that is right for you.
If you haven't been running for a while the table below gives you a good introduction to it.
Only run three times a week following the run times and rest periods and in just over four months you will be able to run for one hour continuously without effort. Have fun.

WEEK	MON	TUESDAY	WED	THURSDAY	FRI	SAT	SUNDAY
1	rest	5 times 1' running +1' walking	rest	5 times 1' running +1 'walking	rest	rest	7 times 1' running +1' walking
2	rest	5 times 2' running +1' walking	rest	8 times 2' running +1' walking	rest	rest	5 times 3' running +1' walking
3	rest	4 times 3' running +1' walking	rest	8 times 2' running +1' walking	rest	rest	5 times 3' running +1' walking
4	rest	3 times 5' running +2' walking	rest	5 times 3' running +2' walking	rest	rest	3 times 5' running +2' walking
5	rest	3 times 6' running +2' walking	rest	5 times 4' running +1' walking	rest	rest	3 times 6' running +2' walking
6	rest	4 times 6' running +2' walking	rest	2 times 8' running +2' walking	rest	rest	3 times 7' running +2' walking
7	rest	3 times 8' running +2' walking	rest	2 times 10' running +3' walking	rest	rest	3 times 7' running +2' walking
8	rest	3 times 10' running +2 ' walking	rest	2 times 10' running +2 'walking	rest	rest	3 times 12' running +2' walking
9	rest	2 times 12' running +3' walking	rest	2 times 10' running +2' walking	rest	rest	2 times 15' running +3' walking
10	rest	20' running	rest	2 times 15' running +2' walking	rest	rest	20' running
11	rest	25' running	rest	2 times 15' running +2' walking	rest	rest	25' running
12	rest	25' running	rest	30' running	rest	rest	30' running
13	rest	30' running	rest	30' running	rest	rest	40' running
14	rest	30' running	rest	40' running	rest	rest	45' running
15	rest	30' running	rest	45' running	rest	rest	45' running
16	rest	40' running	rest	50' running	rest	rest	50' running
17	rest	40' running	rest	50' running	rest	rest	50' running
18	rest	40' running	rest	55' running	rest	rest	55' running
19	rest	45' running	rest	55' running	rest	rest	1h running

fig.311B - How to plan your running.

DON'T FORGET ALWAYS PUSH OR PULL TO UNBALANCE.

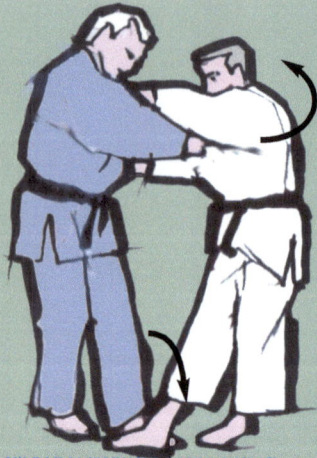

DE ASHI BARAI (FORWARD FOOT SWEEP)
THE MOMENT HE IS ABOUT TO PUT HIS WEIGHT ON THE ADVANCING FOOT, SWEEP HIS ANKLE, PULLING SIDEWAYS TO UNBALANCE HIM FURTHER.

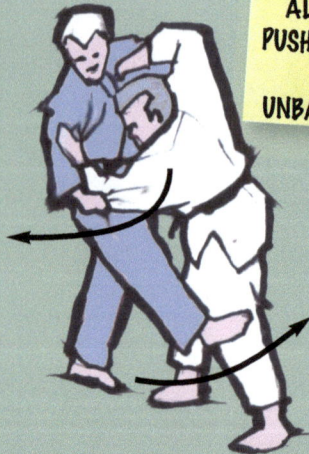

HIZA GURUMA (KNEE WHIRL) PULL HIM TO UNBALANCE ONTO THE SAME KNEE YOU WILL THEN PUT YOUR FOOT ON TO THROW HIM.

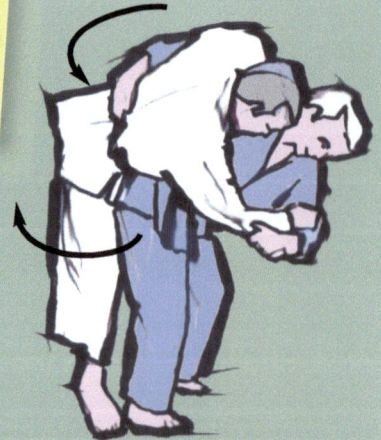

O-GOSHI (HIP ROLL) PULL HIM OFF BALANCE TOWARDS YOU AND THEN SWING ARM AROUND HIS BACK AS YOU PIVOT, JOIN BODIES, BEND KNEES, RAISE HIM ON YOUR HIPS, NOW THROW.

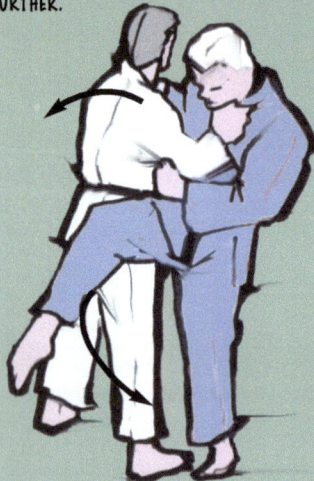

O-SOTO GARI (BIG OUTSIDE CLIP)
UNBALANCE HIM TO THE BACK, SHIFTING HIS WEIGHT ON RIGHT LEG, JOIN BODIES AND SWEEP WITH LARGE MOVEMENT USING YOUR RIGHT LEG.

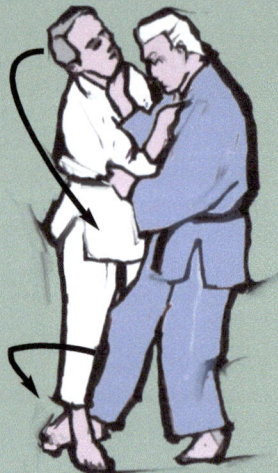

KO UCHI GARI (SMALL INSIDE CLIP)
UNBALANCE HIM TOWARDS THE BACK, CLIP INSIDE OF HIS RIGHT LEG WITH YOUR RIGHT SOLE.

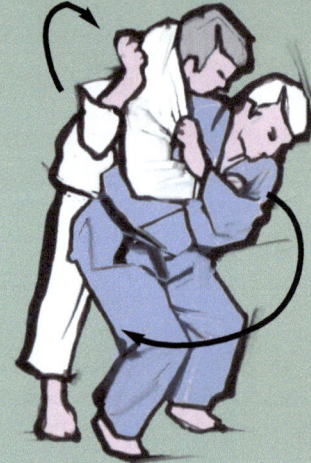

IPPON SEOI NAGE (ONE ARM SHOULDER THROW)
UNBALANCE HIM TOWARDS YOU, BEND YOUR KNEES AS YOU PIVOT, PULLING HIM ON HIS TOES THEN ON YOUR BACK, AS YOU INSERT YOUR RIGHT ARM UNDER HIS ARMPIT PULL HIM ACROSS AND THROW. PUSH YOUR HIPS WELL INTO HIS ABDOMEN.

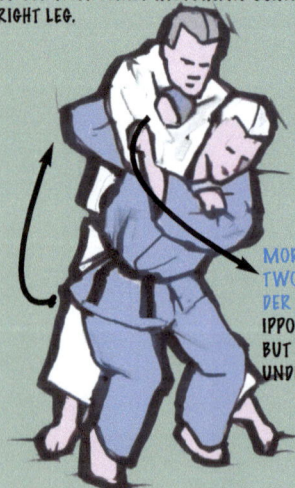

MOROTE SEOI NAGE TWO ARMS (SHOULDER THROW) SEE IPPON SEOI NAGE BUT PUT FOREARM UNDER HIS ARMPIT.

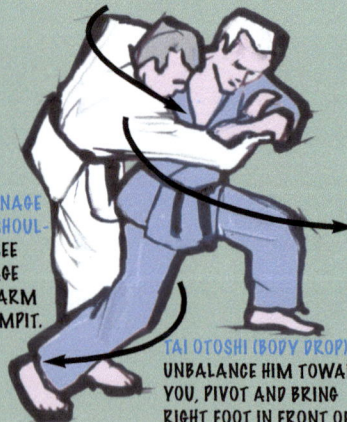

TAI OTOSHI (BODY DROP)
UNBALANCE HIM TOWARDS YOU, PIVOT AND BRING RIGHT FOOT IN FRONT OF BOTH HIS LEGS, PULL HIM ACROSS.

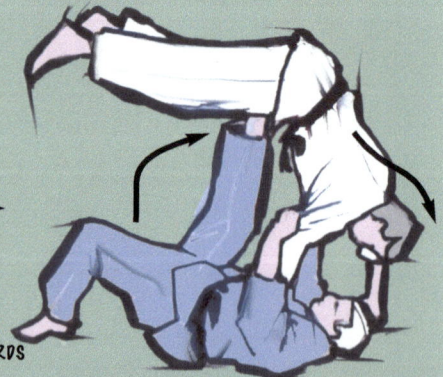

TOMOE NAGE (ROUND THROW)
UNBALANCE HIM TOWARDS YOU, FALL ON YOUR BACK PROPELLING HIM WITH YOUR FOOT

fig.311C

235

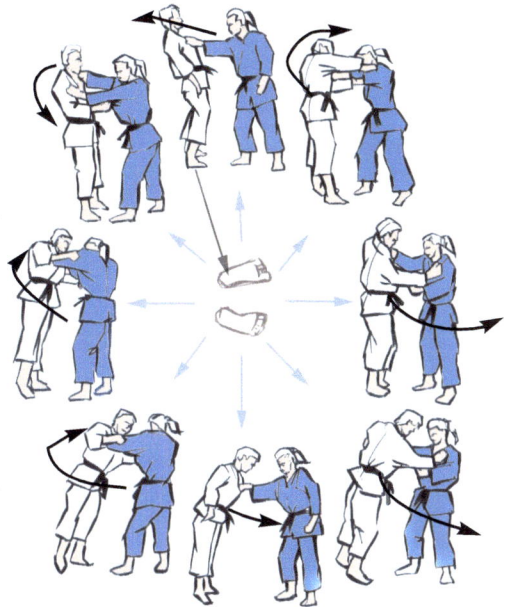

fig.311D - Judo made a science of **KUZUSHI**.

Of all the martial Arts I have practiced in the past, Judo is without a doubt the one that turned out to be the most useful all round in a real life situation. There are many advantages that Judo offers to whoever practices this ancient discipline, not only physical but above all spiritual, giving a mental preparation that will get you out of trouble in many dangerous situations, not necessarily to do with self defence.

Judo is one of the few martial arts where the concept of "sacrifice" is actively practiced (sutemiwaza) to defeat the opponent, the "sutemi" or drop is useful to speed up the action and make the most of gaps between the two opponents, using a window of opportunity that is rarely taken advantage of. Judo incompasses strangulations (shimewaza), joint locks (kansetsuwaza) and striking techniques (atemiwaza), on top of the famous throws (kake).

While everyone is always taken aback by the spectacuar "kake" , in reality the secret of Judo resides in the "kuzushi", breaking your oponent's balance so he becomes easier to throw. A true and in depth understanding of unbalancing techniques can turn most violent attacks into your advantage. An effective unbalancing technique is aledy a successful throw, you just have to add the finishing touch. Kuzushi is the understanding of body's centre of weight and the timing of a sweep, the perfect execution of the push and pull principle. (see fig.311D)

Because Judo puts so much emphasis on learning and perfecting proper falling techniques (ukemiwaza) as well as learning takedowns and throws one can well understand why Judo gives such an amazing preparation.

The techniques that Judokas (Judo practitioners) learn for ground work fighting (newaza) can hugely improve your chances to survive an attack, where the chances of being knocked to the ground are very high. Immobilisation techniques (osaekomi waza) are used by police forces throughout the world and many recently developed martial arts have borrowed plenty of techniques from Judo.

The mental preparation (shin) is what makes Judo a real advantage, constantly reaffirmed throughout training two main principles: "kuzushi" (unbalancing) and "tsukuri" (positioning). These principles are the basis of all effective throws and techniques that every Judoka must master in training and combat (randori). The very same principles that we have insisted so much upon throughout this book. To create or take advantage of that "window of opportunity" counteracting an attack you must enter a frame of mind where unbalancing and positioning yourself in relation to an aggressor makes your defence effective. That is the secret of any effective self defence.

Observing the drawings please note the arrows that indicate the push-pull action that is the most effective way to achieve a successful technique.

THE ONE PERFORMING THE TECHNIQUE IS WEARING BLUE (TORI)

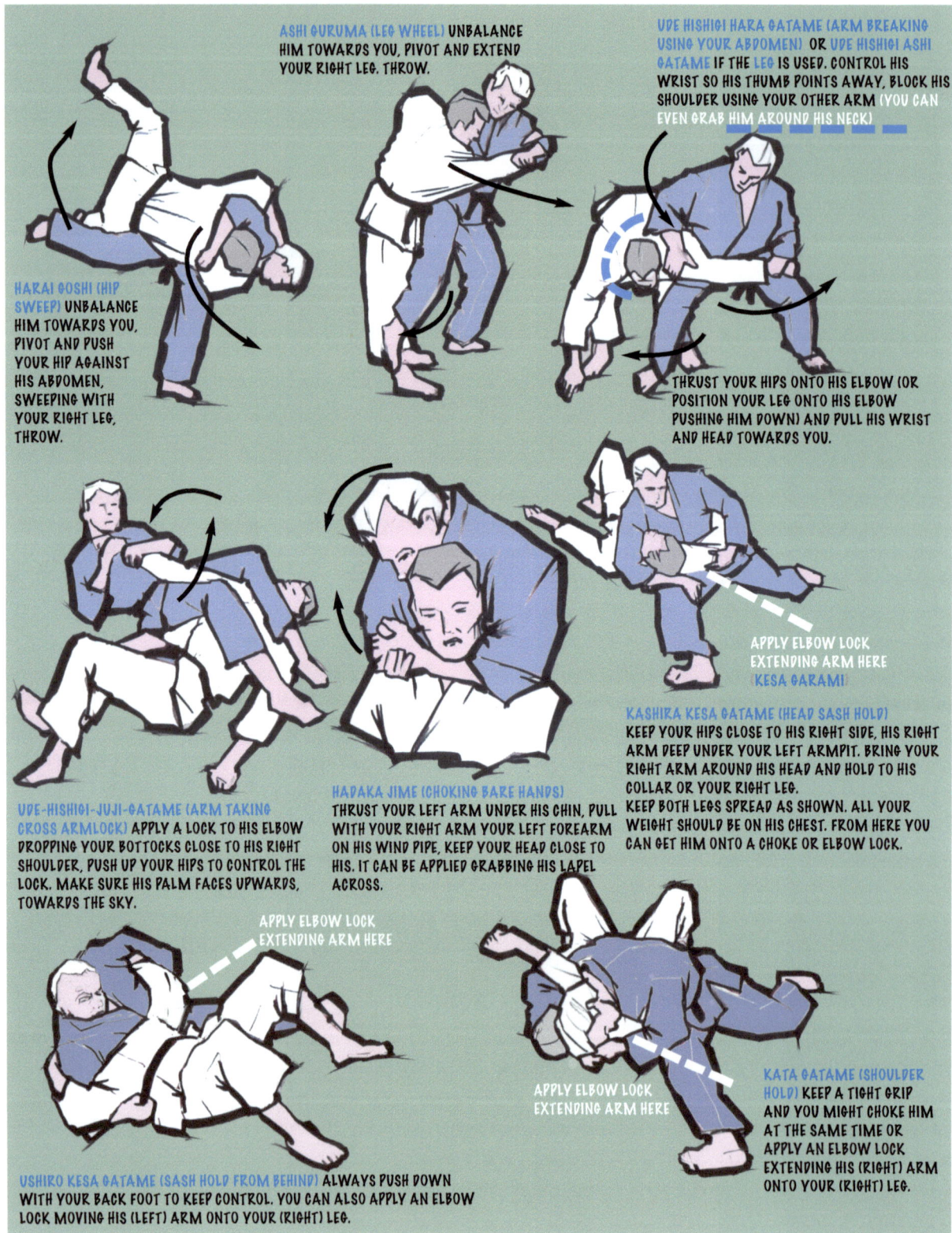

ASHI GURUMA (LEG WHEEL) UNBALANCE HIM TOWARDS YOU, PIVOT AND EXTEND YOUR RIGHT LEG. THROW.

UDE HISHIGI HARA GATAME (ARM BREAKING USING YOUR ABDOMEN) OR UDE HISHIGI ASHI GATAME IF THE LEG IS USED. CONTROL HIS WRIST SO HIS THUMB POINTS AWAY, BLOCK HIS SHOULDER USING YOUR OTHER ARM (YOU CAN EVEN GRAB HIM AROUND HIS NECK)

HARAI GOSHI (HIP SWEEP) UNBALANCE HIM TOWARDS YOU, PIVOT AND PUSH YOUR HIP AGAINST HIS ABDOMEN, SWEEPING WITH YOUR RIGHT LEG, THROW.

THRUST YOUR HIPS ONTO HIS ELBOW (OR POSITION YOUR LEG ONTO HIS ELBOW PUSHING HIM DOWN) AND PULL HIS WRIST AND HEAD TOWARDS YOU.

APPLY ELBOW LOCK EXTENDING ARM HERE (KESA GARAMI)

KASHIRA KESA GATAME (HEAD SASH HOLD) KEEP YOUR HIPS CLOSE TO HIS RIGHT SIDE, HIS RIGHT ARM DEEP UNDER YOUR LEFT ARMPIT. BRING YOUR RIGHT ARM AROUND HIS HEAD AND HOLD TO HIS COLLAR OR YOUR RIGHT LEG.
KEEP BOTH LEGS SPREAD AS SHOWN. ALL YOUR WEIGHT SHOULD BE ON HIS CHEST. FROM HERE YOU CAN GET HIM ONTO A CHOKE OR ELBOW LOCK.

UDE-HISHIGI-JUJI-GATAME (ARM TAKING CROSS ARMLOCK) APPLY A LOCK TO HIS ELBOW DROPPING YOUR BOTTOCKS CLOSE TO HIS RIGHT SHOULDER, PUSH UP YOUR HIPS TO CONTROL THE LOCK. MAKE SURE HIS PALM FACES UPWARDS, TOWARDS THE SKY.

HADAKA JIME (CHOKING BARE HANDS) THRUST YOUR LEFT ARM UNDER HIS CHIN, PULL WITH YOUR RIGHT ARM YOUR LEFT FOREARM ON HIS WIND PIPE, KEEP YOUR HEAD CLOSE TO HIS. IT CAN BE APPLIED GRABBING HIS LAPEL ACROSS.

APPLY ELBOW LOCK EXTENDING ARM HERE

APPLY ELBOW LOCK EXTENDING ARM HERE

KATA GATAME (SHOULDER HOLD) KEEP A TIGHT GRIP AND YOU MIGHT CHOKE HIM AT THE SAME TIME OR APPLY AN ELBOW LOCK EXTENDING HIS (RIGHT) ARM ONTO YOUR (RIGHT) LEG.

USHIRO KESA GATAME (SASH HOLD FROM BEHIND) ALWAYS PUSH DOWN WITH YOUR BACK FOOT TO KEEP CONTROL. YOU CAN ALSO APPLY AN ELBOW LOCK MOVING HIS (LEFT) ARM ONTO YOUR (RIGHT) LEG.

fig.311E

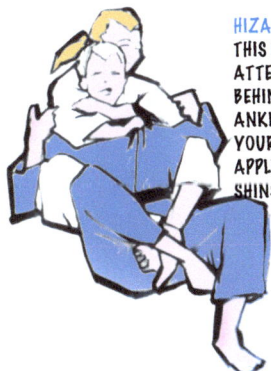

HIZA TORI GARAMI (CROSSED LEGS LOCK)
THIS IS QUITE USEFUL IF SOMEONE IS ATTEMPTING TO CHOKE YOU FROM BEHIND. CROSS YOUR RIGHT LEG OVER HIS ANKLES AND LOCK YOUR FOOT UNDER YOUR LEFT LEG. NOW EXTEND YOUR LEGS APPLYING A VERY PAINFUL LOCK TO HIS SHINS AND ANKLES.

HIZA JIME (KNEE CHOKE) THIS IS A DANGEROUS STRANGLE AND IS FORBIDDEN IN JUDO PRACTICE. IT CAN CAUSE SERIOUS INJURY TO THE SPINE. ONCE YOU SLIDE YOUR LEFT LEG UNDER HIS NECK HOOK YOUR RIGHT LEG ONTO YOUR LEFT AND STRETCH BOTH LEGS OUT. YOU CAN APPLY A JOINT LOCK TO HIS ARM AT THE SAME TIME.

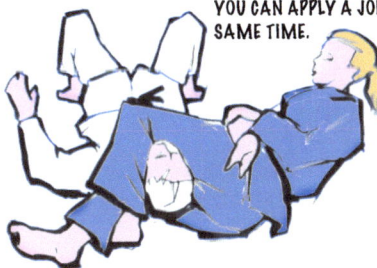

KAMI SHIHO GATAME (UPPER FOUR QUARTER HOLD) ANOTHER EFFECTIVE CONTROL TECHNIQUE ESPECIALLY WHEN USED AS A TRANSITION FROM ANOTHER. THE MAIN THING IS TO KEEP HOLD OF THE SIDES OF YOUR OPPONENT, BELT OR CLOTHING, SPREADING YOUR KNEES AND SINKING YOUR WEIGHT INTO HIS FACE. YOU CAN ALSO SPREAD YOUR LEGS INSTEAD OF KNEELING.

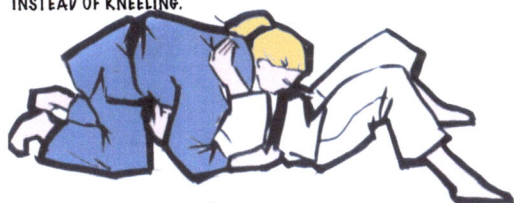

YOKO SHIHO GATAME (SIDE HOLD) IS ONE OF MANY GROUND HOLD SIMILAR IN EXECUTION. THIS IS A VERY USEFUL HOLD WHEN CHANGING POSITION FOR WHATEVER RASON AS YOU RESTRAIN SOMEONE TO THE GROUND. HOLD HIS BELT OR TROUSERS WITH ONE HAND. IN SELF DEFENCE YOU CAN SQUEEZE HIS GENITALS WITH YOUR ARM, OR EVEN BITE HIS STOMACH.

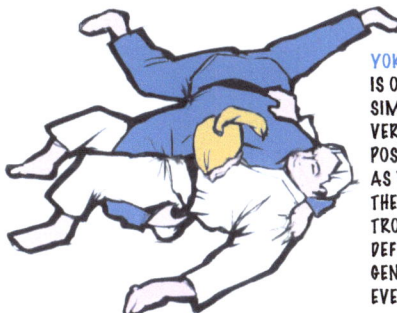

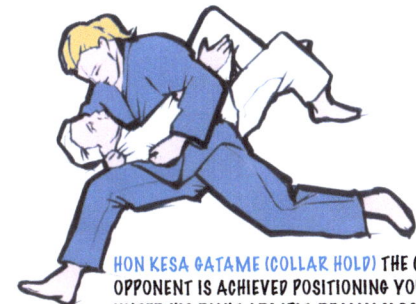

HON KESA GATAME (COLLAR HOLD) THE CONTROL OF YOUR OPPONENT IS ACHIEVED POSITIONING YOURSELF IN THE GAP UNDER HIS RIGHT ARMPIT, REALLY CLOSE AND TIGHT TO HIS CHEST. TRAP HIS RIGHT ARM UNDER YOUR LEFT HOLDING TO HIS CLOTHING AND FOLD YOUR RIGHT ARM AROUND HIS NECK HOLDING HIS COLLAR OR YOUR LEG. THIS HOLD IS VERY DIFFICULT TO ESCAPE AND ALLOWS JOINT LOCKS. SE ALSO KASHIRA KESA GATAME AND KATA GATAME (OPPOSITE PAGE)

RYO HIZA GATAME (DOUBLE KNEE LOCK) OR DOJIME (BODY SQUEEZE) USEFUL IF OPPONENT IS TRYING TO STRANGLE YOU. HOLD HIS ARMS AND SQUEEZE YOUR LEGS JUST BELOW HIS SHOULDERS. IF THE LEGS ARE SQUEEZED AROUND THE TORSO WITH A SCISSOR MOVE, JUST EXTENDIG THEM WHILE HOOKED TOGETHER. IT CAN TURN INTO KANI JIME (CRAB CHOKE) IF THE PERSON ON THE GROUND GRABS THE COLLAR WITH BOTH HANDS AND AT THE SAME TIME THE LEGS ARE USED TO PRESS ON THE ARMS.

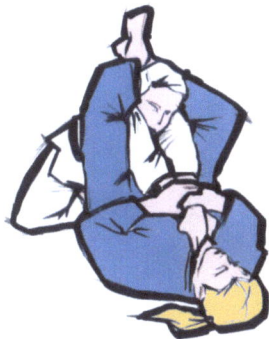

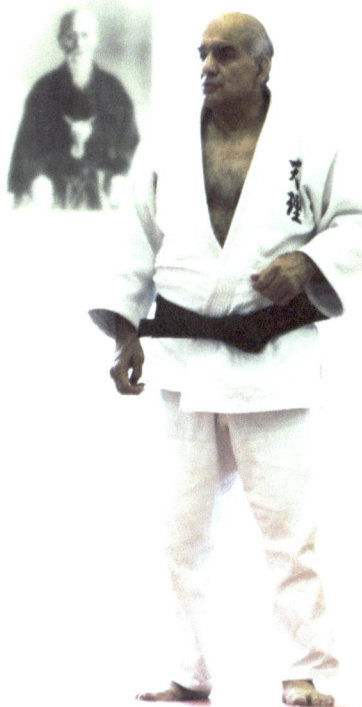

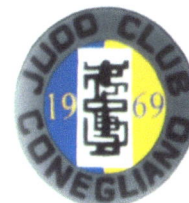

fig.312 - *Practicing Judo will keep you fit and supple. Sensei Carmeni in the Dojo.*

JUDO CLUB
CONEGLIANO
19 69

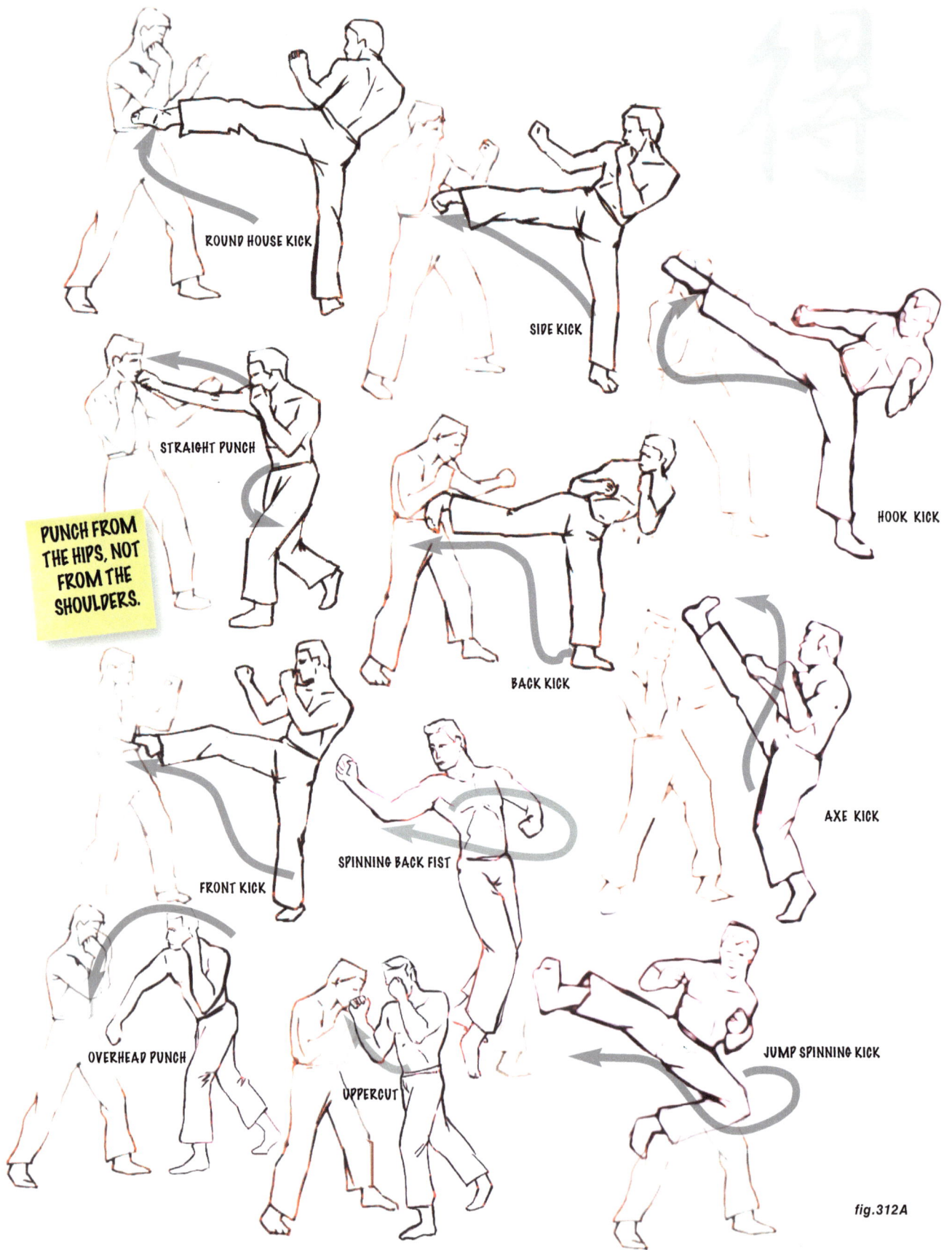

ROUND HOUSE KICK

SIDE KICK

HOOK KICK

STRAIGHT PUNCH

PUNCH FROM THE HIPS, NOT FROM THE SHOULDERS.

BACK KICK

AXE KICK

FRONT KICK

SPINNING BACK FIST

OVERHEAD PUNCH

UPPERCUT

JUMP SPINNING KICK

fig.312A

239

kickboxing

Repeating one hundred times makes it perfect.

To read about the origin of KICKBOXING see GLOSSARY (page 198).

The secret of effective kicking or punching is a perfectly executed technique performed with incredible speed and carried with awesome power. All well understandable, but how do you achieve that? Unfortunately, with very few extremely rare natural talents, there is no secret in how to succeed, in any contact sport such as Kickboxing (but it is true for many other sports or martial arts) the answer is repeating the same technique over and over with increasing speed and perfecting the movement until everything comes together beautifully.

Endless repetitions of kicking techniques make the execution of a kick almost as natural as throwing a punch. The foot reaches the target in no time with maximum power.

There are many combinations that can produce a KO, but always remember that any winning combination develops in a crescendo making the most of how the body is moving and how the momentum is progressing. Great combinations also take into consideration overshooting your strike or any pars or moves that your opponent might put into practice reacting to your strike.

For instance a right hook will make your opponent flinch to your left and if you have a left uppercut coming almost immediately afterwards chances are that you'll catch him on his jaw with it as he moves away and lowers himself, and failing that a straight punch crossed to your left will almost surely catch him again full in the face. Now imagine adding kicks and sweeps and you will understand why kickboxing can be so effective in a violent confrontation.

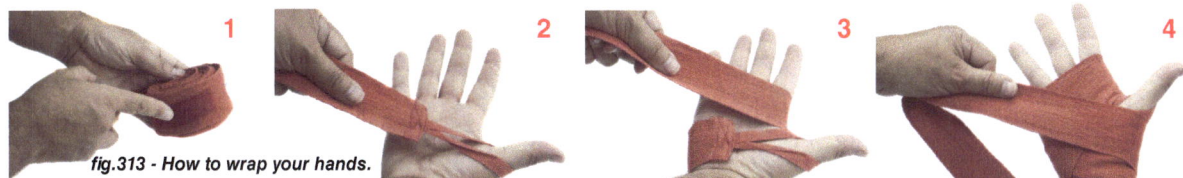

fig.313 - How to wrap your hands.

Unroll the wrap. One end has Velcro and the other end has a loop. Some have "this side down." Place loop around your thumb (2), pull the wrap to the outside of your hand. Wrap around your wrist tightly so that the wrist cannot bend and your arm can absorb the impact. Continue wrapping up your knuckles, spread you fingers out as you do it, if the fingers are too close together, knuckles are constricted. Tie around a couple of times.

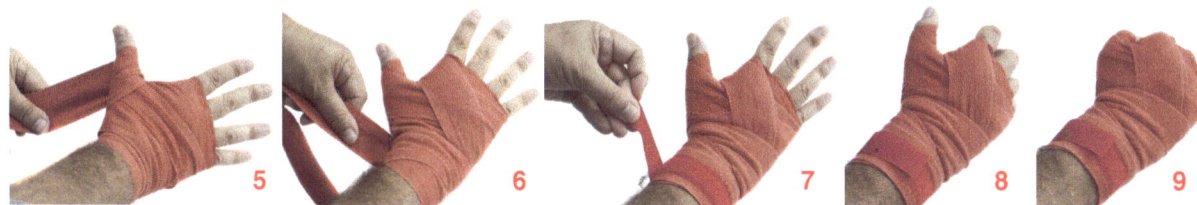

Pull the wrap to the thumb, like this (5). Continue wrapping diagonally as shown in order to cement the wrap. Do not wrap too tightly or you will cut off blood circulation to the thumb. Once done secure strap to wrist to avoid flexing, go around wrist to make sure. Wrap knuckles once more diagonally as shown. then go down to the wrist, wrapping it until the wrap runs out. Secure the velcro, make a fist to make sure it is not too tight. Wear gloves and start hitting.

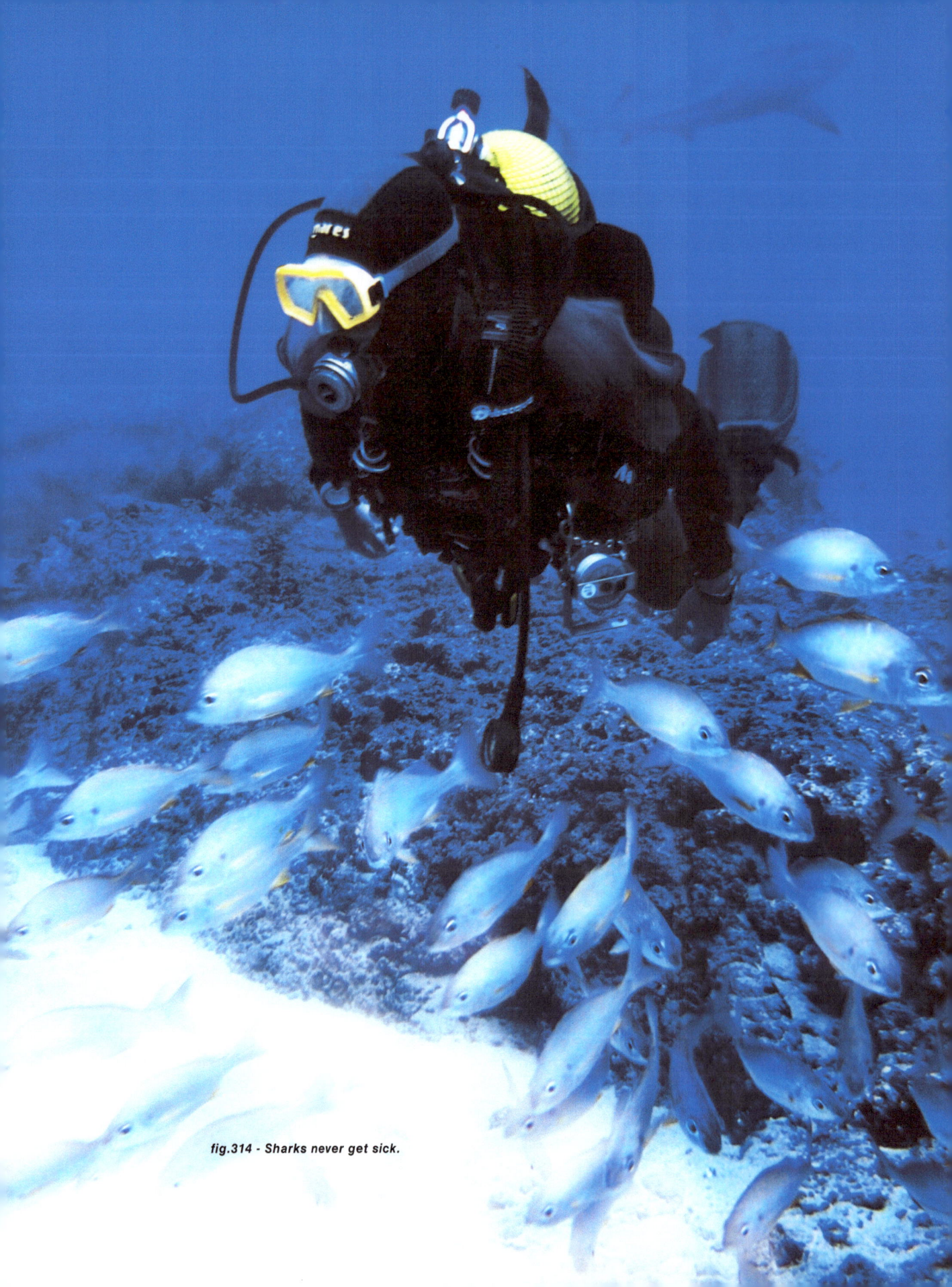

fig.314 - Sharks never get sick.

Sharks are the only animals that never get sick. It seems that they are immune to every known disease including cancer.

The probability of being struck by **lightening** in your lifetime is one in ten million.

Spiral staircases in some medieval castles are built clockwise so attackers would find fighting their way up really difficult, because holding their sword with the right they'd be impeded by the wall.

Sumo wrestlers (rikishi) throw salt in the arena (dohyo) before starting the match. It symbolizes the wish to avoid injury and purification. In practice it kills germs and hardens the dirt.

A person will die from total **lack of sleep** sooner than from starvation. Death will occur in about 10 days without sleep, while starvation takes a few weeks.

The average person falls **asleep** in seven minutes.

It takes 17 muscles to **smile**, 43 to frown. Or so they say.

The human body has over 600 **muscles**, 40% of the body's weight.

Though it makes up only 2 percent of our total body weight, the **brain** demands 20 percent of the body's oxygen and calories.

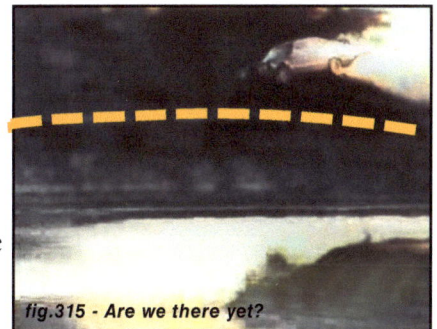

fig.315 - Are we there yet?

Stunt Coordinator Dave Judge and Franz Pagot drove a **car in water jumping a ramp** in Moscow in May 2001. The distance covered airborne was **250 feet/72.2 meters.** Nobody has beaten that record yet. (fig. 315 and also here: www.perfectdefence.com)

Vatican's **Swiss Guard** still wears a uniform designed by Michelangelo in the early 16th century.

Hippos have killed more than 400 people in Africa - more than any other wild animal.

The **blood** of mammals is red, the blood of insects is yellow, and the blood of lobsters is blue.

The **Kiwi**, national bird of New Zealand, cannot fly, lives in a hole in the ground, is almost blind, and lays only one egg each year. Despite this, it has survived for more than 70 million years.

The **shortest war** in history was between Zanzibar and Great Britain in 1896. Zanzibar surrendered after 38 minutes.

You burn more **calories** sleeping than you do watching television.

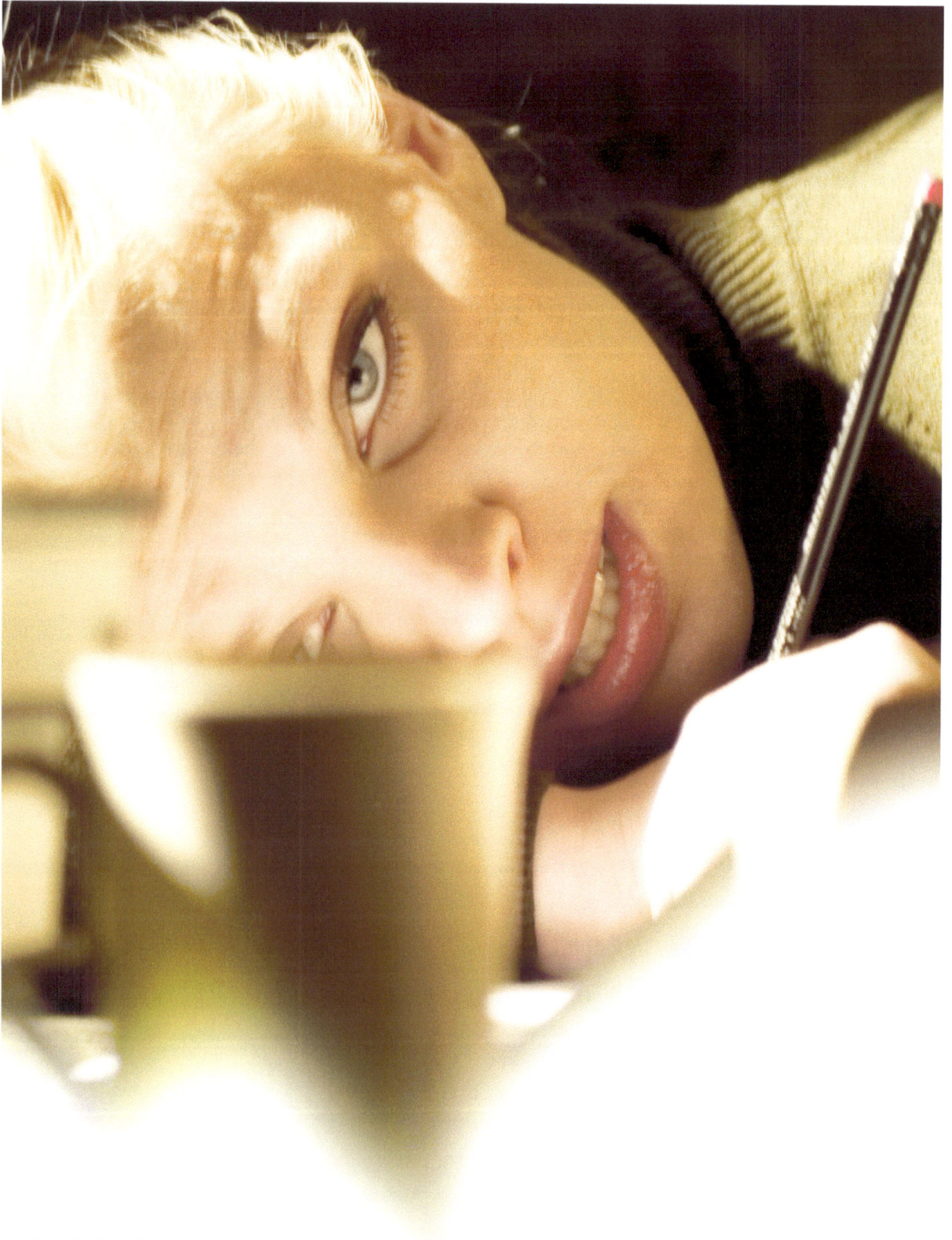

fig.316 - Food for thought.

Books in themselves are of little value without reason. (Confucius)

Even flames are cool for those who clear their minds of unnecessary thoughts. (Anonymous)

An expert fears not even death itself. (Musashi Miyamoto, famous swordsman, 17th century)

Good swimmers are oftenest drowned. (Anonymous)

Respect comes to those who are meek. (Chinese ancient saying)

Prepare for war even in times of peace. (Japanese anonymous)

The only thing we have to fear is fear itself. (Franklin Delano Roosevelt)

It is the unforeseen (unexpected) that always happens. (Latin proverb)

It takes two to make a quarrel. (Proverb, 19th Century)

Threatened men live longer. (Proverb, 16th Century)

He who seeks trouble, never misses. (Herbert, 1640)

The art of living is more like wrestling than dancing. (Marcus Aurelius, Emperor, 2nd Century)

There is no one who does not represent a danger to someone. (Madame De Sevigne, letter, 1675)

If a little knowledge is dangerous, where is the man who has so much as to be out of danger? (T. H. Huxley)

The more you sweat in training the less you bleed in battle. (Anonymous)

Always do what you are afraid to do. (R.W. Emerson)

When you fear everything, you should fear nothing. (T.H. Corneille)

We should fear less those things that scare us most. (Seneca, Latin Pholosopher)

Well begun is half done. Not begun at all until half done. (Anonymous)

Well done is better than well said. (Anonymous)

Beware of the person who has nothing to loose. (Anonymous)

If you want the rainbow you got to put up with the rain. (Anonymous)

If you don't risk anything you risk even more. (Anonymous)

It's better to die on your feet than to live on your knees. (Anonymous)

Luck is a matter of preparation meeting opportunity. (Anonymous)   *Samurai*

Always keep your mistakes around so that may reproach you. (Anonymous)

If you think you are too small to make a difference try sleeping with a mosquito. (Dalai Lama)

To live means to fight. (Seneca)

There is an exponential relationship between reaction time and number of choices. (Anonymous)

Fortune favors the brave. (Terence, Latin writer)

INTERNET FRAUD

www.scamwatch.gov.au Australian scam watch website, very thorough.
www.scamwarners.com Internet anti-fraud centre with plenty of useful advice.
www.ebolamonkeyman.com 419 scam dedicated website, scamming the scammers. Very entertaining reading too.
www.ceop.gov.uk Child Exploitation and Online Protection Centre.
www.thinkuknow.co.uk discusssing safety online, simple but effective advice.
www.stopidfraud.co.uk www.callcredit.co.uk   www.cifas.org.uk identity fraud information sites, CIFAS is the United Kingdom fraud prevention service, if signing for protective registration, they will carry additional checks if anyone applies for anything in your name.
www.equifax.co.uk USA based company managing their customers personal credit information and protecting their identity.
www.e-victims.org/ website dedicated to helping victims of e-crime and online incidents.
www.getsafeonline.org/ A must read for anyone surfing and using the Internet, brilliant advice.
www.escrow.com Escrow service recommended by Ebay. See also the following ebay link: http://pages.ebay.com/help/pay/escrow.html

TRAVEL

www.fco.gov.uk is a website by UK Govermnement advising travellers country by country.
www.rac.co.uk RAC is a UK vehicle recovery service to members. State that you are a woman on your own when stranded with your car and they'll make it a priority to assist you.

SCAMS AND OTHER CRIME

www.crimestoppers-uk.org Crimestoppers is an independent UK charity fighting crime. Providing an anonymous phone number, 0800 555 111, that people can call to pass on information about crime. Callers don't have to give their name or any personal information and calls cannot be traced.
www.cardwatch.org.uk lots of useful advice to prevent fraudulent use of credit cards, debit cards, cheque guarantee cards and charge cards.
www.actionfraud.org.uk UK's fraud reporting centre, helps victims of fraud and gives advice to avoid becoming a victim.

DOMESTIC VIOLENCE

www.helpguide.org/mental/domestic_violence_abuse_types_signs_causes_effects.htm and http://www.opdv.state.ny.us/help/fss/contents.html are both US websites with great expert advice on domestic violence and abuse in relationships.
www.victimsupport.org/UK's charity giving free and confidential help to victims of crime and anyone else affected by it. Telephone 0845 3030 900
www.nspcc.org.uk NSPCC's aim is to end cruelty to children in the UK. They also provide ChildLine on 08001111, a dedicated telephone line that children can call asking for help and the NSPCC Helpline on 08088005000, if an adult is worried about the welfare of a child or wants to report suspected abuse to children.
www.mensadviceline.org.uk Telephone 0808 801 0327 for men experiencing domestic violence

fig.317 - Children look up to us for help.

VIOLENCE AGAINST WOMEN

www.refuge.org.uk Refuge is a UK charity for women suffering domestic violence, providing accommodation and emotional support, helping women and their children enjoing a future free from physical and emotional abuse.

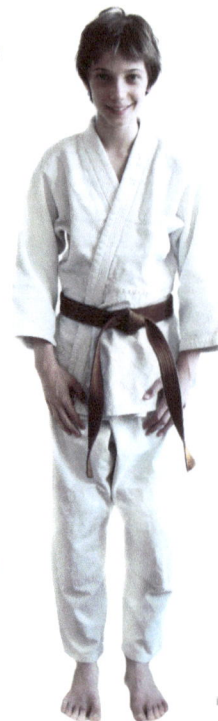

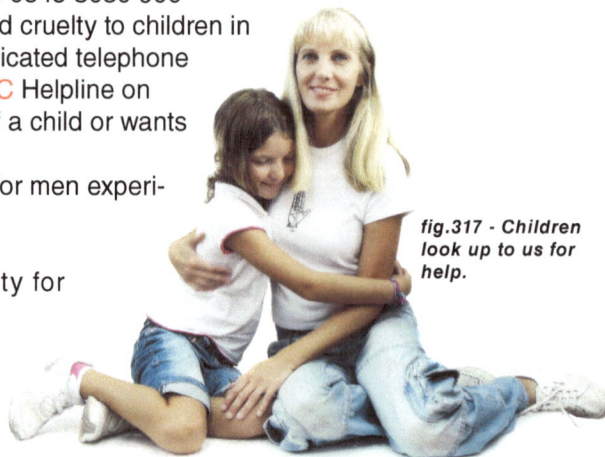

Table XI -HELP-

Friendship

X

help

UK National Domestic Violence Helpline 0808 2000 247 Freephone 24 hour (run in partnership between Women's Aid and Refuge).

www.rapecrisis.org.uk helps women and girls, who have experienced sexual violence.

www.shelter.org.uk Shelter is a charity that works to alleviate the distress caused by homelessness and bad housing. Telephone 0808 800 4444

www.clsdirect.org.uk Community Legal Service. Telephone 0845 345 4 345

www.ncdv.org.uk National Centre for Domestic Violence. Telephone 0844 8044 999

www.broken-rainbow.org.uk Telephone 0300 999 5428 or 08452 60 44 60 Support for lesbian, gay, bisexual, transexual people.

www.getconnected.org.uk provides a free, confidential helpline to under 25s that gives support and information to decide what to do next. Telephone 0808 808 4994

http://www.fco.gov.uk/en/global-issues/human-rights/forced-marriage-unit/ Foreign and Commonwealth Office Forced Marriage Unit. Telephone 020 7008 0151

www.refugeecouncil.org.uk The Refugee Council is the largest organisation in the UK working with asylum seekers and refugees. Telephone 020 7346 6777

www.iasuk.org Immigration Advice Service. Telephone 020 7357 6917

Asylum Aid: Telephone 020 7247 8741

Southall Black Sisters: 020 8571 9595

www.mwhl.org Muslim Women's Helpline: Telephone 020 8904 8193 / 020 8908 6715

www.jwa.org.uk Jewish Women's Aid Helpline: Telephone 0800 59 12 03

Somalian Women's Centre: Telephone 020 8752 1787

www.nawp.org Newham Asian Women's Project: Telephone 020 8552 5524

www.rdlogo.com/cwp/kawa/ Asian Women's Aid: Telephone 020 8558 1986

www.ciac.co.uk Chinese Information and Advice Centre: Telephone 020 7692 3697

Step Out, Black Association of Women: Telephone 029 2043 7390

WOMEN ABUSE

GENERAL ADVICE

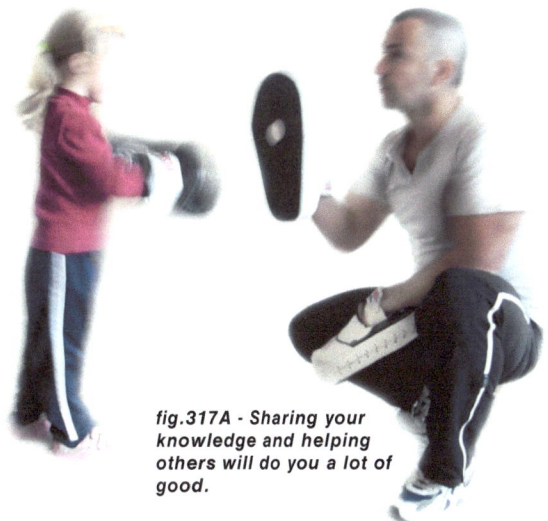

www.amauk.co.uk Amateur Martial Association encompassing many different martial arts styles.

www.secretstoragebooks.com US based company that makes hollow books as hidden safety.

www.yalelock.co.uk one of the oldest international brands, Yale is among the best-known and most respected names in the lock industry.

www.banham.co.uk highly respected company when it comes to securing home or business.

www.met.police.uk/crimeprevention/ The Metropolitan Police gives here simple but thorough information to help protecting yourself and your property. This is highly reccommended reading.

www.crimereduction.gov.uk Crime reduction UK Government initiative.

CAUTION We are not responsible for the content of external websites. This is because we do not produce them or maintain/update them, we cannot change them, they can be changed without our knowledge or agreement. Some of the links offer commercial services, such as online purchases. The inclusion of a link to an external website from us should not be understood to be an endorsement by us of that website or the site's owners.

fig.317A - Sharing your knowledge and helping others will do you a lot of good.

Humane Pressure Point Self-Defence: Dillman Pressure Point Method for Law Enforcement, Medical Personnel, Business Professionals, Men and Women by George Dillman and Chris Thomas (2001)

Aikido and the Dynamic Sphere: An Illustrated Introduction (Tuttle Martial Arts) by Adele Westbrook and Oscar Ratti (2001)

The Way of Energy: Mastering the Chinese Art of Internal Strength with Chi Kung Exercises by Lam Kam Chuen (26 Nov 1999)

How to Handle Bullies, Teasers, and Other Meanies: A Book That Takes the Nuisance Out of Name Calling and Other Nonsense by Kate Cohen-Posey and Betsy A. Lampe (1995)

Mind Control: The Ancient Art of Psychological Warfare by Haha Lung (2007)

Speed Training: How to Develop Your Maximum Speed for Martial Arts by Loren W. Christensensen (1996)

Streetwise: The Complete Manual of Personal Security and Self Defence by Peter Consterdine (1997)

Real world self defence by Jerry Vancook

The Art of Peace (Shambhala Pocket Classics) by Morihei Ueshiba and John Stevens (1993)

Kodo: Ancient Ways. Lessons in the Spiritual Life of the Warrior/Martial Artist. by Kensho Furuya (1996)

The Pyjama Game: A Journey into Judo by Mark Law (2008)

Writing

The Art of Killing: The Story of Tae Kwon Do by Gillis and Alex (2008)

Kick Boxing: A Framework for Success by Pat O'Keeffe (1999)

How to Spot a Dangerous Man Before You Get Involved: by Sandra L. Brown (2005)

You Can't Say That to Me: Stopping the Pain of Verbal Abuse - An 8-Step Program by Suzette Haden Elgin 1995)

Tongue Fu! by S. Horn (1997)

The Verbally Abusive Relationship: How to Recognize it and How to Respond by Patricia Evans (2002)

Kill or Get Killed by Rex Applegate

All-in Fighting by W.E. Fairbairn

Watch My Back: The Geoff Thompson Story by Geoff Thompson

The Mixed Martial Arts Instruction Manual: The Science of Striking by Anderson Silva and Erich Krauss (2008)

Kodokan Judo by Jigoro Kano (1994)

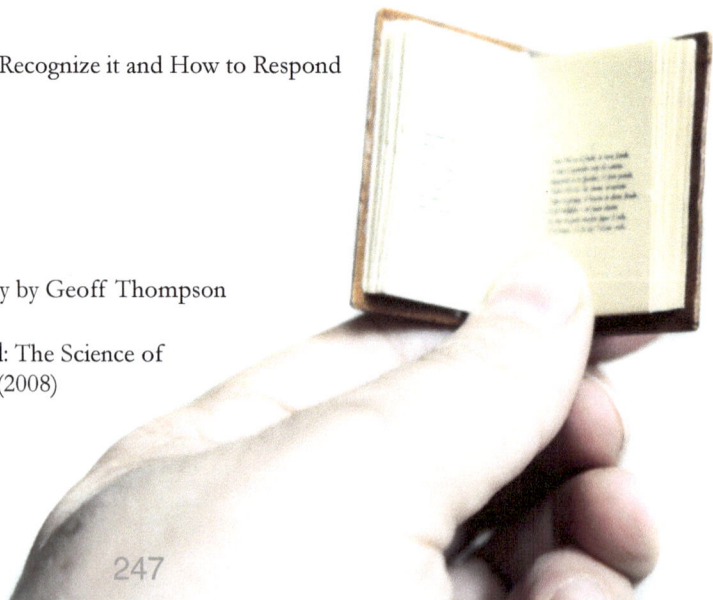

Table XI -ESSENTIAL READING-

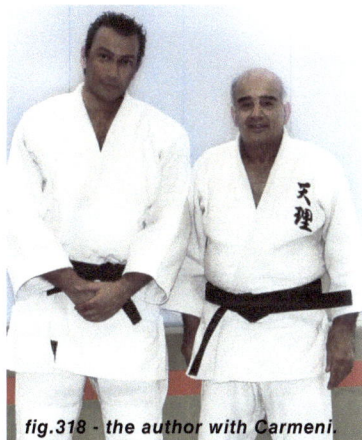

fig.318 - the author with Carmeni.

The Soul of a Butterfly by Muhammad Ali (2005)

Bushido: The Way of the Samurai (Square One Classics) by Tsunetomo Yamamoto, Justin F. Stone, and Minoru Tanaka (2002)

The Lone Samurai: The Life of Miyamoto Musashi by William Scott Wilson (2004)

Osaekomi (Judo Masterclass Techniques) by Katsuhiko Kashiwazaki (1997)

Jujitsu Nerve Techniques: The Invisible Weapon of Self-Defence by George Kirby, R. Horwitz, and J. Wilson (2001)

Stretching Scientifically: A Guide to Flexibility Training by Tom Kurz (2003)

The Art of Shaolin Kung Fu: The Secrets of Kung Fu for Self-defence, Health and Enlightenment by Wong Kiew Kit (2001)

Dead or Alive: The Definitive Self-Protection Handbook (Summersdale Martial Arts): The Choice Is Yours - The Definitive Self-protection Handbook by Geoff Thompson (2004)

Comprehensive Asian Fighting arts by Don F.Draeger and Robert W.Smith, E. Kodansha, Tokyo, 1969

Got Fight?: The 50 ZEN Principles of Hand-toface Combat by Forrest Griffin and Erich Krauss (2009)

Jiu-jitsu University by Saulo Ribeiro and Kevin Howell (2008)

Fighter's Fact Book: Street Fighting Essentials: No. 2 by Loren W. Christensen (2007)

Pre-empt, Prevent, Protect by Chris Holt (2007)

Krav Maga : How to Defend Yourself Against Armed Assault (Paperback) by Imi Sde-Or (Author), Eyal Yanilov

Strong on Defence: Survival Rules to Protect You and Your Family from Crime by Sanford Strong (Author)

The Close-combat Files of Colonel Rex Applegate by Rex Applegate

Meditations on Violence: A Comparison of Martial Arts Training and Real World Violence by Sgt. Rory Miller (2009)

1. Do not ignore your instinct: if it feels wrong it is wrong and if he seems creepy he is a creep.
2. Do not stop to answer a request for information/directions/time, not even if the person asks nicely.
3. Do not hitch hike or accept lifts from strangers ever, especially by people you have just met.
4. Do not talk on the phone for long while walking, without paying attention to your surroundings.
5. Do not listen to music through headphones while walking; it makes you oblivious of your surroundings.
6. Do not stare at a group of youths loitering in the street/park, do not walk into them, avoid.
7. Do not swear at anyone who cuts you up while driving, and do not make obscene gestures either.
8. Do not leave personal details/address in car; keep house key separate from car key.
9. Do not forget to lock yourself in immediately after getting inside car, not a moment later.
10. Do not park you car away from public areas or in a dark spot, remote section, near vans or hidden from view.
11. Do not return to you car without paying attention to surroundings: the highest risk is as you open the door.
12. Do not forget to keep a maglite type torch in your car in good working order.
13. Do not walk to your car with keys in your bag; hold them in your hand.
14. Do not park straight into a parking space; reverse into it, it will be easier to get out and easier to spot trouble.
15. Do not carry too many bags, full hands makes you vulnerable, a trolley can be used as shield.
16. Do not be oblivious to surrounding while loading groceries/luggage/shopping into car.
17. Do not hang around in the car, doing make up, checking sms, on the phone but drive away immediately.
18. Do not feel embarrassed about asking for help of security staff/shop assistant/bus driver/public.
19. Do not trust people using a cane or with an arm in plaster asking for help to load stuff into their van/car.
20. Do not open your main door coming back home oblivious of who is around you. Check behind you.
21. Do not open the door without checking who is calling; be wary of gas/electricity reading requests.
22. Do not open the door to anyone with an excuse that your roof is falling, even if they hold a tile, brick or debris.
23. Do not get out of the car if you spot a casualty on a deserted road, call emergency services first.
24. Do not walk alone at night along porches, alley ways, hidden entrances, cars, vans, big tree, and bushes.
25. Do not take shortcuts through park, field, alley, underpass unless lot of people around. Never!
26. Do not drive your car, even during the daytime, without locking all the doors, put valuables on front floor.
27. Do not sit on a bus/train away from view or next to windows, choose an aisle seat for a quick exit.
28. Do not sit in an empty carriage; always sit where there are a lot of people or next alarm/driver/exit.
29. Do not sit on a passenger seat or diagonally behind the driver in a taxi, always behind the driver.
30. Do not talk loudly in a public space on the phone revealing details of your personal life to everyone.
31. Do not mediate between two people arguing vehemently; call the police if the situation is escalating.
32. Do not ignore objects that surround you or that you have on you to use as a defensive weapon.
33. Do not continue on the same route if you sense danger/problem/risk, change route/direction.
34. Do not wear conspicuous jewellery when walking alone; do not keep your mobile phone inside your bag.
35. Do not look submissive or intimidated, look confident and assertive: chin up, walk tall.
36. Do not stop your car in a deserted road even if someone points at your tyre saying it is flat or similar problems.
37. Do not walk with the traffic, always against the flow so that you can spot trouble in advance.
38. Do not continue in the same direction if you are followed, turn back or ask for help/ring a doorbell.
39. Do not keep your walks to the same routine, change at least your walking times with the dog for instance.
40. Do not assume your area is safe only because you have lived there for many years, things change.
41. Do not trust anyone; even blood stained, asking to open the door to call emergency services, say you'll do it.
42. Do not give personal information to phone callers, even if sounding like an official body/institution/bank.
43. Do not give your details to "researchers" on the street asking to fill in forms for statistics/surveys.
44. Do not have oms on your answering machine saying "I am not in" instead have "I can't take your call right now..."
45. Do not write your name on your doorbell, specifying Ms. have only your initial and surname.
46. Do not have your name and address in full view on your luggage tags, advertising you are going away.
47. Do not reveal to the taxi driver who picked you up from your home address how long you'll be away for.
48. Do not get picked up from your home address, but at a neighbour's next door.
49. Do not walk around unknown surroundings with a map in your hands, if you need to check it do so inside a bar.
50. Do not stay in the far corner of a lift, stay near buttons/door. Leave if someone makes you uneasy.
51. Do not trust anyone who accidentally spills ice cream/ketchup/drink on you; move out of the way immediately.
52. Do not hire a car with signs/labels/writings that shouts hired car to anyone.

53 Do not necessarily trust someone just because they are wearing a uniform or flashing a badge, be alert.

54 Do not leave the "please make my room" sign on hotel door, tell housekeeping/concierge instead.

55 Do not trust the lock of your hotel room door, jam chair or door stop onto it at night.

56 Do not open your hotel room door to people knocking as if they are room service, check with the concierge first.

57 Do not take unlicensed taxis thinking it will save you money, it will not and it may actually harm you.

58 Do not follow anyone posing as a police officer/security/official into a secluded area, stay in public view.

59 Do not follow into a car/van/house/hidden spot because someone threatens you with a weapon. Run!

60 Do not refuse giving up your valuables if you are threatened. Throw them and run the opposite way.

61 Do not hold back if you need to hit someone, use your strong points and hit hard and fast many times.

62 Do not hit only one point of your attackers' body, hit many points many times.

63 Do not use arms or hands against a knife attack, keep kicking furiously.

64 Do not forget to keep a good distance if feeling uneasy when necessary.

65 Do not be careless on the internet; behave as if you are on the street.

66 Do not throw away documents/statements/bills/letters without prior destruction (burn/shred).

67 Do not forget to fit timers to operate lights/radio when you are away.

68 Do not forget to change all locks when moving into a new property or if your handbag has been stolen.

69 Do not use ATM/CASH MACHINE alone or isolated/late at night, be alert, do not count money, be quick.

70 Do not enter your home if you find any signs of a break in; go to a neighbour/call police.

71 Do not use public toilets alone; never send a child alone to a public toilet.

72 Do not fight if you can run, yell as loud as possible while running.

73 Do not fall asleep while on public transport/taxi if alone.

74 Do not tell anyone you are travelling alone, wear a wedding ring in some countries such as in Asia.

75 Do not walk alone when drunk, on medication, or while upset/fragile emotional state/after a quarrel.

76 Do not underestimate the effectiveness of distracting your attacker to strike or flee.

77 Do not strike half minded, use full force and commit fully, you might have one chance to succeed.

78 Do not stop until your attacker is totally incapacitated or after reaching safety, do not overstay.

79 Do not strike at random, try to hit as many different vital points as you can as strongly as you can.

80 Do not give away your intention to strike, better to fake submission or hide your reaction.

81 Do not keep still when start to fight, move all the time, keep your hands moving, shift position.

82 Do not remain on the ground if thrown; get up safely as quickly as possible keeping sight of your attacker.

83 Do not wait for your attacker to hit you first, if you are under threat strike first as hard as possible.

84 Do not interrupt a choke until your attacker loses consciousness, then release immediately and flee.

85 Do not rely on strength alone; use the centre of your weight manipulation and your attacker's momentum.

86 Do not rely on technique alone; remember the principle so the technique will follow.

87 Do not use complicated moves; simplicity is the most effective way to succesful strikes.

88 Do not shift your weight to the forward foot, you are more vulnerable.

89 Do not cross your feet as you move, shift them in the direction you want to go.

90 Do not square up to your opponent, move to his side to be in an advantageous position.

91 Do not hesitate to gauge your attacker's eyes, not very nice, but a real life saver.

92 Do not forget to strike using your entire body behind the blow, twisting your hips as you punch.

93 Do not think that proximity is a disadvantage; in fact it reduces the power of your opponent's blows.

94 Do not tackle someone with a knife if you can flee, if you have no choice use your legs first.

95 Do not apply one action to a move, but combine many actions: pull/push, pull/rotate, grab/pull/rotate, etc.

96 Do not parry or deflect a strike unless you are also prepared to strike back immediately as you parry.

97 Do not forget to use whatever is at hand to strike, sand, gravel, a belt, a bag, and coins.

98 Do not underestimate that a strike to the throat can seriously incapacitate anyone, no matter how big.

99 Do not expect a fair fight in a self defence situation, be ruthless and merciless.

100 Do not get over confident or careless because you now know a few self defence moves or read this book.

DONTs ARE EASIER TO REMEMBER THAN DOs.

HIT FIRST AT WHATEVER IS WITHIN YOUR REACH.

DO NOT FEEL EMBARASSED TO CALL FOR HELP OR THE POLICE IF SENSING TROUBLE.

DO NOT ABSORB A FALL WITH YOUR BODY, ROLL AS YOU LAND.

Aknowledgements:
I would like to thank the following people (from left, standing): Courtney Starr (performer), Sirle Von Schihver (performer), Ann Alasi (make up and hair), Nadege Sundi (performer), Giulia Milan (performer), Martin Qesku (sound recordist), Ed Bowen Carpenter (cameraman), Keiko Nagai (performer)- front row crouching from left: Franz, Dave Tett, (additional photography with the following images: fig.3, 4A, 8, 9, 15, 16, 22, 23, 26, 33, 35, 36, 37, 38, 39, 43, 44, 44A, 45, 46, 47, 50, 57, 59, 60, 62, 63, 64, 65, 71, 72, 74, 75, 75A, 76, 77, 78, 79, 80, 81, 82, 83, 84, 85, 86, 89, 90, 91, 92, 93, 94, 95, 96, 97, 98, 99, 100, 101, 102, 103, 104, 106, 106A, 109, 111, 112, 113, 114, 115, 116, 117, 121, 128, 129, 130, 131, 132, 133, 134, 135, 136, 137, 138, 139, 140, 141, 142, 143, 145, 148, 149, 150, 151, 152, 154, 156, 157, 158, 159, 160, 162, 165, 166, 167, 168, 169, 170, 171, 173, 174, 177, 179, 181, 184, 186, 187, 188, 191A, 193, 196, 197, 206, 206A, 206B, 210, 211, 212, 255, 271).
Also a big thank you to Alessandro Manente (web designer), Silvia Righetti (graphic supervision), Vincent Garnier (performer) Loris Arduino (performer) Faye (performer) Lisa Buckland (performer) Ryan Buckland (performer) Kerry Kisses Dunn (performer) Max Oppenheim (studio hire) Roberta Bononi (video editor) Lisa Cole (copy editor) the rabbit Pebble and Diva, the dog.

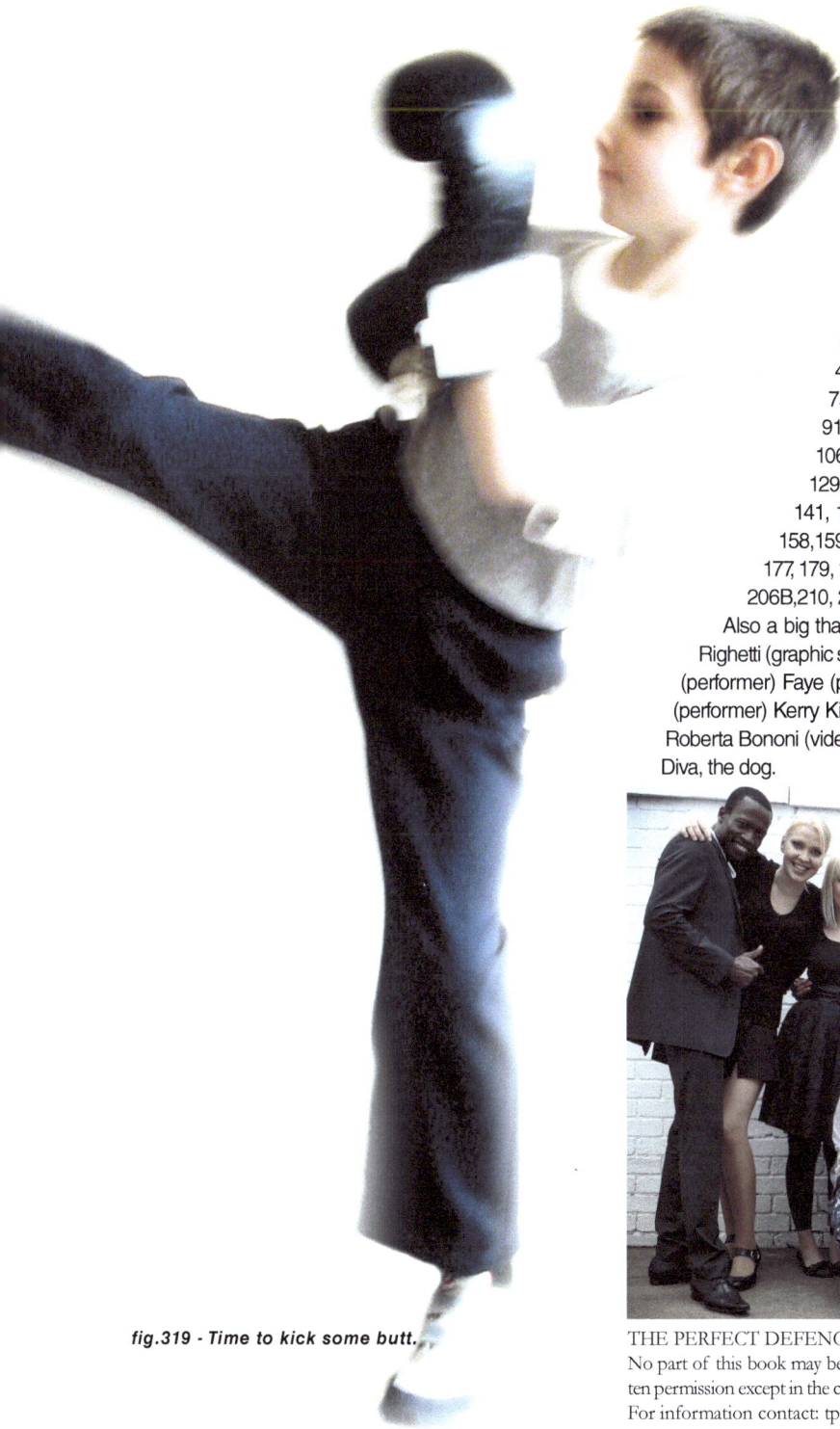

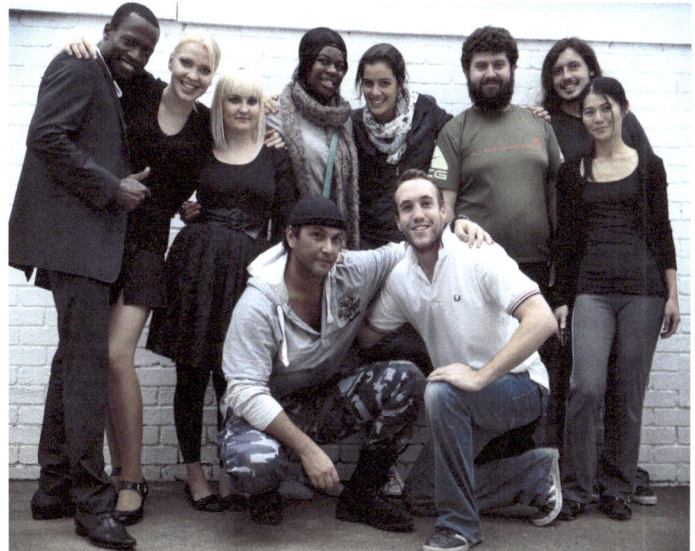

fig.319 - Time to kick some butt.

Cover photo and design by Franz Pagot. Library of Congress Cataloguing-in-Publication data has been applied for.   ISBN 978-0-9568180-0-3

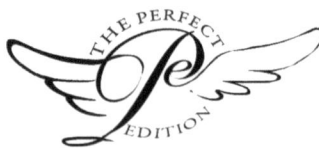

The Perfect Edition publishing company
London
United Kingdom

www.theperfectedition.com
www.theperfectdefence.com